UROLOGIC CLINICS

OF NORTH AMERICA

New Approaches in the Treatment of Advanced Prostate Cancer

GUEST EDITORS
Joseph A. Smith, Jr, MD
and Sam S. Chang, MD

CONSULTING EDITOR
Martin I. Resnick, MD

May 2006 • Volume 33 • Number 2

SAUNDERS

An Imprint of Elsevier, Inc.
PHILADELPHIA   LONDON   TORONTO   MONTREAL   SYDNEY   TOKYO

W.B. SAUNDERS COMPANY
A Division of Elsevier Inc.

1600 John F. Kennedy Boulevard • Suite 1800 • Philadelphia, Pennsylvania 19103-2899

http://www.theclinics.com

UROLOGIC CLINICS OF NORTH AMERICA   Volume 33, Number 2
May 2006   ISSN 0094-0143
Editor: Catherine Bewick   ISBN 1-4160-3563-X

Urologic Clinics of North America (ISSN 0094-0143) is published quarterly by W.B. Saunders, 360 Park Avenue South, New York, NY 10010-1710. Months of publication are February, May, August, and November. Business and Editorial Offices: 1600 John F. Kennedy Blvd., Suite 1800, Philadelphia, PA 19103-2899. Accounting and Circulation Offices: 6277 Sea Harbor Drive, Orlando, FL 32887-4800. Periodicals postage paid at New York, NY and additional mailing offices. Subscription prices are $210.00 per year (US individuals), $325.00 per year (US institutions), $240.00 per year (Canadian individuals), $390.00 per year (Canadian institutions), $280.00 per year (foreign individuals), and $390.00 per year (foreign institutions). Foreign air speed delivery is included in all *Clinics* subscription prices. All prices are subject to change without notice. **POSTMASTER:** Send address changes to *Urologic Clinics of North America*, Elsevier, Periodicals Customer Service, 6277 Sea Harbor Drive, Orlando, FL 32887-4800. **Customer Service: 1-800-654-2452 (US). From outside the US, call 1-407-345-4000.**

Urologic Clinics of North America is covered in *Index Medicus, Excerpta Medica, Current Contents/ Clinical Medicine, Science Citation Index,* and *ISI/BIOMED.*

Printed in the United States of America.

CONSULTING EDITOR

MARTIN I. RESNICK, MD, Lester Persky Professor and Chairman, Department of Urology, Case Western Reserve University, School of Medicine/University Hospitals, Cleveland, Ohio

GUEST EDITORS

JOSEPH A. SMITH, JR, MD, Professor and Chair, Department of Urologic Surgery, Vanderbilt University, Nashville, Tennessee

SAM S. CHANG, MD, Associate Professor, Department of Urologic Surgery, Vanderbilt University, Nashville, Tennessee

CONTRIBUTORS

CHRISTOPHER L. AMLING, MD, FACS, Professor and Director, Division of Urology, University of Alabama, Birmingham, Alabama

EARLE F. BURGESS, MD, Department of Medicine, Division of Hematology/Oncology, Vanderbilt University Medical Center, Vanderbilt-Ingram Cancer Center, Nashville, Tennessee

SAM S. CHANG, MD, Associate Professor, Department of Urologic Surgery, Vanderbilt University, Nashville, Tennessee

PETER E. CLARK, MD, Assistant Professor of Urology, Wake Forest University School of Medicine, Winston-Salem, North Carolina

MICHAEL S. COOKSON, MD, Associate Professor, Department of Urologic Surgery, Vanderbilt University Medical Center, Nashville, Tennessee

JUANITA CROOK, MD, FRCPC, Professor of Radiation Oncology, University of Toronto/Princess Margaret Hospital, Toronto, Ontario, Canada

PRATIK DESAI, MD, SUO Urologic Oncology Fellow, Department of Urology, Indiana University School of Medicine, Indianapolis, Indiana

THOMAS A. GARDNER, MD, Associate Professor of Urology, Microbiology, and Immunology, Walther Oncology Center, Department of Urology, Indiana University School of Medicine, Indianapolis, Indiana

SCOTT M. GILBERT, MD, Health Services Research and Urologic Oncology Fellow, Department of Urology, University of Michigan, Ann Arbor, Michigan

M. CRAIG HALL, MD, Professor of Urology and Director of Urologic Oncology, Wake Forest University School of Medicine, Winston-Salem, North Carolina

CELESTIA S. HIGANO, MD, Associate Professor, Division of Medical Oncology, Department of Medicine, University of Washington, Seattle, Washington

JEFFREY M. HOLZBEIERLEIN, MD, Assistant Professor of Urology, Department of Urology, University of Kansas Medical Center, Kansas City, Kansas

MARCIA JAVITT, MD, Professor of Radiology, Uniformed Services University of the Health Sciences, Bethesda, Maryland; Section Head of Body MRI and Genitourinary Radiology, Walter Reed Army Medical Center, Washington, District of Columbia

JUAN A. JIMÉNEZ, Graduate student, Department of Urology, Indiana University School of Medicine, Indianapolis, Indiana

PIL S. KANG, MD, Department of Diagnostic Radiology, Walter Reed Army Medical Center, Washington, District of Columbia

CHINGHAI KAO, PHD, Associate Professor of Urology, Microbiology, and Immunology, Walther Oncology Center, Department of Urology, Indiana University School of Medicine, Indianapolis, Indiana

SUSAN KASPER, PhD, Assistant Professor, Department of Urologic Surgery, Vanderbilt University Medical Center, Nashville, Tennessee

LAURENCE KLOTZ, MD, Division of Urology, Sunnybrook and Women's College Health Sciences Centre, University of Toronto, Toronto, Ontario

WILLIAM R. KREUGER, DO, Department of Diagnostic Radiology, Walter Reed Army Medical Center, Washington, District of Columbia

DANIEL W. LIN, MD, Assistant Professor, Department of Urology, University of Washington, Seattle, Washington

WILLIAM T. LOWRANCE, MD, Resident, Department of Urologic Surgery, Vanderbilt University Medical Center, Nashville, Tennessee

MICHAEL J. MANYAK, MD, Vice President of Medical Affairs, Cytogen Corporation, Princeton, New Jersey; Professor of Urology, Engineering, Microbiology, and Tropical Medicine, The George Washington University, Washington, District of Columbia

JAMES M. MCKIERNAN, MD, Assistant Professor, Department of Urology, Columbia University College of Physicians & Surgeons, New York, New York

J. DANIELL RACKLEY, MD, Resident, Department of Urology, Wake Forest University School of Medicine, Winston-Salem, North Carolina

BRUCE J. ROTH, MD, Professor of Medicine and Urologic Surgery, Department of Medicine, Division of Hematology/Oncology, Vanderbilt University Medical Center, Vanderbilt-Ingram Cancer Center, Nashville, Tennessee

ERIK S. STORM, DO, Department of Diagnostic Radiology, Walter Reed Army Medical Center, Washington, District of Columbia

JONATHAN L. WRIGHT, MD, MS, Senior Resident, Department of Urology, University of Washington, Seattle, Washington

CONTRIBUTORS

CONTENTS

Medical advances will be driven by the enhancement of imaging for diagnosis, refinement of treatment, and evaluation of treatment efficacy. The convergence of technology in materials science, biology, and the computer industry has greatly advanced diagnostic imaging. Precision in control of the spatial and temporal properties of light and its heterogeneous scattering properties have extended our capability for imaging. Refinements in radioimmunoscintigraphy for image acquisition, fusion of images, and outcome data now suggest use for image-guided therapy. Novel MRI agents appear to provide significant imaging capabilities to detect malignant lymph nodes. Future applications of optical coherence tomography, electron paramagnetic resonance imaging, nanotechnology, molecular imaging, and hyperspectral spectroscopy promise further refinements to image tissues for diagnosis.

The quoted incidence of biochemical recurrence (BCR) after localized treatment varies significantly and depends on numerous well-known prognostic factors; however, it likely occurs in at least 30%-40% of patients who receive localized treatment. Because the clinical significance of BCR is often unclear, and depends in many cases on unknown factors, it is difficult to select the best treatment and determine when best to institute that therapy. This review examines some of the issues associated with BCR and attempts to shed some light on this common but controversial clinical scenario. Some treatment strategies discussed in this article include salvage radiotherapy after radical prostatectomy, salvage therapy after radiotherapy, and hormonal therapy.

The use of combined androgen blockade therapy in prostate cancer management remains controversial. This article reviews the effect of the different non-steroid androgens in blocking androgen-independent activation of the androgen receptor in the androgen-depleted environment, and the potential benefit of bicalutamide in comparison to the first generation of anti-androgens (flutamide and nilutamide). An estimate of the benefit of combined therapy with bicalutamide suggests there is a high probability that bicalutamide 50 mg as combined therapy provides a survival advantage over castration alone. This treatment must be balanced against the potential for an increase in side-effects and a consequent adverse effect on the patient's quality of life.

Prostate cancer is more frequently being diagnosed at an earlier age, men are dying of prostate cancer at an older age, and men are now treated with androgen deprivation for biochemical relapse. As a result, the amount of time that patients are potentially subjected to androgen deprivation is increasing. Intermittent androgen deprivation (IAD) has been investigated as a potential alternative to continuous androgen deprivation (CAD) in order to improve quality of life and potentially delay the progression to androgen independence. Along with the increased use of primary hormonal therapy in clinically localized prostate cancer, IAD may supplant the traditional surgical or radiotherapy options, specifically in men who have underlying co-morbidities and decreased life expectancy. There are ongoing multi-institutional, randomized trials that will lend insight into the utility, efficacy, and feasibility of IAD versus CAD. This article discusses the theoretical benefits and rationale of IAD and reviews the completed and ongoing IAD trials. Finally, the controversies, practical applications, and future directions of IAD are addressed.

With the increase in the number of prostate cancer cases seen in the United States, the use of androgen deprivation therapy (ADT) as a form of treatment has continued to rise. With the increasing use of ADT, it is important for the urologist to recognize the potential side effects from the use of ADT and ways in which to minimize or eliminate the risks from these side effects. This article describes the potential complications of ADT and the recommendations for treatment or prevention of these complications. In addition, we examine the role of nontraditional forms of ADT and the potential benefits they offer.

Androgen deprivation therapy (ADT) is associated with a significant decrease in bone mineral density (BMD), and continued exposure seems to increase the risk of osteoporotic fracture in men who have prostate cancer treated with this strategy. Men who have prostate cancer may have low BMD before initiation of ADT. Bisphosphonates are pyrophosphate analogs that decrease bone resorption primarily through direct inhibition of osteoclast activity and proliferation. Several bisphosphonates have been evaluated in randomized clinical trials, and the cumulative data show that these medications increase or maintain BMD in men receiving ADT for prostate cancer. The effect on clinical fractures has not been assessed adequately, but bisphosphonates offer an important potential treatment modality to reduce the risk of osteoporotic fracture in this population of men.

GOAL STATEMENT

The goal of *Urologic Clinics of North America* is to keep practicing urologists and urology residents up to date with current clinical practice in urology by providing timely articles reviewing the state of the art in patient care.

ACCREDITATION

Urologic Clinics of North America is planned and implemented in accordance with the Essential Areas and Policies of the Accreditation Council for Continuing Medical Education (ACCME) through the joint sponsorship of the University of Virginia School of Medicine and Elsevier. The University of Virginia School of Medicine is accredited by the ACCME to provide continuing medical education for physicians.

The University of Virginia School of Medicine designates this educational activity for a maximum of 15 AMA PRA Category 1 Credits™ Physicians should only claim credit commensurate with the extent of their participation in the activity.

The American Medical Association has determined that physicians not licensed in the US who participate in this CME activity are eligible for 15 AMA PRA Category 1 Credits™.

Category 1 credit can be earned by reading the text material, taking the CME examination online at http://www.theclinics.com/home/cme, and completing the evaluation. After taking the test, you will be required to review any and all incorrect answers. Following completion of the test and evaluation, your credit will be awarded and you may print your certificate.

FACULTY DISCLOSURE/CONFLICT OF INTEREST

The University of Virginia School of Medicine, as an ACCME accredited provider, endorses and strives to comply with the Accreditation Council for Continuing Medical Education (ACCME) Standards of Commercial Support, Commonwealth of Virginia statutes, University of Virginia policies and procedures, and associated federal and private regulations and guidelines on the need for disclosure and monitoring of proprietary and financial interests that may affect the scientific integrity and balance of content delivered in continuing medical education activities under our auspices.

The University of Virginia School of Medicine requires that all CME activities accredited through this institution be developed independently and be scientifically rigorous, balanced and objective in the presentation/discussion of its content, theories and practices.

All authors/editors participating in an accredited CME activity are expected to disclose to the readers relevant financial relationships with commercial entities occurring within the past 12 months (such as grants or research support, employee, consultant, stock holder, member of speakers bureau, etc.). The University of Virginia School of Medicine will employ appropriate mechanisms to resolve potential conflicts of interest to maintain the standards of fair and balanced education to the reader. Questions about specific strategies can be directed to the Office of Continuing Medical Education, University of Virginia School of Medicine, Charlottesville, Virginia.

The authors/editors listed below have identified no professional or financial affiliations for themselves or their spouse/ partner:
Christopher L. Amling, MD, FACS; Catherine Bewick, Acquisitions Editor; Earle F. Burgess, MD; Peter E. Clark, MD; Juanita Crook, MD, FRCPC; Pratik Desai, MD; Scott M. Gilbert, MD; M. Craig Hall, MD, FACS; Celestia S. Higano, MD; Juan Antonio Jiménez, MD; Pil S. Kang, MD, CPT, USA; Chinghai Kao, PhD; Susan Kasper, PhD; Laurence Klotz, MD; William R. Kreuger, DO; Daniel W. Lin, MD; William T. Lowrance, MD; J. Daniel Rackley, MD; Martin I. Resnick, MD, Consulting Editor; Joseph Smith, Jr., MD; Erik S. Storm, DO, CPT, MC, USA; and, Jonathan L. Wright, MD, MS.

The authors/editors listed below identified the following professional or financial affiliations for themselves or their spouse/partner:
Sam S. Chang, MD is on the speakers' bureau for Novartis and participated in a clinical trial with Amgen.
Michael S. Cookson, MD is a consultant for Sanofi-Aventis, GlaxoSmithKline, Envisioeering Medical Technologies; is on Aeterna Zentaris Solvay's Advisory Board; is an investigator and on the speakers' bureau for Sanofi-Aventis. He has a scientific study with Photocure, NIH, Sanofi-Aventis, and GTX.
Thomas A. Gardner, MD is on the speakers' bureau and advisory board for Pfizer.
Jeffrey M. Holzbeierlein, MD is an independent contractor for Merck, on the Advisory Committee for Pfizer and Dendreon, and is on the speakers' bureau for Pfizer.
Marcia C. Javitt, MD is on the speakers' bureau for Cytogen, Advanced Magnetics, and TAP Pharmaceuticals.
Michael J. Manyak, MD is on the Advisory Board for Imalux Corporation, Metastatin Pharmaceuticals, and Endocare, Inc. He is a consultant for Imalux Corporation, and Endocare, Inc.; has stock ownership in Cytogen Corporation and has stock and holds a patent for Metastatin Pharmaceuticals; he is an employee of Cytogen Corporation.
Bruce J. Roth, MD is on the Advisory Committee for Bristol-Myers Squibb and Novartis.

Disclosure of Discussion of non-FDA approved uses for pharmaceutical products and/or medical devices:
The University of Virginia School of Medicine, as an ACCME provider, requires that all faculty presenters identify and disclose any "off label" uses for pharmaceutical and medical device products. The University of Virginia School of Medicine recommends that each physician fully review all the available data on new products or procedures prior to instituting them with patients.

TO ENROLL

To enroll in the Urologic Clinics of North America Continuing Medical Education program, call customer service at 1-800-654-2452 or visit us online at www.theclinics.com/home/cme. The CME program is available to subscribers for an additional fee of $195.00

FORTHCOMING ISSUES

RECENT ISSUES

THE CLINICS ARE NOW AVAILABLE ONLINE!

Access your subscription at:
http://www.theclinics.com

UROLOGIC CLINICS
of North America

Urol Clin N Am 33 (2006) xi

Foreword

New Approaches in the Treatment of Advanced Prostate Cancer

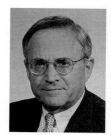

Martin I. Resnick, MD
Consulting Editor

Over the past two decades, there have been significant advances in the evaluation and management of patients with localized carcinoma of the prostate. The routine use of prostate-specific antigen test determinations has resulted in a marked increase in the diagnosis of men with disease localized to the prostate, and significant advances have occurred in radial prostatectomy and radiation therapy, so that the morbidity associated with these treatments has been greatly reduced. Additionally, follow-up studies have clearly demonstrated enhanced survival, with reduced recurrence in those patients treated for early localized disease.

Unfortunately, progress in the management of patients with either recurrent or advanced disease has not been as dramatic. Imaging to detect recurrent disease has improved, and enhanced understanding of androgen deprivation therapy has resulted in its use in different manners, including primary continuous therapy, intermittent therapy, or in association with radiation therapy. As documented in this issue of *Urologic*

Clinics of North America, new approaches have been utilized in patients who have either failed hormonal therapy or presented with advanced disease. These developments have resulted in the reduction of skeletal complications and in the improved management of those patients who have developed hormone-resistant disease. The advances have had a significant impact on these patients and, as noted in the last article on future innovations, there is more to come. For these reasons, it is likely that the next decade will witness improved treatment modalities for those patients whose disease has progressed to an advanced stage.

Martin I. Resnick, MD
Department of Urology
Case Western Reserve University
School of Medicine/University Hospitals
Cleveland, OH, USA

E-mail address: martin.resnick@case.edu

UROLOGIC
CLINICS
of North America

Urol Clin N Am 33 (2006) xiii

Preface

New Approaches in the Treatment of Advanced Prostate Cancer

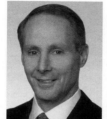
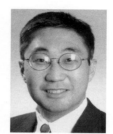

Joseph A. Smith, Jr, MD   Sam S. Chang, MD
Guest Editors

Screening and early detection have transformed the face of prostate cancer at the time of presentation. Although it was common in the era before prostate-specific antigen testing for men to present with advanced or even metastatic prostate cancer, only a small proportion of patients in contemporary series have disease outside the prostate at the time of detection. Coupled with early detection programs, effective treatment strategies have led to a recent trend showing a decrease in the number of men dying from prostate cancer. Despite these advances, carcinoma of the prostate remains the second most common cause of cancer death in men in this country.

Treatment of advanced carcinoma of the prostate remained relatively stagnant for almost half a century after the pioneering work of Huggins showed the link between androgens and prostate cancer progression. Although hormonal manipulation is still a mainstay of treatment, the last decade has seen the emergence of effective chemotherapy, improvements in radiation therapy, exploration of immune-based therapy, and the possibility of better imaging and targeting of therapy.

The field of knowledge is changing rapidly and it is important for clinicians to stay abreast of new developments. Multidisciplinary management strategies have brought together urologic surgeons, medical oncologists, and radiation oncologists as never before. Further, the translational potential of basic science research makes it incumbent for clinicians to work even more closely with their basic science colleagues.

This issue of the *Urologic Clinics of North America* provides a concise yet comprehensive overview of the current state of the art in the treatment of advanced carcinoma of the prostate. Leading investigators from multiple disciplines have contributed, and we are indebted to all of them for their work. Patients with advanced prostate cancer have new treatment options today and even more promising therapy on the horizon.

Joseph A. Smith, Jr, MD
Sam S. Chang, MD
Department of Urologic Surgery
Vanderbilt University
Nashville, TN, USA

E-mail addresses: joseph.smith@vanderbilt.edu
sam.chang@vanderbilt.edu

ELSEVIER
SAUNDERS

Urol Clin N Am 33 (2006) 133–146

UROLOGIC
CLINICS
of North America

The Evolution of Imaging in Advanced Prostate Cancer

Michael J. Manyak, MD[a,b,*], Marcia Javitt, MD[c,d],
Pil S. Kang, MD[d], William R. Kreuger, DO[d], Erik S. Storm, DO[d]

[a]Cytogen Corporation, Princeton, NJ, USA
[b]Engineering, Microbiology, and Tropical Medicine, The George Washington University, Washington, DC, USA
[c]Uniformed Services University of the Health Sciences, Bethesda, MD, USA
[d]Department of Diagnostic Radiology, Walter Reed Army Medical Center, Washington, DC, USA

The paradigm for prostate cancer presentation has shifted over the last 15 years since the introduction of prostate specific antigen (PSA) testing. Educational programs and greater focus on screening have led to a decrease in the number of patients who present initially with advanced disease. The recently reported data from the National Cancer Institute Surveillance, Epidemiology, and End Results Program (SEER) demonstrate that approximately 90% of patients, regardless of race, were diagnosed with localized prostate cancer between 1995 and 2000 [1]. This represents almost a 20% drop in patients who presented with distant disease in the SEER database reported in 1997 [2].

After the diagnosis of prostate cancer, it is critical to determine the extent of the disease in order to select appropriate therapy. It is possible to make some prediction of disease stage because of accumulated clinical knowledge about biopsy histopathological characteristics and tumor markers such as PSA, especially in their extremes [3,4]. Although the nomograms are robust for determination of local extension or seminal vesicle involvement, they are less accurate for prediction of lymph node metastasis, because the databases rely on tissue samples from a limited area of possible lymphatic spread. Several factors suggest that underestimation of nodal disease is worse than previously expected. In a recent study of patients who underwent abdominoperineal resection for colorectal carcinoma, perirectal lymph nodes contained prostate cancer in 4.5% of the patients [5]. The increased survival rates that result from extended pelvic lymph node dissection in patients who have small volume metastatic lymph node deposits, are tempered by the 39% (4 year) and 43% (5 year) progression-free rates, which again demonstrate the wider extent of the disease [6,7]. Stratification by risk category is useful for prognostication, but lymph node involvement is still underestimated, even in the low-risk prostate cancer population [7].

Various forms of noninvasive imaging have been used to evaluate patients who have prostate cancer, but the clinical utility of standard cross-sectional imaging is limited because a relatively large volume of disease is generally required for detection. However, several advances in imaging technology, the introduction of new modalities for molecular imaging, and the diagnostic use of light sources provide enhanced accuracy of prostate cancer localization and significant promise for future improvements in imaging capabilities.

Imaging for locally advanced disease

Transabdominal ultrasound is not currently useful for evaluation of regional or distant

* Corresponding author. 2322 Blaine Drive, Chevy Chase, MD 20815.
E-mail address: mmanyak@cytogen.com (M.J. Manyak).

0094-0143/06/$ - see front matter © 2006 Elsevier Inc. All rights reserved.
doi:10.1016/j.ucl.2005.12.014

prostate cancer. However, conventional two-dimensional (2-D) sonographic imaging of the prostate has been used for decades. The prostate can be visualized by way of the transabdominal and transrectal approaches, but transrectal ultrasound (TRUS) is preferred because it provides the clearest view of the prostate. TRUS is currently the most common imaging modality in prostate cancer, and is used almost universally during initial staging to assist with transrectal prostate biopsy. It is also useful for overall anatomic assessment, assessment of brachytherapy seed placement, and guidance for cryotherapy techniques [8].

The development of higher frequency (≥ 7.5 MHz transducers) has improved sonographic evaluation of the prostate. The classical appearance of a prostate tumor is hypoechoic, but many cancers are isoechoic, or rarely, hyperechoic. A discrete hypoechoic area does not preclude systematic biopsies because cancer frequently co-exists in adjacent or separate areas with an isoechoic signal. Conventional TRUS is an imprecise technique for detection and staging of prostate cancer: up to 80% of hypoechoic prostate lesions do not represent prostate cancer and 50% of nonpalpable prostate cancers >1 cm are not visualized by sonography. Sonographic findings that suggest extracapsular extension of cancer include irregularity along capsular borders, invasion of tumor into periprostatic fat, and posterior thickening or loss of bulging of seminal vesicles [8]. Directed transrectal sonography has been reported to be more sensitive than MRI for detection of rectal wall involvement by prostate cancer in patients who undergo salvage pelvic exenteration or cystoprostatectomy [9].

Three-dimensional (3-D) TRUS generates a series of superimposed sequential images, and produces a high-quality, high-resolution final image. Some studies suggest that 3-D TRUS is a superior tool for depiction of tumor presence as well as for identification of extra-glandular disease, and overall staging accuracy is reported to be as high as 94% (versus 72% with 2-D TRUS) [10,11].

Color Doppler (CDUS) and power Doppler (PDUS) ultrasound techniques, which are based on the premise of increased or altered microvessel blood flow within cancerous areas, have been inconclusive for cancer detection within the gland [12]. Some studies, however, suggest that cancers visible with CDUS are more likely to be aggressive or have extracapsular extension or seminal vesicle invasion [13]. It has been reported that PDUS demonstrated high specificity (94%) for detection of extracapsular extension of prostate cancer with detection of a vessel crossing the capsule [14].

Fluorocarbon microbubble sonographic contrast agents have been evaluated as a method to increase the amplitude of a reflected signal in the blood pool, thereby helping to accentuate areas on CDUS or PDUS that have increased microvessel density (Fig. 1) [15,16]. Microbubble sonographic contrast significantly increased sensitivity but did not change specificity for detection of cancer within the gland. The contrast-enhanced, CD-guided biopsies provided a 2.6 times greater chance of detecting cancer in the 230 patients tested [16]. Whether this modality has utility for detection of locally advanced disease remains to be determined, but investigations with fusion of microbubble images and radioimmunoscintigraphy may provide more information about local extension of disease.

Use of MRI for detection of locally advanced disease has provided mixed results. The concensus of investigators is that the use of an endorectal coil (ERC) may enhance detection rates in intermediate and high-risk groups [17]. In one recent study that compared presurgical ERC MRI with prostatectomy specimens, the high specificity (89%) and positive predictive value (81%) for extracapsular extension was balanced by a low sensitivity (43%) and negative predictive value (59%) [18]. ERC MRI may be useful to detect location of local recurrence following prostatectomy, which has implications for salvage external beam dosimetry [19]. MRI spectroscopy is under evaluation for detection of localized tumors within the

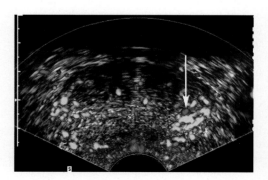

Fig. 1. Fluorocarbon microbubble contrast-enhanced PDUS image of a prostate cancer lesion (*white arrow*) that is not evident on standard gray scale ultrasound. (Courtesy of E. Halpern, MD, Philadelphia, PA.) Supported by Department of the Army grant # DAMD17-01-1-0061.

prostate, and it is unknown whether this will be more advantageous for detection of locally advanced disease compared with other modalities.

Detection of distant metastasis

Skeletal scintigraphy

Standard radiography for evaluation of osseous involvement by prostate cancer has long been known to be poorly sensitive. Radionuclide skeletal scintigraphy has been the mainstay for evaluation of osseous metastases and detects bone metastases in 25% of patients who have normal skeletal surveys. Nearly 50% of bone marrow must be replaced before detection of metastases by skeletal survey, but scintigraphy can detect lesions with only 10% marrow replacement (Fig. 2) [20]. Limitations of skeletal scintigraphy Technetium 99m (Tc99m)-labeled bisphosphonate agents are now more clearly recognized. The diagnosis of prostatic adenocarcinoma is most frequently established by TRUS-guided biopsy after an elevated or rapidly increasing PSA. In the pre-PSA era, when diagnosis resulted from an abnormal digital rectal exam or presentation with an extraprostatic manifestation, bone scintigraphy was nearly always obtained. Because most prostate cancer is now found at earlier stages, the incidence of osseous metastases on initial staging is very low, and most researchers advocate skeletal evaluation by scan only when the serum PSA level is > 10 ng/mL, and in some cases ≥ 20 ng/mL, in the presence of well-differentiated primary tumors [21].

Scintigraphy has less of a role in the evaluation of osseous disease in patients who have biochemical recurrence after definitive therapy. Patients who have biochemical recurrence after radical prostatectomy have a low probability of a positive bone scan (9.4%) within 3 years of biochemical recurrence. Most patients who have a positive bone scan have a high PSA level and a high PSA velocity defined as > 0.5 ng/mL/mo [22].

Therapy with bisphosphonates for osseous metastases is being used more frequently and scintigraphy has been shown to correlate well with

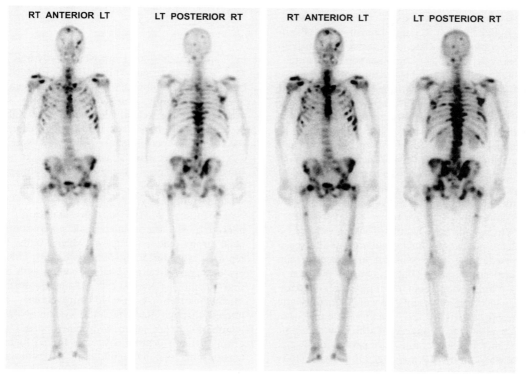

Fig. 2. Skeletal scintigraphy with delayed images in anterior and posterior projections after intravenous administration of Tc99m-hydroxydisphosphonate, which demonstrates multifocal increased uptake consistent with osteoblastic metastatic prostate cancer.

response (a 2% false-positive rate and a 12% false-negative rate) compared with pathological confirmation in an autopsy series [23]. Another potential use for skeletal scintigraphy is in the androgen insensitive patient population. Pretherapy diagnostic Tc99 scans have now been used to estimate absorbed doses of 186Re-1,1-hydroxyethylidene diphosphonate (186Re-HEDP) in conjunction with peripheral stem cell support in hormone-refractory prostate cancer patients who have skeletal metastases [24].

Cross-sectional imaging with CT and MRI

The limitations of both CT and MRI to detect prostate cancer and lymph node metastasis are recognized. Conventional CT and MRI use size criteria to declare metastases in lymph nodes (threshold dimensions >10 mm in the short axis diameter of an elongated node or 8 mm in diameter if the lymph node is round), but use of size criteria has low sensitivity. Several studies cite that the sensitivity of CT for lymph node metastases ranges from 25% to 78%, and specificity ranges from 77% to 98% [25–28]. In one of the few studies that showed tissue confirmation of radiographic findings, CT had a sensitivity of 4% in a cohort of intermediate to high-risk patients [29]. CT may fail to detect lymphadenopathy because the nodes are beneath the size threshold for detection, may contain microscopic tumor foci without enlargement, or because of technical performance of the scan and interobserver variability in interpretation [30]. When adenopathy is detected, CT does not distinguish between inflammatory and neoplastic involvement [31]. Therefore, standard CT is best reserved for patients who have clinical stage T3 or T4 disease and for radiotherapy pretreatment planning [8]. CT also remains useful as a conformal study for image coregistration.

Whole-body MR imaging, which is used to evaluate patients for metastatic disease, has been reported to be more sensitive and specific than skeletal scintigraphy (Fig. 3), but in the past it took a long time to acquire an image on the scanner, which can adversely affect image quality and therefore sensitivity [32]. A sliding table platform, which allows for imaging of different anatomic parts in rapid succession, may permit rapid, efficient whole-body MR imaging [33]. A recent study reported that all cerebral, pulmonary, and hepatic metastatic disease deposits >6 mm in diameter could be identified when the sliding table platform was used for MR imaging. The detection of

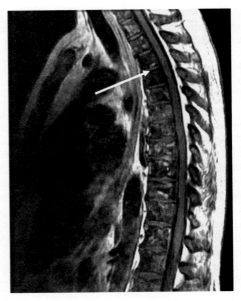

Fig. 3. Sagittal T2 weighted images of the thoracic spine. Areas of marrow replacement correspond to osteoblastic metastatic disease (*white arrow*). Osteoblastic metastatic disease tends to be dark on both T1 and T2 images, much like normal cortical bone.

pulmonary nodules on these whole-body MR images is inferior to conventional CT of the chest, but the missed pulmonary nodules did not change overall therapeutic strategies. Whole-body MR was superior to skeletal scintigraphy and CT in detecting skeletal and liver metastatic disease, respectively. The per-patient sensitivity and specificity values were 100% when compared with standard reference imaging (contrast-enhanced CT of the brain, chest, abdomen and pelvis, and skeletal scintigraphy).

The utility of MRI may be significantly enhanced by the use of ultrasmall superparamagnetic iron oxide particles, which were first reported in a murine model in 1990 [34]. The 20-nm hexagonal iron oxide cores coated with dextran (Combidex, Advanced Magnetics, Boston, Massachusetts) are injected intravenously and filtered through the lymphatic system. Normal lymph nodes are laden with macrophages and areas of tumor deposit have very few. A high-intensity signal is noted in all lymph nodes initially, but macrophage phagocytosis in areas of normal lymph node architecture creates a very dark signal caused by the nanoparticle paramagnetic properties and, therefore, eliminates the high intensity signal on repeat MRI 24 hours later. Lymph nodes that have metastatic disease demonstrate a continued high-intensity signal in areas of tumor (Fig. 4). In the recently published study on incidence of lymph node involvement with prostate cancer, performance characteristics of the MRI with lymphotrophic particles when compared with MRI alone were: sensitivity 96% versus 29%, specificity 99% versus 87%, positive predictive value 96% versus 29%, and negative predictive value 99% versus 87% in lymph nodes between 5 mm and 1 cm. In lymph nodes < 5 mm, sensitivity and positive predictive value were 41% and 78% versus 0% for MRI alone [35]. Furthermore, several noncontiguous positive lymph nodes were detected, which corroborated previous work that reported up to 17% of patients who had a solitary iliac metastasis and 7% to 14% of patients who had a solitary presacral or presciatic metastasis outside of the conventional area for lymph node dissection [36,37]. This is also consistent with the findings that even modestly extended lymph node dissection detects unsuspected disease [6,7]. MRI with lymphotropic superparamagnetic nanoparticles correctly identified all patients who had nodal metastases [35].

The tissue-confirmed results of this study are striking and strongly suggest that this modality will be highly useful to determine treatment regimens. The advantage of this imaging with this contrast agent is that it is independent of tumor metabolic activity, unlike positron emission tomography (PET) which requires high metabolic activity to detect a signal. This changes the paradigm for evaluation of lymph nodes from one of size alone to one of signal intensity characteristics which denote functional activity regardless of size. Although this imaging agent is not available for general use in the United States at the time of this publication, it has been demonstrated in preliminary clinical trials to be useful for many other types of tumor lymph node metastases as well.

Positron emission tomography

Positron emission tomography measures metabolism of a radio-labeled analog in tissue where the higher metabolic rate of neoplasia registers an increased scintigraphic signal, which is especially noted in rapidly progressive tumors. Although the most commonly used radiotracer for PET is ^{18}F-fluoro-2-deoxyglucose (FDG), this analog is not particularly useful to evaluate prostate cancer [38]. PET is unable to differentiate between tumor and hyperplasia, and is also less sensitive than bone scintigraphy for detection of osseous metastases (Fig. 5) [38].

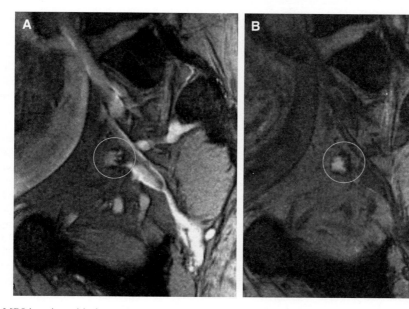

Fig. 4. MRI imaging with dextran-coated iron oxide nanoparticles shows pre-contrast high-intensity signal (*A*) which persists in the post-contrast phase (*B*). This 7-mm metastatic lymph node did not meet morphologic or size criteria for diagnosis of metastasis on standard MRI. (Courtesy of M. Harisinghani, MD, Boston, MA.)

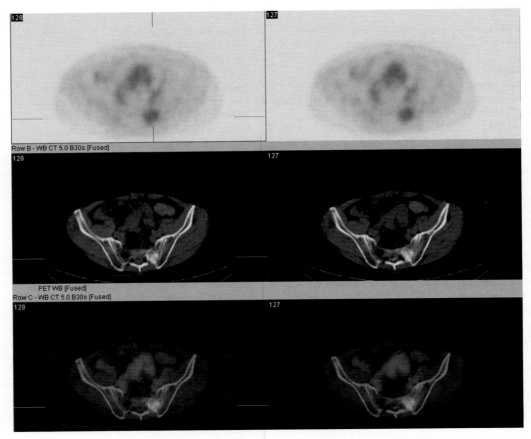

Fig. 5. Co-registered PET and CT scans after administration of FDG. The focus of mildly increased glucose metabolism within the left sacrum corresponded to an obvious osteoblastic focus on skeletal scintigraphy.

FDG-PET has shown variable results for lymph node assessment and its use may be hampered because of a relatively low glycolytic rate in prostate cancer and its metastases [39]. However, several newer positron-emitting agents have shown utility for prostate cancer imaging not solely based on tumor metabolism. Though the mechanism of action is not completely understood, it appears that ^{11}C-acetate is incorporated into the lipid pool of neoplastic tissues that have low oxidative metabolism and a high rate of lipid synthesis, and choline-derived agents undergo intracellular phophorylation and are incorporated into cell membranes [40]. The ^{11}C-methionine analog is incorporated in intracellular proteins and the ^{18}F-derivative of dihydrotestosterone uses a hormonal-based pathway [41]. The ^{11}C derivatives of methionine, acetate, and choline avoid renal excretion, unlike ^{18}F-FDG; therefore, the detection of juxtavesicular disease in the pelvis is not hindered by an artifactual signal in the bladder as it is with ^{18}F-FDG [40]. A recent study that used PET with ^{11}C-choline yielded a sensitivity of 80%, specificity of 96%, and accuracy of 93% without tissue confirmation in 67 patients [42]. In another report, ^{11}C-acetate, significantly outperformed both FDG-PET and CT [43]. Co-registration of PET images with anatomic CT data improves anatomic localization with many tumors and may be the best use of PET scans for prostate cancer.

Although these studies are encouraging, perhaps the next major leap for use of PET imaging will occur with the introduction of small, high-resolution PET scanners for the prostate (Fig. 6), which have achieved a threefold increase in resolution over conventional PET scanners in tissue (I. Weinberg, MD, personal communication, 2002). This prototype scanner has two heads, similar to standard PET scanners, but one of the gamma

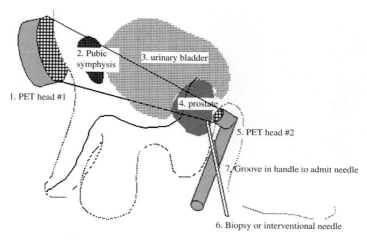

Fig. 6. Prototypical miniaturized PET scanner which can provide greater resolution through transrectal access. (Courtesy of I. Weinberg, PhD, Rockville, MD.)

heads is a miniature handheld camera for insertion into the rectum. This unit uses specialized proprietary Monte Carlo-based computer algorithms that incorporate position-sensing technology needed to obtain images from the handheld PET geometry.

Radioimmunoscintigraphy

Radioimmunoscintigraphy has long held promise for diagnostic applications in staging malignancy. In contrast to anatomic imaging, this modality acquires images through use of a radiolabeled antibody that recognizes prostate tissue. The antigen that has stimulated the most interest is prostate-specific membrane antigen (PSMA), which is expressed in prostate cells and upregulated in higher grade cancer, androgen insensitive cancer, and metastatic deposits [44–48]. The most intensively studied monoclonal antibody conjugate to PSMA is capromab pendetide (ProstaScint, Cytogen Corp., Princeton, New Jersey), which is a 100 kd type II transmembrane glycoprotein that recognizes an intracellular epitope [49]. Several other candidates have been evaluated, including those to extracellular epitopes, but none have been approved for general use [50]. Despite controversy about the utility of an antibody to an internal epitope, and the question of whether this antibody recognizes live tissue, capromab pendetide has been shown to bind to live cells and there are several studies that show a high correlation of pathological specimens to scan results [29,51–53].

The pivotal clinical trial demonstrated a 63% sensitivity (compared with 4% for CT and 15% for MRI) and a 92% negative predictive value with tissue confirmation of scan results [29]. The ProstaScint scan, however, was not widely adopted at that time because of erratic scan results at clinical sites. Mixed reports about accuracy resulted from differences in camera technology used for image acquisition and from lack of experienced readers for scan interpretation. It has taken major advances in image acquisition and the advent of image co-registration to significantly enhance and standardize the accuracy of disease detection. The functional imaging with radioimmunoscintigraphy differs from and is synergistic with anatomic imaging such as CT or MRI. Although PET scans have not proven useful for prostate cancer imaging with the current metabolic imaging analogs, the fusion of PET and CT for other tumors has raised awareness of the enhanced resolution one can obtain from fused anatomical and functional scans. By combining dual head gamma cameras with fusion of the functional single photon emission tomography (SPECT) and an anatomical image, the 7E-11 radioimmunoconjugate has made a dramatic difference for prostate cancer detection (Fig. 7) [53–55]. Localization accuracy has doubled and tissue confirmation of scan results now demonstrate an accuracy of 83% with fused images [54–55].

The emergence of clinical outcomes data related to PSMA and capromab pendetide scan results strengthen the case for the use of this radioimmunoconjugate. Patients who have

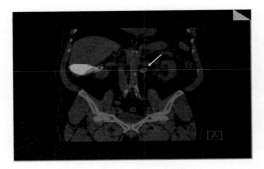

Fig. 7. Fused SPECT and CT scan with capromab pendetide which demonstrates a solitary renal perihilar lymph node (*white arrow*) in an intermediate-risk patient who has prostate cancer confirmed on biopsy to be metastatic disease. Fused scans have doubled localization accuracy for prostate cancer. (Courtesy of B. Prestidge, MD, San Antonio, TX.)

prostate cancer and who overexpress PSMA in the prostate gland have been shown to have twice the recurrence rate and a faster time to recurrence compared with those who have normal expression in the gland [56]. The dramatically improved resolution with fused scans has been correlated with step-sectioned prostatic pathological evaluation which shows an 80% overall accuracy and 79% sensitivity, specificity of 80%, positive predictive value of 68%, and negative predictive value of 88% for detection of cancer within the prostate gland [57]. This preliminary study was the basis for focal image-guided brachytherapy for intermediate- to high-risk prostate cancer patients where the treatment field was altered on the basis of the scan (Fig. 8) [58]. The 7 year follow-up data on 239 patients demonstrated superior results across all risk categories compared with the 5 year metanalysis of brachytherapy patients (96%

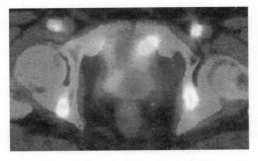

Fig. 8. Fused SPECT and CT scan in which increased signal intensity suggests localized prostate cancer. (Courtesy of R. Ellis, MD, Cleveland, OH.)

versus 87% low risk, 87% versus 74% intermediate risk, and 73% versus 50% high risk) [59]. Furthermore, patients with a ProstaScint scan positive outside of the pelvis, showed a threefold increase in biochemical disease recurrence regardless of risk category. This suggests that the scan results can be used both to predict better outcomes based on the absence of distant signal intensity and to direct increased dosimetry to focal areas of increased uptake within the prostate gland. Future studies will address focal image-guided therapy for localized prostate cancer with cryotherapy on the basis of these data.

Patients who have a rising PSA after prostatectomy have also been evaluated with capromab pendetide. Reports have shown mixed results. Some investigators demonstrate a durable complete biochemical response rate to external beam radiotherapy over a nearly 5-year period, although others claim there is no advantage for the use of the scan [60–63]. The latter studies used images obtained in the era before the introduction of dual-head cameras and fused images, when image quality varied among institutions and depended on how the image was acquired and skill of the reader. In the modern era of fused images from higher resolution cameras, investigators report the value of radioimmunoscintigraphy [64]. These data suggest that the fused scans will be more suitable for patient selection and localization for targeted therapy (Fig. 9).

The future of prostate cancer imaging

The next quantum leap in medical advances will be driven by our enhancement of imaging for diagnosis, for refinement of treatment, and for sophisticated evaluation of treatment efficacy. The convergence of technology in the fields of material science, biology, and the defense and communications industries have greatly advanced diagnostic imaging. Precision in control of the spatial and temporal properties of light along with understanding of light and its heterogeneous scattering properties within tissue have extended our capability for imaging. Radioimmunoscintigraphy has been used for a decade for prostate cancer imaging and refinements in image acquisition, fusion of images, and outcome data which provide better clinical information, now suggest a use for image-guided therapy. Optical coherence tomography (OCT) uses diffuse reflectance to image subepithelial structures to identify neurovascular tissue and radiation effects. The introduction of

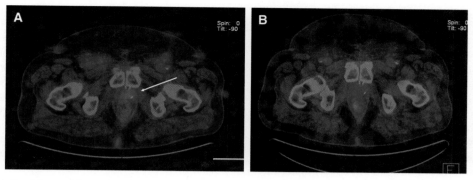

Fig. 9. A fused ProstaScint and CT scan for a patient who had PSA recurrence 2 years after radical prostatectomy and a postoperative undetectable PSA, which demonstrates an increased signal in the prostatic fossa (*white arrow*) (*A*). A repeat fused scan demonstrates no signal 6 months after external beam radiotherapy and a return to undetectable PSA levels (*B*). Signal intensity is noted in the rectal lumen caused by excretion of the radioimmunoconjugate, which demonstrates the need for fused scans for accurate anatomical localization. (Courtesy of B. Prestidge, MD, San Antonio, TX.)

newer MRI agents, such as the dextran-coated iron oxide nanoparticles, appears to provide significant imaging capabilities to detect malignant lymph nodes. Future applications of electron paramagnetic resonance imaging and hyperspectral imaging promise further refinements of our ability to image tissues for diagnosis.

Technologies on the horizon

Electron paramagnetic resonance

A functional imaging modality that is promising for prostate cancer evaluation uses electron paramagnetic resonance (EPR) to correlate tumor presence with hypoxia. It has been reported that localized prostate cancer is characterized by marked hypoxia and significant heterogeneity in oxygenation [65–67]. Overhauser enhanced MRI (OMRI) combines two spectroscopic techniques, Nuclear Magnetic Resonance (NMR) and Electron Paramagnetic Resonance (EPR) to provide high-resolution MR images at low magnetic fields ($\sim$10 mT). Although NMR detects species that have magnetic nuclei such as water protons, EPR detects species that have unpaired electrons such as paramagnetic molecules. Infusion with the paramagnetic agent before scanning with both the EPR frequency and the NMR frequency yields MR images that have high spatial resolution [66]. Image resolution is poor without the contrast agent consistent with the low magnetic fields used, but significantly enhanced resolution is evident after infusion with the paramagnetic

agent. Very small probes are used that require about 650-fold less energy than standard MRI (Fig. 10). In vivo studies demonstrate that tumor accumulates significant amounts of the contrast agent yet large areas of the tumor are severely hypoxic. This unique, small, portable OMRI technique is capable of providing anatomically co-registered images of oxygen distribution, which again demonstrates the value of image fusion.

Diagnostic light technology

Light is increasingly being used in various forms to gather information about biological systems and there are implications for use in prostate cancer. Diagnosis using light varies in

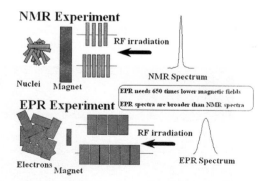

Fig. 10. High-resolution MR images can be obtained at low magnetic fields with EPR to measure tumor hypoxia. This small portable MR technology requires approximately 650-fold less energy than standard MRI. (Courtesy of M. Krishna, PhD, Bethesda, MD.)

one fundamental respect from therapeutic applications of light sources, such as lasers. Therapeutic uses of light are determined by the effect of light on tissue; diagnostic uses of light generally detect changes that result from the effect of tissue on light [68]. The rapid, non-invasive determination of tissue characteristics, such as scattering and absorption, is essential to process information received from the light interaction in tissue during a diagnostic procedure. These are the fundamental principles governing diagnostic light use in tissue for the emerging modalities such as optical coherence tomography and hyperspectral imaging.

Optical coherence tomography

Optical coherence tomography (OCT) is an intriguing application of diffuse reflectance spectroscopy, the same principle used in pulse oximetry. OCT was originally used to image human tissue in 1991 and uses continuous wave light (instead of sound waves) to obtain images in a manner analogous to B-mode ultrasonography. However, OCT does not require a conducting medium and can therefore image through air or water with far greater resolution than ultrasound [69]. Reflected light, generated in the near infrared spectrum by a superluminescent diode, is measured by interferometry to produce 2-D images. OCT images tissue in situ and in real time, and provides resolution on the order of 5–20 μm, which is comparable to traditional confocal microscopic analysis. Cellular features detected by OCT include mitotic activity, nuclear-to-cytoplasmic ratios, and cellular migration [70]. In addition, OCT is relatively inexpensive, portable, and can be used with existing endoscopic instrumentation [71].

OCT technology was initially used to image the transparent ocular structures in vitro but quickly expanded to include imaging of the retina and macula in vivo, with resolution of 10 μm [72,73]. After initial studies demonstrated the ability to image the nearly transparent ocular structures, OCT efforts focused on imaging solid tissue [74]. Successful in vivo imaging of dermatologic structures was followed by endoluminal imaging of vascular tissue components [75]. OCT produced resolution over six times greater than the highest available frequency intravascular ultrasound [76]. Endoscopic OCT in the human gastrointestinal tract has detected inflammatory, neoplastic, metaplastic, and cancerous processes of the esophagus, colon, and endometrium [77,78].

OCT imaging of human genitourinary tissue was first demonstrated in 1997. In vitro OCT images from biopsies of prostate, bladder and ureter were compared with standard preparations with hematoxylin and eosin staining. OCT images provided axial resolution of 16 μm and demonstrated differentiation between the prostatic urethra and prostate, visualization of the neurovascular bundle and the prostate-adipose border, visualization of the prostatic capsule, and differentiation of the anatomic layers in the bladder and ureter [79]. A recent report has demonstrated the feasibility and high sensitivity for determination of early bladder tumor invasion (Fig. 11) [80]. OCT is currently being used to evaluate effects on prostate tissue from ionizing radiation and to locate neurovascular tissue during radical prostatectomy. Improvements in the ability to obtain OCT images strongly suggest that greater depth of tissue penetration will be possible and there will be greater implications for solid tissue evaluation.

Hyperspectral imaging

Diffuse reflectance spectroscopy from different wavelengths of light can be used to gather

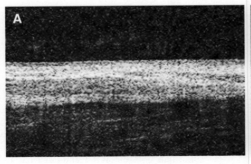
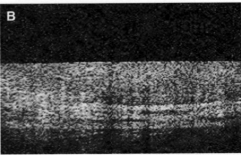

Fig. 11. OCT demonstrates excellent resolution in superficial normal tissue (*A*) and carcinoma in situ (*B*). OCT is under evaluation to identify neurovascular tissue during surgical procedures and to monitor radiation effects.

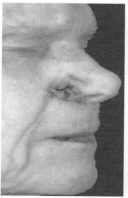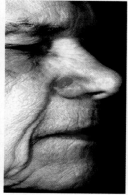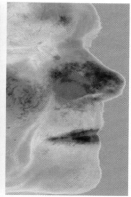

Fig. 12. Hyperspectral analysis with diffuse reflectance spectroscopy from different wavelengths of light identifies a unique spectral signature in areas of neoplasia. Fusion of images from this type of technology with other non-invasive modalities holds promise for solid tissue evaluation. (Courtesy of S.J. Spear, PhD, Hancock, MS).

a composite image of tissue and identify abnormalities. This hyperspectral imaging has been used for evaluation of diverse problems that range from oxygen saturation and tissue perfusion to wound extent and neoplasia [81–84]. Evaluation of cutaneous lesions by analysis of full-thickness dermal specimens yielded distinct spectral signatures for regions of interest in the epidermis, normal dermis, and abnormal dermal areas (Fig. 12). The rapid scan of the regional surface area using these hyperspectral signatures revealed an exclusionary, pseudo-color pattern, which consistently defined a central abnormal area that had a unique spectral signature. An algorithm that compared abnormal hyperspectral areas with histopathological findings showed no significant variation from standard bright-field microscopy. These data indicate that hyperspectral analysis may provide a high-throughput alternative for tissue evaluation that approximates standard bright-field image analysis. Although this technology has not been used for prostate cancer, the ability to perturb tissue with a variety of wavelengths delivered by an optical fiber holds promise for solid tissue evaluation, especially in combination with other minimally invasive diagnostic imaging technologies. The combination of these types of diagnostic techniques with other imaging information is the wave of the future.

Summary

Prostate cancer imaging has evolved from morphological mapping on 2-D images to tissue characterization through use of tissue-specific agents, molecular imaging, and nanotechnology. Sensor fusion and co-registration enhance detection and provide unique tissue signatures once thought impossible. A cooperative effort to achieve definitive tissue sampling, noninvasive image-guided therapy, and surveillance with 3-D imaging in real time will provide clinical data that should lead to real breakthroughs in patient management of this enigmatic disease.

References

[1] Jemal A, Murray T, Ward E, et al. Cancer statistics, 2005. CA Cancer J Clin 2005;55:10–30.

[2] Parker SL, Tong T, Bolden S, et al. Cancer statistics, 1997. CA Cancer J Clin 1997;47:5–27.

[3] Khan MA, Partin AW, Mangold LA, et al. Probability of biochemical recurrence by analysis of pathologic stage, Gleason score, and margin status for localized prostate cancer. Urology 2003;62:866–71.

[4] Kattan MW, Eastham JA, Wheeler TM, et al. Counseling men with prostate cancer: a nomogram for predicting the presence of small, moderately differentiated, confined tumors. J Urol 2003;170:1792–7.

[5] Murray SK, Breau RH, Guha AK, et al. Spread of prostate carcinoma to the perirectal lymph node basin: analysis of 112 rectal resections over a 10-year span for primary rectal adenocarcinoma. Am J Surg Pathol 2004;28:1154–62.

[6] Allaf ME, Palapattu GS, Trock BJ, et al. Anatomical extent of lymph node dissection: impact on men with clinically localized prostate cancer. J Urol 2004;172:1840–4.

[7] Bader P, Burkhard FC, Markwalder R. Disease progression and survival of patients with positive lymph

nodes after radical prostatectomy. Is there a chance of cure? J Urol 2003;169(3):849–54.

[8] Purohit RS, Shinohara K, Meng MV, et al. Imaging clinically localized prostate cancer. Urol Clin N Am 2003;30:279–93.

[9] Leibovici D, Kamat AM, Do KA, et al. Transrectal ultrasound versus magnetic resonance imaging for detection of rectal wall invasion by prostate cancer. Prostate 2005;62:101–4.

[10] Hamper UM, Trapanotto V, DeJong MR, et al. Three-dimensional US of the prostate: early experience. Radiology 1999;212:719.

[11] Garg S, Fortling B, Chadwick D, et al. Staging of prostate cancer using 3-dimensional transrectal ultrasound images: a pilot study. J Urol 1999;162: 1318–21.

[12] Okihara K, Kojima M, Nakanouchi T, et al. Transrectal power Doppler imaging in the detection of prostate cancer. BJU Int 2000;85:1053–7.

[13] Ismail M, Peterson RO, Alexander AA, et al. Color Doppler imaging in predicting the biologic behavior of prostate cancer: correlation with disease-free survival. Urology 1997;50:906–12.

[14] Sauvain JL, Palascak P, Bourscheid D, et al. Value of power doppler and 3D vascular sonography as a method for diagnosis and staging of prostate cancer. Eur Urol 2003;44:21–31.

[15] Eckersley RJ, Sedelaar JP, Blomley MJ, et al. Quantitative microbubble enhanced transrectal ultrasound as a tool for monitoring hormonal treatment of prostate carcinoma. Prostate 2002; 51(4):256–67.

[16] Frauscher F, Klauser A, Volgger H, et al. Comparison of contrast enhanced color Doppler targeted biopsy with conventional systematic biopsy: impact on prostate cancer detection. J Urol 2002;167:1648–52.

[17] Adusumilli S, Pretorius ES. Magnetic resonance imaging of prostate cancer. Semin Urol Oncol 2002;20: 192–210.

[18] Brassell SA, Krueger WR, Choi JH, et al. Correlation of endorectal coil magnetic resonance imaging of the prostate with pathologic stage. World J Urol 2004;22:289–92.

[19] Sella T, Schwartz LH, Swindle PW, et al. Suspected local recurrence after radical prostatectomy: endorectal coil MR imaging. Radiology 2004;231:379–85.

[20] Montie JE, et al. Staging systems for prostate cancer. In: Vogelzang NJ, Scardino PT, Shipley WU, et al, editors. Genitourinary oncology. 2nd edition. Philadelphia: Lippincott Williams and Wilkins; 2000. p. 673–9.

[21] Gomez P, Manoharan M, Kim SS, et al. Radionuclide bone scintigraphy in patients with biochemical recurrence after radical prostatectomy: when is it indicated? BJU Int 2004;94:299–302.

[22] Kane CJ, Amling CL, Johnstone PA, et al. Limited value of bone scintigraphy and computed tomography in assessing biochemical failure after radical prostatectomy. Urology 2003;61:607–11.

[23] Roudier MP, Vesselle H, True LD, et al. Bone histology at autopsy and matched bone scintigraphy findings in patients with hormone refractory prostate cancer: the effect of bisphosphonate therapy on bone scintigraphy results. Clin Exp Metastasis 2003;20:171–80.

[24] Binnie D, Divoli A, McCready VR, et al. The potential use of 99mTc-MDP bone scans to plan high-activity 186Re-HEDP targeted therapy of bony metastases from prostate cancer. Cancer Biother Radiopharm 2005;20:189–94.

[25] Golimbu M, Morales P, Al-Askari S, et al. CAT scanning in staging of prostate cancer. Urology 1981;18:305–8.

[26] Oyen RH, Van Poppel HP, Ameye FE, et al. Lymph node staging of localized prostatic carcinoma with CT and CT-guided fine-needle aspiration biopsy: prospective study of 285 patients. Radiology 1994; 190:315–22.

[27] Rorvik J, Halvorsen OJ, Albrektsen G, et al. Lymphangiography combined with biopsy and computer tomography to detect lymph node metastases in localized prostate cancer. Scand J Urol Nephrol 1998;32:116–9.

[28] Weinerman PM, Arger PH, Coleman BG, et al. Pelvic adenopathy from bladder and prostate carcinoma: detection by rapid sequence computed tomography. AJR Am J Roentgenol 1983;140:95–9.

[29] Manyak MJ, Hinkle GH, Olsen JO, et al. Immunoscintigraphy with [111] In-capromab pendetide: evaluation before definitive therapy in patients with prostate cancer. Urology 1999;54:1058–63.

[30] Ferguson JK, Oesterling JE. Patient evaluation if prostate-specific antigen becomes elevated following radical prostatectomy or radiation therapy. Urol Clin North Am 1994;21:677–85.

[31] Platt JF, Bree RL, Schwab RE. The accuracy of CT in the staging of cancer of the prostate. Am J Radiol 1987;149:315–20.

[32] Ghanem N, Altehoefer C, Hogerle S, et al. Comparative diagnostic value and therapeutic relevance of magnetic resonance imaging and bone marrow scintigraphy in patients with metastatic solid tumors of the axial skeleton. Eur J Radiol 2002;43:256–61.

[33] Lauenstein TC, Goehde SC, Herborn CU, et al. Whole-body MR imaging: evaluation of patients for metastases. Radiology 2004;233:139–48.

[34] Weissleder R, Elizondo G, Wittenberg J, et al. Ultrasmall superparamagnetic iron oxide: an intravenous contrast agent for assessing lymph nodes with MR imaging. Radiology 1990;175:494–8.

[35] Harisinghani MG, Barentsz J, Hahn PF, et al. Noninvasive detection of clinically occult lymph-node metastases in prostate cancer. N Engl J Med 2003; 348:2491–9.

[36] McLaughlin AP, Saltzstein SL, McCullough DL, et al. Prostatic carcinoma: incidence and location of unsuspected lymphatic metastases. J Urol 1976; 115:89–94.

[37] Golimbu M, Morales P, Al-Askari S, et al. Extended pelvic lymphadenectomy for prostate cancer. J Urol 1979;121:617–20.

[38] Hain SF, Maisey MN. Positron emission tomography for urological tumours. BJU Int 2003;92: 159–64.

[39] Shvarts O, Han KR, Seltzer M, et al. Positron emission tomography in urologic oncology. Cancer Control 2002;9:335–42.

[40] Schoder H, Larson SM. Positron emission tomography for prostate, bladder, and renal cancer. Sem Nucl Med 2004;34:274–92.

[41] Larson SM, Morris M, Gunther I, et al. Tumor localization of 16beta-18F-fluoro-5alpha-dihydro-testosterone versus 18F-FDG in patients with progressive, metastatic prostate cancer. J Nucl Med 2004;45:366–73.

[42] de Jong IJ, Pruim J, Elsinga PH, et al. Preoperative staging of pelvic lymph nodes in prostate cancer by 11C-choline PET. J Nucl Med 2003;44:331–5.

[43] Oyama N, Miller TR, Dehdashti F, et al. 11C-acetate PET imaging of prostate cancer: detection of recurrent disease at PSA relapse. J Nucl Med 2003;44:549–55.

[44] Horoszewicz JS, Kawinski F, Murphy GP. Monoclonal antibodies to a new antigenic marker in epithelial prostatic cells and serum of prostatic cancer patients. Anticancer Res 1987;7:927–35.

[45] Israeli RS, Powell CT, Fair WR, et al. Molecular cloning of a complementary DNA encoding a prostate-specific membrane antigen. Cancer Res 1993;53: 227–30.

[46] Wright GL Jr, Grob BM, Haley C, et al. Upregulation of prostate-specific membrane antigen after androgen-deprivation therapy. Urology 1996;48: 326–34.

[47] Silver DA, Pellicer I, Fair WR, et al. Prostate-specific membrane antigen expression in normal and malignant human tissues. Clin Cancer Res 1997;3:81–5.

[48] Rochon YP, Horoszewicz JS, Boynton AL, et al. Western blot assay for prostate-specific membrane antigen in serum of prostate cancer patients. Prostate 1994;25:219–23.

[49] Troyer JK, Beckett ML, Wright GL Jr. Location of prostate-specific membrane antigen in the LNCaP prostate carcinoma cell line. Prostate 1997;30: 232–42.

[50] Smith-Jones P, Vallabhajosula S, Navarro V, et al. Radiolabeled monoclonal antibodies specific to the extracellular domain of prostate-specific membrane antigen: preclinical studies in nude mice bearing LNCaP human prostate tumor. J Nucl Med 2003; 44:610–7.

[51] Barren RJ, Holmes EH, Boynton AL, et al. Monoclonal antibody 7E11.C5 staining of viable LNCaP cells. Prostate 1997;30:232–42.

[52] Hinkle GH, Burgers JK, Neal CE, et al. Multicenter radioimmunoscintigraphic evaluation of patients with prostate carcinoma using indium-111 capromab pendetide. Cancer 1998;83:739–47.

[53] Sodee DB, Nelson AD, Faulhaber PF, et al. Update on fused capromab pendetide imaging of prostate cancer. Clin Prostate Cancer 2005;3: 230–8.

[54] Schettino CJ, Kramer E, Noz M, et al. Impact of fusion of Indium-111 capromab pendetide volume data sets with those from MRI or CT in patients with recurrent prostate cancer. AJR 2004;183: 519–24.

[55] Wong TZ, Turkington TG, Polascik TJ, et al. ProstaScint (capromab pendetide) imaging using hybrid gamma camera-CT technology. AJR Am J Roentgenol 2005;184:676–80.

[56] Ross JS, Sheehan CE, Fisher HA, et al. Correlation of primary tumor prostate-specific membrane antigen expression with disease recurrence in prostate cancer. Clin Cancer Res 2003;9:6357–62.

[57] Ellis RJ, Kim EY, Conant R, et al. Radioimmunoguided imaging of prostate cancer foci with histopathological correlation. Int J Radiat Oncol Biol Phys 2001;49:1281–6.

[58] Ellis RJ, Vertocnik A, Kim EY, et al. Four-year biochemical outcome after radioimmunoguided transperineal brachytherapy for patients with prostate adenocarcinoma. Int J Radiat Oncol Biol Phys 2003;57:362–70.

[59] Ellis RJ, Kim EY, Zhou H, et al. Seven-year biochemical disease-free survival rates following permanent prostate brachytherapy with dose escalation to biological tumor olumes (BTVs) identified with SPECT/CT image fusion. Presented at the 26th Annual Meeting of the American Brachytherapy Society; San Francisco, June 1–3, 2005.

[60] Kahn D, Williams RD, Manyak MJ, et al. 111Indium-capromab pendetide in the evaluation of patients with residual or recurrent prostate cancer after radical prostatectomy. The ProstaScint Study Group. J Urol 1998;159:2041–6.

[61] Kahn D, Williams RD, Haseman MK, et al. Radioimmunoscintigraphy with In-111-labeled capromab pendetide predicts prostate cancer response to salvage radiotherapy after failed radical prostatectomy. J Clin Oncol 1998;161:284–9.

[62] Thomas CT, Bradshaw PT, Pollock BH, et al. Indium-111-capromab pendetide radioimmunoscintigraphy and prognosis for durable biochemical response to salvage radiation therapy in men after failed prostatectomy. J Clin Oncol 2003;21: 1715–21.

[63] Wilkinson S, Chodak G. The role of 111indium-capromab pendetide imaging for assessing biochemical failure after radical prostatectomy. J Urol 2004; 172:133–6.

[64] Jani AB, Blend MJ, Hamilton R, et al. Radioimmunoscintigraphy for postprostatectomy radiotherapy: analysis of toxicity and biochemical control. J Nucl Med 2004;45:1315–22.

[65] Parker C, Milosevic M, Toi A, et al. Polarographic electrode study of tumor oxygenation in clinically localized prostate cancer. Int J Radiat Oncol Biol Phys 2004;58:750–7.

[66] Krishna MC, English S, Yamada K, et al. Overhauser enhanced magnetic resonance imaging for tumor oximetry: coregistration of tumor anatomy and tissue oxygen concentration. Proc Natl Acad Sci USA 2002; 99:2216–21.

[67] Zhao D, Ran S, Constantinescu A, et al. Tumor oxygen dynamics: correlation of in vivo MRI with histological findings. Neoplasia 2003;5:308–18.

[68] Parrish JA, Wilson BC. Current and future trends in laser medicine. Photochem Photobiol 1991;53: 731–8.

[69] Feldchtein FI, Gelikonov GV, Gelikonov VM, et al. Endoscopic applications of optical coherence tomography. Opt Express 1998;3:257–60.

[70] Boppart SA, Bouma BE, Pitris C, et al. In vivo cellular optical coherence tomography imaging. Nat Med 1998;4:861–5.

[71] Manyak MJ, Warner JW. An update on laser use in Urology. Contemp Urol 2003;15:13–28.

[72] Hee MR, Izatt JA, Swanson EA, et al. Optical coherence tomography of the human retina. Arch Ophthalmol 1995;113:325–32.

[73] Puliafito CA, Hee MR, Lin CP, et al. Imaging of macular diseases with optical coherence tomography. Ophthalmology 1995;102:217–29.

[74] Schmitt JM, Knüttel A, Yadlowsky M, et al. Optical-coherence tomography of a dense tissue: statistics of attenuation and backscattering. Phys Med Biol 1994;39:1705–20.

[75] Brezinski ME, Tearney GJ, Bouma BE, et al. Optical coherence tomography for optical biopsy. Properties and demonstration of vascular pathology. Circulation 1996;93:1206–13.

[76] Brezinski ME, Tearney GJ, Weissman NJ, et al. Assessing atherosclerotic plaque morphology: comparison of optical coherence tomography and high frequency intravascular ultrasound. Heart 1997;77: 397–403.

[77] Jackle S, Gladkova N, Feldchtein F, et al. In vivo endoscopic optical coherence tomography of the human gastrointestinal tract—toward optical biopsy. Endoscopy 2000;32:743–9.

[78] Pitris C, Goodman A, Boppart SA, et al. High-resolution imaging of gynecologic neoplasms using optical coherence tomography. Obstet Gynecol 1999;93: 135–9.

[79] Tearney GJ, Brezinski ME, Southern JF, et al. Optical biopsy in human Urologic tissue using optical coherence tomography. J Urol 1997;157:1915–9.

80 Manyak MJ, Gladkova ND, Makari JH, et al. Evaluation of superficial bladder transitional cell car cinoma by optical coherence tomography. J Endourol 2005;19:570–4.

[81] Khoobehi B, Beach JM, Kawano H. Hyperspectral imaging for measurement of oxygen saturation in the optic nerve head. Invest Ophthalmol Vis Sci 2004;45:1464–72.

[82] Zuzak KJ, Gladwin MT, Cannon RO 3rd, et al. Imaging hemoglobin oxygen saturation in sickle cell disease patients using noninvasive visible reflectance hyperspectral techniques: effects of nitric oxide. Am J Physiol Heart Circ Physiol 2003;285: H1183–9.

[83] Shah SA, Bachrach N, Spear SJ, et al. Cutaneous wound analysis using hyperspectral imaging. Biotechniques 2003;34:408–13.

[84] Zuzak KJ, Schaeberle MD, Lewis EN, et al. Visible reflectance hyperspectral imaging: characterization of a noninvasive, in vivo system for determining tissue perfusion. Anal Chem 2002;74:2021–8.

ELSEVIER
SAUNDERS

Urol Clin N Am 33 (2006) 147–159

UROLOGIC
CLINICS
of North America

Biochemical Recurrence after Localized Treatment

Christopher L. Amling, MD, FACS

Division of Urology, FOT 1105, University of Alabama, 1530 3rd Avenue, South Birmingham, AL 35294-3411, USA

Before the advent and widespread use of prostate-specific antigen (PSA) testing, recurrence after radical prostatectomy or radiotherapy was usually defined by the postoperative development of a palpable mass in the prostate or in the prostatic fossa, or by evidence of metastatic disease on postoperative imaging studies. With postoperative PSA monitoring, and particularly with the use of ultrasensitive PSA assays, biochemical recurrence can now be detected many years before the development of clinically evident disease. The quoted incidence of biochemical recurrence (BCR) after localized treatment varies significantly and depends on numerous well-known prognostic factors; however, it likely occurs in at least 30%–40% of patients who receive localized treatment. It is estimated that more than 50,000 men per year in the United States will develop a PSA-only relapse [1]. This number will probably increase because of the trend toward diagnosis and treatment of prostate cancer in progressively younger men.

The health management of these men represents a diagnostic and treatment dilemma. Because many of these men have long life expectancies at the time of BCR, the benefits of further therapy must be balanced against the potential for treatment-related quality-of-life compromises over a much longer period of time. The localization (local or distant) of recurrent cancer in this setting is challenging, and makes selection of the best treatment problematic. Because the clinical significance of BCR is often unclear, and depends in many cases on unknown factors, it is difficult to select the best treatment and determine when best to institute that therapy. This review examines some of these issues and

attempts to shed some light on this common but controversial clinical scenario.

Defining biochemical recurrence

Radical prostatectomy

To date, there has been no general consensus on what represents the best definition of PSA recurrence after radical prostatectomy (RP). Although some RP series use any detectable PSA level as evidence of treatment failure, most define some selected PSA threshold to indicate recurrence. Biochemical outcomes after RP are dependent to some degree on the PSA threshold used to define failure. In a large surgical series from the Mayo Clinic, the impact of varying definitions of recurrence on outcome reporting was investigated [2]. A PSA cut point ≥ 0.2 ng/mL was compared with a cut point of ≥ 0.4 ng/mL, and a 14% and 16% improvement in PSA progression-free survival at 5 and 10 years respectively, was seen, which favored the higher PSA cut point. A definition that required a PSA value of 0.4 ng/mL or greater was compared to a definition that required two such values, and a 7% and 18% difference in recurrence rate was seen at 5 in 10 years respectively. The better reported outcomes occurred when two abnormal values were required. Because it takes longer for two PSA values above a given threshold to occur, progression is delayed and reported outcomes are better using these definitions.

Although it is generally assumed that any detectable PSA level after RP represents persistent or progressive disease, this may not always be the case. Some men develop detectable but stable PSA levels that do not appear to progress further. These low stable PSA levels are probably a result of residual benign tissue left behind at the time of RP, particularly at the prostatic apex or bladder

E-mail address: camling@surg.uab.edu

0094-0143/06/$ - see front matter © 2006 Elsevier Inc. All rights reserved.
doi:10.1016/j.ucl.2005.12.002

neck [3–6]. Low stable levels could also be attributed to periurethral glands that produce PSA [7]. In the Mayo Clinic RP series, only 49% of patients who reached a PSA threshold of 0.2 ng/mL progressed to a higher PSA value over a 3-year period [2]. It wasn't until the PSA value reached 0.4 ng/mL that most patients demonstrated a subsequent PSA increase, which suggests that this threshold would be an appropriate definition for failure. In a smaller but similar study of 358 men who underwent RP at the West Los Angeles Veterans Medical Center, a PSA cut point of 0.2 ng/mL was associated with a 100% risk of an increasing PSA over the subsequent 3-year period [8]. These investigators suggested that a cut point of 0.2 ng/mL was the most appropriate for use in defining BCR.

The definition of biochemical recurrence after radical prostatectomy is further complicated by the use of ultrasensitive PSA assays. The most important potential utility of ultrasensitive PSA assays would be to identify recurrent disease earlier in its course. Stamey and coworkers [9] used a PSA assay that had a biological detection limit for serum PSA of 0.07 ng/mL, to study serum samples from 22 patients who had RP and later developed recurrent cancer, which was evident by a detectable PSA level > 0.3 ng/mL. Recurrence was detected a mean of 310 days earlier using the ultrasensitive assay. In another study that used an ultrasensitive assay and that had a 0.08 ng/mL level of detectability, it was calculated that recurrent disease could be identified 22 months sooner than with conventional PSA assays [10]. Other studies have shown similar ability to predict biochemical recurrence much earlier than standard assays [11–13].

One recent study examined the utility of nadir PSA as detected by ultrasensitive assay with lower limit of detection < 0.01 ng/mL to detect early relapse after RP, defined as two consecutive post-nadir PSA levels ≥ 0.1 ng/mL [14]. In multivariate analysis, nadir PSA was an important predictor of eventual BCR; the lowest recurrence rates were seen in subjects who had nadir values < 0.01 ng/mL. BCR occurred in 89% of subjects whose PSA nadir was 0.04 to 0.1 ng/mL. It is undoubtedly true than higher nadir values are associated with higher recurrence rates, however, does identification of BCR at an earlier point in time, yet within the undetectable level of standard assays, provide any benefit for the efficacy of further treatment? It is accepted that radiation to the prostatic fossa for local recurrence after RP is most beneficial when the PSA is low, but there is no current evidence that this therapy is more effective when disease is detected at ultrasensitive PSA levels.

The ideal definition of BCR after RP would be one that is clearly associated with progression to clinically evident metastatic disease. There are some patients who develop BCR that have an indolent course and others who harbor a more malignant tumor type that is destined to progress to metastatic disease. These patients can often be differentiated by consideration of the pathologic tumor characteristics, the timing of recurrence, and PSA kinetics [15]. Thus far, it has been difficult to devise a definition of BCR that encompasses all of these considerations. Consensus on a definition is important for consistent outcome comparisons between surgical series and varied patient populations. A consensus, however, has not been reached, and the most appropriate definition of BCR after RP continues to be debated.

Radiotherapy

Because the prostate gland is left in situ after radiotherapy, the decrease in PSA after treatment depends on the effect of radiation on the cancer as well as the cellular effects of radiation on normal prostate tissue. Although radical prostatectomy results in nadir—usually undetectable PSA values within weeks of surgery, PSA levels may decrease quite slowly after radiation, and nadir levels are usually not achieved until at least 18 months after completion of treatment [16]. The rapidity and magnitude of the PSA decrease also depends on prostate size and the type of radiation (external beam versus brachytherapy) that is administered. Several studies have shown that PSA levels are usually < 0.5 ng/mL in men who receive pelvic radiotherapy for nonprostatic malignancies and a rising PSA in this setting is unusual [17,18]. Thus, a rising PSA after radiotherapy for prostate cancer may be a good marker of persistent recurrent disease. Nadir PSA level is also an important prognostic factor to predict eventual biochemical recurrence, but nadir values indicative of successful cancer eradication vary according to prostate size and type of radiation. For example, lower PSA levels are expected after brachytherapy or combined brachytherapy-external beam therapy [16]. In contrast to RP, in which a simple cutpoint can be used, there are many other factors to consider when defining recurrence after radiation therapy.

A consensus panel of the American Society for Therapeutic Radiology and Oncology (ASTRO) was convened in 1996 to determine the best PSA surrogate endpoint to define recurrence after irradiation and it remains the most widely used failure definition [19]. This definition defines biochemical recurrence as three consecutive PSA increases after the post-radiation nadir is achieved and the date of failure is backdated to the midpoint between the post-radiation nadir and the first of the three consecutive PSA rises. The ASTRO definition has been criticized for several reasons including the bias associated with backdating the failure date, the significant impact of follow-up interval on outcome estimates, and the considerable difference between this and surgical failure definitions [16,20,21].

To investigate how the ASTRO definition might affect reported biochemical recurrence rates when applied to radical prostatectomy patients, this definition was applied to radical prostatectomy patients in two large surgical series [2,22]. The requirement for consecutive PSA increases was shown to delay the event time significantly, and backdating made late recurrence much less likely. If the ASTRO definition is compared to the failure definition used in the Mayo Clinic series (0.4 ng/mL), the result is a 19% advantage at a 10-year recurrence rate with the ASTRO definition [2]. In the Johns Hopkins series, censoring patients who had fewer than three consecutive PSA increases yielded biochemical no-evidence-of-disease (bNED) rates that were superior to the actuarial surgical definition rate by nearly 20% at 15 years [22]. Backdating the event time to between the nadir and the first of these rising PSA levels produced an apparent increase in survival from 68% to 80% percent at 15 years. When both the requirement for three consecutive rising PSA values and backdating were combined, biochemical failure was eliminated after 5 years. These comparisons illustrate how differences in the definition of biochemical failure between radical prostatectomy and radiation series make it difficult to compare biochemical outcome between these groups.

As criticisms of the ASTRO definition emerged, several alternative definitions were proposed. Thames and coworkers used a large multi-institutional database of 4839 men who received external beam radiotherapy with a median follow-up of 6.3 years, to test the sensitivity and specificity of 102 candidate PSA failure definitions for their ability to reliably predict clinical failure [20]. Three definitions were found to have the highest sensitivity and

specificity and were superior to the ASTRO definition for predicting ultimate clinical failure: (1) two PSA rises of at least 0.5 ng/mL backdated, (2) PSA level at or greater than the absolute nadir value plus 2 ng/mL not backdated, and (3) a PSA increase of 2 or 3 ng/mL from the previous value at any point, not backdated. Surgical type failure cut-points based on PSA levels greater than 0.2 or 0.5 ng/mL were inferior to other definitions. Backdating introduced a bias that overestimated freedom from biochemical failure and resulted in increasingly better outcome estimates with shorter median follow-up times. In a recent follow-up study using the same database, Kuban and coworkers [21] demonstrated significant differences in PSA disease-free survival estimates for seven alternative definitions. In comparison to the ASTRO definition, within the first 5 years post-radiation, differences of up to 13% with PSA rise definitions and up to 44% with surgical type definitions were seen.

The ASTRO definition will probably change to one of the alternative definitions that is easier to use and removes some of the bias associated with backdating. However, there are significant differences between radiation and surgical definitions of PSA recurrence which make it nearly impossible to accurately compare treatment outcomes between these two modalities. Although it would be ideal to have a universal failure definition that could be applied to all forms of therapy for localized prostate cancer, the significant differences in the mechanism of tumor eradication between these treatments makes it unlikely that a universally applied definition of biochemical failure will be found.

Diagnostic evaluation

It is important to distinguish between local and systemic disease in BCR in order to select the most appropriate treatment. In most cases, digital rectal examination is not helpful since the prostatic fossa after radical prostatectomy is usually unremarkable and the prostate after radiotherapy it difficult to interpret because of radiation induced changes. Biopsy of the prostatic fossa after radical prostatectomy, although performed commonly to rule out local recurrence in the past, is usually negative. More importantly, a negative prostatic fossa biopsy does not rule out local disease and a positive biopsy does not necessarily mean that regional or distant disease is not also present. Thus, many men with biochemical recurrence undergo abdominal-pelvic computed tomography (CT) and radionuclide bone scan in an attempt to locate the site of recurrence. Unfortunately, however, the yield of these studies is low in this setting, particularly when the PSA level is low.

Bone scan and computed tomography

The utility of bone scan in the setting of biochemical recurrence after radical prostatectomy was first assessed by Cher and coworders [23] in a series of 93 men undergoing 144 bone scans. In the absence of adjuvant therapy, the lowest PSA associated with a positive bone scan was 46 ng/mL. Unless the PSA was > 40 ng/mL and the PSA velocity was > 5.0 ng/mL/month, the probability of a positive bone scan was less than 5%. In multivariate analysis, only absolute PSA value and PSA velocity were predictive of a positive scan. In a retrospective analysis of the Center for Prostate Disease Research (CPDR) database, Kane and coworkers [24] reviewed the utility of bone scan and CT in the setting of BCR in 131 patients. Scans performed within 3 years of recurrence were analyzed. Of the 127 bone scans performed, 12 were positive, but only 2 patients with a positive bone scan had a PSA velocity (PSAV) < 0.5 ng/mL/month. Of the 86 CT scans performed, 12 were positive, but in most instances these scans were not used to assist clinical decision making. It was concluded that there is a low probability of positive scans within 3 years of biochemical recurrence and that only patients with higher PSA and PSAV levels should be considered for these imaging studies.

In a more recent study, the utility of pelvic CT scan and bone scan were assessed in 128 patients with biochemical recurrence after radical prostatectomy [25]. In this study, 11 of 97 bone scans (11%) and 5 of 71 CT scans (7%) were positive. This study examined using PSA doubling time (PSADT) in conjunction with serum PSA level to determine when it would be most appropriate to perform these studies. Men with PSADT less than 6 months were at increased risk of a positive bone scan but the risk was also related to the PSA level at the time the study was obtained. Despite a relatively short PSADT of less than 6 months, the probability of a positive bone scan or CT scan was low when the PSA level was < 10 ng/mL, but it was as high as 57% for pelvic CT and 46% for bone scan if the PSA was > 10 ng/mL.

Taken together, these studies demonstrate the limited clinical utility of bone scan and CT scan in early BCR. In the asymptomatic man, bone scan is rarely positive when the PSA is < 10 ng/mL. A bone scan should probably be withheld until the PSA level reaches 10–20 ng/mL. Similarly, CT scan is also rarely useful until the PSA reaches values exceeding 20 ng/mL. Short PSADT, particularly those less than 6 months, may identify individuals in which an earlier bone scan or CT should be considered, although the likelihood of a positive scan is still very low until the PSA exceeds 10 ng/mL.

Prostascint Scan

The Prostascint Scan (indium-111 capromab pendetide; Cytogen Corporation, Princeton, NJ) uses a radio-labeled monoclonal antibody targeted to the intracellular epitope of the prostate-specific membrane antigen (PSMA). PSMA is expressed on prostate epithelial cells, both malignant and benign but its expression appears to be increased in metastatic and hormone-refractory cancers [26]. Prostascint is FDA approved for the evaluation of postprostatectomy patients who have rising PSA levels and who are suspected to have metastatic disease. Since standard imaging studies are often negative, particularly in early BCR, it was hoped that this study would help to discriminate between local and distant recurrence in this setting.

Early studies assessed Prostascint scans in the setting of BCR by using prostatic fossa biopsy as the gold standard for a positive finding. In a multi-institutional study of 181 men who had BCR after RP, Kahn and coworkers [27] reported that in 60% of patients with interpretable scans, 42% had positive extraprostatic fossa scans, which suggested metastatic disease, and prostatic fossa biopsy was positive in 50% of those with positive fossa scans. Since extraprostatic fossa sites were not pathologically confirmed and because prostate biopsy is often falsely negative, it was difficult to interpret the results of this study. In a more recent study, Prostascint scans were used to evaluate 255 men who had early BCR (PSA ≤ 4.0 ng/mL) [28]. A positive scan was seen in 72% of patients; 31% had local (prostatic fossa) uptake only. The authors concluded that there is no minimal PSA level required for a positive Prostascint scan. However, the clinical utility of the study was not assessed because there was no pathologic confirmation of scan findings and because follow-up of response to salvage therapy was too short.

It has been suggested that Prostascint scans may help predict who will respond most effectively to salvage radiotherapy by limiting radiation to patients who do not shoe evidence of extraprostatic disease. In the first study to evaluate this idea, a "durable" response to salvage radiotherapy was seen in 70% of subjects who had a normal extraprostatic scan, compared with 22% of subjects who had a positive scan outside the prostatic fossa [29]. Unfortunately, the median follow-up time in this study was only 13 months. More recent studies have questioned the utility of Prostascint scans for the selection of appropriate salvage radiotherapy candidates. In a study of 30 men who had 34.5 months follow-up after salvage radiotherapy, there was no difference in the 2-year probability of PSA control between those with or without a positive extraprostatic fossa scan [30]. Another recent study also failed to show the utility of Prostascint scan for predicting salvage radiotherapy response [31]. Of 16 subjects undergoing salvage radiotherapy, 15 had isolated uptake in the prostatic fossa. However, only 7 (47%) had a durable response to salvage radiotherapy.

The specificity of the Prostascint scan may be improved upon by fusion of its images with simultaneous cross-sectional imaging studies such as CT and MRI. In a recent study by Schettino and coworkers [32], 58 patients underwent simultaneous Prostascint and technetium-99m blood pool imaging. Volume data sets from these scans were then fused with images from CT and MRI scans of the pelvis. Seventy-four of 161 perfusion-positive sites were found to be negative after fusion, identified primarily as bowel, vessel, or bone marrow uptake. In two patients, nodal disease not seen on initial scans was identified on the fusion images and 25 patients thought to have positive nodes appeared to have only local disease after fusion. Thus, fusion of CT and MRI images with the Prostascint scan appears to significantly improve its overall specificity and promises to add considerably to its clinical applicability.

The monoclonal antibody on which the Prostascint scan is based targets the intracellular domain of the PSMA antigen. As such, cellular death or lysis is necessary for it to take up the antibody. This may be one of the primary reasons for the limited accuracy of the Prostascint study. An antibody that targets the extracellular domain of PSMA, J591, is currently undergoing clinical trials. In phase I studies, this antibody accurately targeted metastatic lesions in 42 of 43 (98%) patients [33]. An additional advantage of J591 is its ability to target bone lesions as well as soft tissue metastases. As such, imaging studies based on this antigen can potentially image both bone and soft tissue lesions simultaneously.

Natural history of progression

It is clear that many men who develop biochemical recurrence after definitive therapy do not go on to death from prostate cancer. The first and only study to examine the untreated natural history of disease progression in men with BCR was the study of the Johns Hopkins RP population reported by Pound and coworkers [34]. Of 1997 patients who underwent RP and were observed for a mean of 5.3 years, 315 developed BCR and 304 were observed expectantly without additional therapy until the development of metastatic disease. As a group, the median time to disease progression was 8 years and death from prostate cancer occurred approximately 5 years later. Although this may be the best-case scenario given the careful selection of patients for RP at Johns Hopkins, it demonstrates convincingly that there are many men who have an indolent course of disease after PSA-detected recurrence. In this series, time to PSA recurrence, pathologic Gleason grade, and PSADT were all found to be significant predictors of progression to metastatic disease. In a recent update to this series (mean follow-up 10.5 years), PSADT and Gleason score remained significant predictors but time-to-recurrence became less useful [35].

There is a growing body of evidence that PSA kinetics may be the most clinically useful indicator of disease aggressiveness in men who have BCR [15]. The value of PSADT and PSAV was first recognized in the early 1990s in both the post-RP and post-radiotherapy settings [36–38]. After RP and radiotherapy, the rate of rise in PSA was initially investigated as a potential tool to distinguish between local and distant recurrence. It was consistently found that shorter PSADT and higher PSAV were associated with progression to systemic disease and slower rises in PSA were more often indicative of local recurrence [39–41]. A PSADT < 6 months was more consistent with distant failure after radiotherapy in the series by Sartor and coworkers [41], and longer doubling times were more likely to be associated with local recurrence. In the series by Pound and colleagues

[34], a PSADT of < 10 months was found to be a significant predictor. Patel and colleagues [39] found a PSADT of < 6 months to be strongly associated with clinical recurrence regardless of when after prostatectomy the PSA became detectable. In a large series of 2809 patients undergoing RP at the Mayo Clinic between 1987 and 1993, Roberts and coworkers [42] confirmed the strong prognostic value of PSADT. For PSADT > 1 year, the actuarial progression-free probability was more than 95% compared with only 64% if PSADT was < 6 months. In multivariate analysis, PSADT was the only significant factor that predicted systemic progression after BCR.

Although these studies all demonstrated the value of PSADT for predicting systemic progression, only recently has PSADT been confirmed as a predictor of prostate cancer death as well. D'Amico and colleagues [43] examined the value of PSADT in 8669 men who underwent both RP (n = 5918) and radiation therapy (n = 2751) between 1988 and 2002. A PSADT of < 3 months was associated with a statistically significant increased risk of death from prostate cancer. Men who had a PSADT of < 3 months were 19.6 times more likely than others to die from prostate cancer. The median time to cancer-related death was 6 years. In another recent report, Freedland and coworkers [44] demonstrated the importance of postoperative PSADT for predicting prostate cancer-specific death after RP. In this study, PSADT, Gleason score, and time to recurrence after surgery were all significant independent predictors of death from prostate cancer. In a population based cohort of 1136 men who underwent surgery and radiation therapy, Albertsen and coworkers [45] reported that a post-treatment PSADT of < 2 months was associated with a high risk of death from prostate cancer within 10 years of diagnosis.

It is clear from these studies that short PSADT may help to define a higher risk population in patients who develop BCR. It may also be a marker of the biological aggressiveness of the cancer even before treatment is initiated. Pruthi and colleagues [46] performed a multivariate analysis on 94 patients who developed BCR after prostatectomy and found that postoperative PSADT could be predicted by worse pathologic findings at the time of surgery. In two recent studies, D'Amico and colleagues [47,48] demonstrated the importance of PSA velocity before treatment as a predictor of ultimate death from prostate cancer. In both RP and radiation therapy patients, a pretreatment PSAV of > 2.0 ng/mL/year was

significantly associated with prostate cancer death. Particularly striking was that this finding held true even for patients considered to have low-risk pretreatment tumor characteristics (PSA < 10 ng/mL, Gleason score < 7, and clinical tumor stage < T2b).

PSA kinetics may be the most important factor in discriminating between significant and insignificant recurrent disease, and may help in the selection of patients for additional treatment. In a recently reported series of 1011 men who underwent RP at a single institution, men with a preoperative PSA < 10 ng/mL, a non-palpable cancer with Gleason score < 7, and a preoperative PSA increase that did not exceed 0.5 ng/mL/year, either did not recur or had a postoperative PSADT of > 12 months [49]. The authors suggested that because a PSADT longer than 12 months is rarely associated with prostate cancer death, these men might be safely observed without salvage treatment. In addition, these patients may be able to be identified preoperatively.

Treatment strategies

Salvage radiotherapy after radical prostatectomy

Salvage radiotherapy remains the only potentially curative therapy in men who develop recurrence after RP. The real challenge in this setting is determining which patients harbor isolated local recurrence, because these are the men who are most likely to benefit from this therapy. Many urologists are reluctant to recommend salvage radiotherapy because of the perception that it is ineffective, particularly for cancers that have more aggressive features, and that it might induce additional morbidity in the post-prostatectomy setting. This may be linked to the general perception that most men with PSA recurrence have occult metastatic disease. In a recent assessment of secondary treatment in men who experience biochemical recurrence after radical prostatectomy from the CaPSURE database, only 43% received salvage radiotherapy and 57% were treated with hormonal therapy [50]. Although hormonal therapy provided adequate disease control in many of these men, it is not curative and has the potential for significant adverse affects, particularly with chronic use.

The reported success rate of salvage radiotherapy ranges from 10% to 50%, when success is defined as a "durable" biochemical response to treatment [51–60]. Although up to 90% of men will have an initial response to salvage radiotherapy (measured by a fall in PSA level), only half of these men will have a prolonged PSA response. The relatively high number of initial responders suggests that local recurrence is a frequent component of biochemical recurrence. The lower number of long-term responders suggests that there is often a component of distant disease as well. To date, no study has shown that salvage radiotherapy improves survival or prevents the development of distant metastases. Because it is unlikely that local disease control with radiotherapy has any long-term benefit in patients with concomitant micrometastatic disease, it is advantageous to select patients for salvage therapy based on a high likelihood of isolated local recurrence.

Numerous studies have attempted to define factors most predictive of a durable response to salvage radiotherapy. One of the most consistent findings across these studies is that outcome is better when salvage therapy is administered at the earliest evidence of disease progression when serum PSA level is still low. The best PSA threshold below which salvage radiotherapy should be administered, however, is still debated. The American Society for Therapeutic Radiology and Oncology (ASTRO) consensus panel concluded that the most appropriate PSA cut-point seemed to be 1.5 ng/mL based on the available evidence. Other authors have recommended PSA cut-points ranging from 0.6 to 4.0 ng/mL. The most recent publications on this topic suggest that initiating therapy at PSA levels ≤ 0.6 ng/mL may be optimal [58–60]. There is a risk of overtreatment if salvage radiotherapy is initiated at very low PSA levels since some men with low stable PSA levels after prostatectomy fail to progress. As such, it is important to confirm that PSA level is increasing before initiating treatment.

A recent large retrospective review of salvage radiotherapy administered to 501 men at five US academic medical centers attempted to delineate who may benefit from salvage radiotherapy by identifying variables associated with a durable response [60]. The initial complete response rate to salvage therapy was 67% and with a median follow-up of 45 months, the overall 4-year progression-free probability (PFP) was 45% (95% CI, 40%–50%). In multivariate analysis, adverse predictors of progression were a Gleason score of 8 to 10, pre-radiotherapy PSA level of > 2.0 ng/mL, negative surgical margins, PSADT of 10 months or less, and seminal vesicle invasion. In patients with none of these adverse features, PFP was 77%. In patients who had a PSA level < 2.0 ng/mL, significantly better outcomes were seen in those with levels ≤ 0.6 ng/ml. A recent large series from the Mayo Clinic also demonstrated the importance of PSADT in predicting outcome in this setting [59]. Consistent with many previous studies, positive surgical margins were a powerful predictor of a durable response to salvage radiotherapy as well. Although at first this may seem counterintuitive, since positive margins are often associated with adverse clinical and pathologic tumor features, a positive surgical margin is often associated with surgical technique and makes it more likely that recurrence is caused by residual pelvic disease.

Another important finding of the study by Stephenson and colleagues [60] was the result of salvage radiotherapy in patients who had tumor characteristics often associated with distant micrometastatic disease. Of the patients who were free of PSA progression for a minimum of 4 years after salvage therapy, 15% had Gleason scores of 8 to 10, 38% had a PSADT of <10 months, and 70% recurred within 12 months of RP. In fact, for patients with Gleason scores of 8 to 10 in whom overall 4-year PFP was only 29%, if pre-radiotherapy was ≤ 2.0 ng/mL, surgical margins were positive and PSADT was >10 months, a 4-year PFP of 81% was observed. These findings suggest that there are a subset of patients with high-risk tumor features whose locally recurrent disease may be effectively treated with radiation therapy if it is given early in the course of recurrent disease before progression to distant metastases. Traditionally, these patients were rarely considered for salvage radiotherapy. Although the findings of this study should be confirmed in a randomized prospective trial, these results suggest that salvage radiotherapy should at least be considered in any patient with positive margins who develops biochemical recurrence, even those with high-grade tumors or rapid PSADT.

Salvage therapy after radiotherapy

Because local failure after radiotherapy has been found to be a strong predictor of distant metastasis, several secondary treatment modalities have been assessed for their ability to cure locally persistent or recurrent disease after radiotherapy [61]. There are three treatment modalities that have been used in this setting: (1) salvage radical prostatectomy, (2) cryotherapy, and (3) brachytherapy. Although salvage brachytherapy has been used as a salvage option after failed external beam radiotherapy, experience with this technique is limited and reported complications have been relatively frequent [62,63]. Preliminary biochemical disease-free outcomes at 5-years range from 34% to 53% depending on the definition used. As higher external beam radiation doses are delivered with current conformal techniques, the applicability of this technique may be even more limited than it is presently.

There has been an increased interest in the use of salvage cryotherapy with the advent of third-generation prostate cryotherapy equipment. These newer systems use argon gas, smaller cryoprobes, and more precise probe placement by way of a brachytherapy-like template, to improve upon the relatively high morbidity associated with the older machines. In modern series with limited follow-up (19–21 months), disease-free survival approximates 40% depending on the definition used [64,65]. In one of the largest series (n = 131) with adequate follow-up (median 4.8 years) reported by Izawa and colleagues [66], the 5-year actuarial disease-free survival (defined as PSA $\leq$ 2 ng/mL above nadir) was 40%. In a recently reported multicenter experience with third-generation cryotherapy in 106 men with at least one year of follow-up, 18 patients received salvage cryotherapy [67]. At 12 months, PSA was < 0.4 ng/mL in 13 of 17 patients (77%). Like most salvage cryotherapy series, impotence rates were high (86%) but the rates of tissue sloughing (11%), incontinence requiring pads (11%), and urge incontinence without pads (6%), were less than those reported in earlier series. In general, the reported complication rates of salvage cryotherapy are higher than those of primary cryotherapy, and this is especially true for incontinence rates and pelvic pain [61]. Longer follow-up is needed to accurately assess cancer control in the salvage setting.

Salvage prostatectomy has not gained wide acceptance as a treatment for recurrence after radiotherapy because of the challenges of operating in a radiated field and the significant complications reported in historical series. However, salvage prostatectomy may be the only treatment in this setting that can provide a durable cure and recent reports suggest that the complication rates may be decreasing. Candidates for salvage prostatectomy should have a positive prostate biopsy to confirm locally recurrent and persistent disease, and a negative metastatic imaging workup which should include a CT scan, chest radiograph, and bone scan. Given the relatively high morbidity of this procedure, patient selection is critical. The ideal patient has a long life expectancy (at least 10 years) with few if any co-morbidities and tumor parameters that make locally confined disease most likely. These include a low PSA level at the time of salvage surgery and before radiotherapy (under 4 ng/mL best, but at least <10 ng/mL), and clinical stage $\leq$ T2 both before radiotherapy and at the time of recurrence. Patients must also be highly motivated and accepting of the increased morbidity.

The long-term oncologic outcomes of salvage radical prostatectomy were recently updated in two large series from the Memorial Sloan-Kettering Cancer Center (MSKCC) and the Mayo Clinic [68,69]. In the 100 consecutive patients with 5-year median follow-up from MSKCC, disease progression was defined as a PSA $\geq$ 0.2 ng/mL or the initiation of androgen deprivation therapy [68]. The 5-year progression-free probability (PFP) was 55% (95% CI, 46%–64%) and the 10-year cancer-specific survival rate was 73%. The 5-year PFP was 77% with pathologically organ-confined disease and 86% if PSA level at the time of salvage surgery was < 4 ng/mL. In the Mayo Clinic series, both prostatectomy and cysto-prostatectomy patients were included (n = 199) [69]. Considering only the salvage RP patients (n = 138) in this series, 5-year PFP (defined as PSA $\geq$ 0.4 ng/mL) was 63% and cancer-specific survival at 10 years was 77%. In multivariate analysis, PSA <10 ng/mL was a significant independent predictor of PFP and localized disease was the best predictor of cancer-specific survival. These two large series show that salvage prostatectomy can result in reasonably good oncologic outcomes; 5-year PFP can exceed 60% in carefully selected patients.

These two series also suggest that the morbidity of salvage prostatectomy may be decreasing in more recently treated patients [69,70]. In the MSKCC series, the major complication rate decreased significantly (from 33% to 13%; P = .02) since 1993 [70]. In particular, the rectal injury rate decreased from 15% before 1993 to 2% in more recently treated patients. Urinary continence (one pad or less per day) was 68% at 5 years; 39% required no pads. This rate improved from 57% before 1993 to 68% after but this difference did not reach statistical significance. Anastomotic stricture rates were high (30%) and did not improve over time. In previously potent men getting nerve-sparing surgery, the 5-year potency rate (erections satisfactory for penetration with or without sildenifil) was 45%. In the Mayo series, the rectal injury rate was 5% and bladder neck contracture occurred in 22% of patients [69]. Since 1990, complete continence (0 pads) improved from 43% to 56% and an additional 20% required one or fewer pads daily.

Despite these recent reports, however, salvage prostatectomy remains a technically challenging procedure and carries the potential for significant morbidity. These are important considerations when contemplating salvage prostatectomy. It does, however, offer the carefully selected patient a viable treatment option with the best opportunity for cure in this setting. As experience with salvage prostatectomy at major medical centers increases, and with a growing population of younger men being treated with radiotherapy, it may become a more commonly used treatment for radiation failure.

Hormonal therapy

Hormonal therapy of various forms is the most commonly used treatment for men who have BCR after localized treatment. In an analysis of men in the CaPSURE database who required secondary treatment after RP, hormonal therapy was the initial therapy used in 57% of men [50]. Although traditional hormonal therapy (LHRH agonist with or without an antiandrogen) is used most commonly, nontraditional forms of hormonal therapy have also been used. These unconventional hormonal therapies include antiandrogen monotherapy with bicalutamide or flutamide, 5α-reductase inhibitor therapy with finasteride or dutasteride, and combined antiandrogen and 5α-reductase therapy [71]. Intermittent traditional hormonal therapy is also used in this setting. By limiting the adverse affects associated with traditional hormonal therapy, these unconventional approaches offer potential advantages. The disadvantages to these approaches are the potential for other side effects specific to these drugs (eg, breast pain and gynecomastia) and the lack of knowledge regarding the long-term efficacy of these therapies.

Despite the widespread use of hormonal therapy in men with BCR, there remain many uncertainties regarding its appropriate use because of the lack of any significant study of hormonal therapy in the BCR population. To date, there are no prospective trials specifically evaluating the use of traditional hormonal therapy in patients with BCR and only one small study examining the use of finasteride [72]. Retrospective studies suffer from selection bias, lack of sufficient follow-up and the relatively benign natural history characterizing many of these recurrences. We are left then to make treatment recommendations based on extrapolation from studies of hormonal therapy in other stages of advanced prostate cancer. Whether or not this extrapolation is valid or applicable continues to be the source of ongoing debate.

One of the most challenging clinical questions regarding the use of hormonal therapy in BCR is how to determine the optimal timing for therapy. On the one hand, many men will have an indolent disease course that requires no therapy at al, yet on the other hand, many men will request or receive treatment as a result of the anxiety brought on by a rising PSA level. There is a growing body of evidence in favor of the early administration of hormonal therapy in men who have other stages of advanced prostate cancer. The Medical Research Council study compared early and later administration of traditional hormonal therapy in men who had locally advanced or metastatic prostate cancer and reported improved survival and fewer complications with earlier therapy [73]. This advantage seemed to be more pronounced in men without radiographic evidence of metastatic disease which suggests that hormonal therapy may be more effective with lesser overall tumor burden. If men with BCR have unrecognized micrometastatic disease, the results of the ECOG study of early versus delayed hormonal therapy in men who have positive lymph nodes at the time of radical prostatectomy may apply [74]. This study demonstrated an overall and cancer-specific survival advantage in the early hormonal therapy group. It has been suggested that the improved survival seen with the addition of hormonal therapy to radiotherapy in locally advanced disease is because of early administration of hormonal therapy.

It is uncertain whether the results of these investigations in men who have more advanced prostate cancer can be extrapolated to the setting of BCR, because they likely represent very different disease states. However, there may be subsets of men with BCR who would benefit from the earlier administration of hormonal therapy. In a retrospective analysis of the CPDR database, Moul and coworkers [75] attempted to define a group of men with BCR who benefited from early hormonal therapy. Of the 1352 men with

BCR, 103 (7.6%) developed clinical metastases during follow-up. Although early hormonal therapy (administered at a PSA level of 5 ng/mL or less) had no advantage overall, it was associated with a delay to the development of clinical progression in men with pathologic Gleason scores of 8 to 10 or PSADT < 12 months ($P = .004$). PSADT has also been used to guide the administration of hormonal therapy in BCR after radiation therapy. D'Amico and colleagues [76] analyzed the outcomes of 94 of 381 men who developed BCR after external beam radiotherapy. PSADT < 12 months was associated with a 5.1 relative risk of death from prostate cancer compared with those with longer PSADT. An increase in disease-specific and overall survival was seen when hormonal therapy was initiated before radiographic evidence of metastatic disease. In another study of BCR after radiation, Pinover and colleagues found that PSADT was a significant predictor of metastasis-free survival [77]. When PSADT was <12 months, earlier administration of hormonal therapy resulted in significantly better 5-year metastasis-free survival (57% versus 78%; $P = .026$). For men with PSADT > 12 months, the timing of hormonal therapy had no impact on metastasis-free survival.

These studies suggest that some men with BCR benefit from early administration of hormonal therapy although the PSA threshold at which to initiate therapy is uncertain. These men may be best identified by a rapid PSADT although other tumor characteristics may also help to define a high risk group. Men who have high-risk features should also be considered for clinical trials that incorporate chemotherapy and newer novel agents as well. For men who request hormonal therapy despite apparent low-risk disease, unconventional approaches including intermittent hormonal therapy, antiandrogen monotherapy, and 5α-reductase inhibitor therapy can be considered, although the benefit of these therapies is unproven. Further study of the optimal form and timing of hormonal therapy in this setting is obviously needed.

References

[1] Moul JW. Variables in predicting survival based on treating "PSA-only" relapse. Urol Oncol 2003;21: 292–304.

[2] Amling CL, Bergstralh EJ, Blute ML, et al. Defining prostate specific antigen progression after radical prostatectomy: what is the most appropriate cut point? J Urol 2001;165:1146–51.

[3] Ravery V. The significance of recurrent PSA after radical prostatectomy: benign versus malignant sources. Semin Urol Oncol 1999;17:127–9.

[4] Fowler JE Jr, Brooks J, Pandey P, et al. Variable histology of anastomotic biopsies with detectable prostate specific antigen after radical prostatectomy. J Urol 1995;153:1011–4.

[5] Wood DP, Peretsman SJ, Seay TM. Incidence of benign and malignant prostate tissue in biopsies of the bladder neck after radical prostatectomy. J Urol 1995;154:1443–6.

[6] Shah O, Melamed J, Lepor H. Analysis of apical soft tissue margins during radical retropubic prostatectomy. J Urol 2001;165:1943–9.

[7] Iwakiri J, Granbois K, Wehner N, et al. An analysis of urinary prostate specific antigen before and after radical prostatectomy: Evidence for secretion of prostate specific antigen by the periurethral glands. J Urol 1993;149:783–6.

[8] Freedland SJ, Sutter ME, Dorey F, et al. Defining the ideal cut point for determining PSA recurrence after radical prostatectomy. Urology 2003;61: 365–9.

[9] Stamey TA, Graves HCB, Wehner N, et al. Early detection of residual prostate cancer after radical prostatectomy by an ultrasensitive assay for prostate specific antigen. J Urol 1993;149:787–92.

[10] Ellis WJ, Vessella RL, Noteboom JL, et al. Early detection of recurrent prostate cancer with an ultrasensitive chemiluminescent PSA assay. Urology 1997; 50(4):573–9.

[11] Witherspoon LR, Lapeyrolerie T. Sensitive prostate specific antigen measurements identify men with long disease free intervals and differentiate aggressive from indolent cancer recurrences within 2 years after radical prostatectomy. J Urol 1997;157:1322–8.

[12] Haese A, Huland E, Graefen M, et al. Ultrasensitive detection of prostate specific antigen in the follow-up of 422 patients after radical prostatectomy. J Urol 1999;161:1206–11.

[13] Yu H, Diamandis EP, Wong PY, et al. Detection of prostate cancer relapse with prostate specific antigen monitoring at levels of 0.001 to 0.1 microG./L. J Urol 1997;157:913–8.

[14] Shen S, Lepor H, Yaffee R, et al. Ultrasensitive serum PSA nadir accurately predicts the risk of early relapse after radical prostatectomy. J Urol 2005; 173:777–80.

[15] Cannon GM, Walsh PC, Partin AW, et al. Prostate-specific antigen doubling time in the identification of patients at risk for progression after treatment and biochemical recurrence for prostate cancer. Urology 2003;62(Suppl 6B):2–8.

[16] Kuban DA, Thames HD, Shipley WU. Defining recurrence after radiation for prostate cancer. J Urol 2005;173:1871–8.

[17] Willett CG, Zietman AL, Shipley WU, et al. The effect of pelvic radiation therapy on serum level of prostate specific antigen. J Urol 1994;151:1579.

[18] Zietman AL, Zehr EM, Shipley WU. The long-term effect on PSA values of incidental prostatic irradiation in patients with pelvic malignancies other than prostate cancer. Int J Radiat Oncol Biol Phys 1999;43:715.

[19] Consensus statement: guidelines for PSA following radiation therapy. American Society for Therapeutic Radiology and Oncology Consensus Panel. Int J Radiat Oncol Biol Phys 1997;37:1035–41.

[20] Thames H, Kuban D, Levy L, et al. Comparison of alternative biochemical failure definitions based on clinical outcome in 4839 prostate cancer patients treated by external beam radiotherapy between 1986 and 1995. Int J Radiat Oncol Biol Phys 2003; 57(4):929–43.

[21] Kuban D, Thames H, Levy L, et al. Failure definition-dependent difference in outcome following radiation for localized prostate cancer: can one size fit all? Int J Radiat Oncol Biol Phys 2005;61(2):409–14.

[22] Gretzer MB, Trock BJ, Han M, et al. A critical analysis of the interpretation of biochemical failure in surgically treated patients using the American Society for Therapeutic Radiation and Oncology criteria. J Urol 2002;168:1419–22.

[23] Cher ML, Bianco FJ, Lam JS, et al. Limited role of radionuclide bone scintigraphy in patients with prostate specific antigen elevations after radical prostatectomy. J Urol 1998;160:1387.

[24] Kane CJ, Amling CL, Johnstone PA, et al. Limited value of bone scintigraphy and computed tomography in assessing biochemical failure after radical prostatectomy. Urology 2003;61:607–11.

[25] Okotie OT, Aronson WJ, Wieder JA, et al. Predictors of metastatic disease in men with biochemical failure following radical prostatectomy. J Urol 2004;171:2260–4.

[26] Brassell SA, Rosner IL, McLeod DG. Update on magnetic resonance imaging, ProstaScint, and novel imaging in prostate cancer. Curr Opin Urol 2005;15: 163–6.

[27] Kahn D, Williams RD, Manyak MJ, et al. 111-Indium-capromab pendatide in the evaluation of patients with residual of recurrent prostate cancer after radical prostatectomy. J Urol 1998;159:2041–7.

[28] Raj GV, Partin AW, Polascik TJ. Clinical utility of indium 111-capromab pendatide immunoscintigraphy in the detection of early, recurrent prostate carcinoma after radical prostatectomy. Cancer 2002;94: 987–96.

[29] Kahn D, Williams RD, Haseman MK, et al. Radio-immunoscintigraphy with In-111-labeled capromab pendetide predicts prostate cancer response to salvage radiotherapy after failed radical prostatectomy. J Clin Oncol 1998;16:284–9.

[30] Thomas CT, Bradshaw PT, Pollock BH, et al. Indium-111-capromab pendetide radioimmunoscintigraphy and prognosis for durable biochemical response to salvage radiation therapy in men after failed prostatectomy. J Clin Oncol 2003;21:1715–21.

[31] Willkinson S, Chodak G. The role of 111-indium-capromab pendetide imaging for assessing biochemical failure after radical prostatectomy. J Urol 2004; 172:133–6.

[32] Schettino CJ, Kramer EL, Noz ME, et al. Impact of fusion of Indium-111 capromab pendetide volume data sets with those of MRI and CT in patiens with recurrent prostate cancer. AJR 2004;183: 519–24.

[33] Bander NH, Trabulsi EJ, Kostakoglu L, et al. Targeting metastatic prostate cancer with radiolabeled monoclonal antibody J591 to the extracellular domain of prostate specific membrane antigen. J Urol 2003;170:1717–21.

[34] Pound CR, Partin AW, Eisenberger MA, et al. Natural history of progression after PSA elevation following radical prostatectomy. JAMA 1999;281: 1591–7.

[35] Partin AW, Rootselaar CV, Epstein JI. Natural history of progression after PSA elevation following radical prostatectomy. J Urol 2003;169:935A.

[36] D'Amico AV, Hanks GE. Linear regressive analysis using prostate-specific antigen doubling time for predicting tumor biology and clinical outcome in prostate cancer. Cancer 1993;72:2638–43.

[37] Pollack A, Zagars GK, Kavadi VS. Prostate specific antigen doubling time and disease relapse after radiotherapy for prostate cancer. Cancer 1994;74: 670–8.

[38] Partin AW, Pearson JD, Landis PK, et al. Evaluation of serum prostate specific antigen velocity after radical prostatectomy to distinguish local recurrence from distant metastasis. Urology 1994;43:649–59.

[39] Patel A, Dorey F, Franklin J, et al. Recurrence patterns after radical retropubic prostatectomy: Clinical usefulness of prostate specific antigen doubling times and log slope prostate specific antigen. J Urol 1997;158:1441–5.

[40] Lee WR, Hanks GE, Hanlon A. Increasing prostate-specific antigen profile following definitive radiation therapy for localized prostate cancer: clinical observations. J Clin Oncol 1997;15:230–8.

[41] Sartor CI, Strawderman MH, Lin XH, et al. Rate of PSA rise predicts metastatic versus local recurrence after definitive radiotherapy. Int J Radiat Oncol Biol Phys 1997;38:941–7.

[42] Roberts SG, Blute ML, Bergstralh EJ, et al. PSA doubling time as a predictor of clinical progression after biochemical failure following radical prostatectomy for prostate cancer. Mayo Clin Proc 2001;76: 576–81.

[43] D'Amico AV, Moul JW, Carroll PR, et al. Surrogate end point for prostate cancer-specific mortality after radical prostatectomy or radiation therapy. J Natl Cancer Inst 2003;95:1376–83.

[44] Freedland SJ, Humphreys EB, Mangold LA, et al. Risk of prostate cancer-specific mortality following biochemical recurrence after radical prostatectomy. JAMA 2005;294:433–9.

[45] Albertson PC, Hanley JA, Penson DF, et al. Validation of increasing prostate specific antigen as a predictor of prostate cancer death after treatment of localized prostate cancer with surgery or radiation. J Urol 2004;171:2221–5.

[46] Pruthi RS, Johnstone I, Tu IP, et al. Prostate-specific antigen doubling times in patients who have failed radical prostatectomy: correlation with histologic characteristics of the primary cancer. Urology 1997; 49(5):737–42.

[47] D'Amico AV, Chen MH, Roehl KA, et al. Preoperative PSA velocity and the risk of death from prostate cancer after radical prostatectomy. N Engl J Med 2004;351:125–35.

[48] D'Amico AV, Renshaw AA, Sussman B, et al. Pretreatment PSA velocity and the risk of death from prostate cancer following external beam radiation therapy. JAMA 2005;294:440–7.

[49] D'Amico AV, Chen MH, Roehl KA, et al. Identifying patients at risk for significant versus clinically insignificant postoperative prostate-specific antigen failure. J Clin Urol 2005;23:4975–9.

[50] Mehta SS, Lubeck DP, Sadetsky N, et al. Patterns of secondary cancer treatment for biochemical failure following radical prostatectomy: data from CaPSURE. J Urol 2004;171:215–9.

[51] Cadeddu JA, Partin AW, DeWeese TL, et al. Long-term results of radiation therapy for prostate cancer recurrence following radical prostatectomy. J Urol 1998;159:173–7.

[52] Pisansky TM, Kozelsky TF, Myers RP, et al. Radiotherapy for isolated serum prostate specific antigen elevation after prostatectomy for prostate cancer. J Urol 2000;163:845–50.

[53] Anscher MS, Clough R, Dodge R. Radiotherapy for a rising prostate-specific antigen after radical prostatectomy: the first 10 years. Int J Radiat Oncol Biol Phys 2000;48:369–75.

[54] Levintis AK, Shariat SF, Kattan MW, et al. Prediction of response to salvage radiation therapy in patients with prostate cancer recurrence after radical prostatectomy. J Clin Oncol 2001;19:1030–9.

[55] Song DY, Thompson TL, Ramakrishnan V, et al. Salvage radiotherapy for rising or persistent PSA after radical prostatectomy. Urology 2002;60:281–7.

[56] Katz MS, Zelefsky MJ, Venkatraman ES, et al. Predictors of biochemical outcome with salvage conformal radiotherapy after radical prostatectomy for prostate cancer. J Clin Oncol 2003;21:483–9.

[57] Liauw SL, Webster WS, Pistenmaa DA, et al. Salvage radiotherapy for biochemical failure of radical prostatectomy: a single-institution experience. Urology 2003;61:1204–10.

[58] MacDonald OK, Schild SE, Vora SA, et al. Radiotherapy for men with isolated increase in serum prostate specific antigen after radical prostatectomy. J Urol 2003;170:1841–2.

[59] Ward JF, Zincke H, Bergstralh EJ, et al. Prostate specific antigen doubling time subsequent to radical prostatectomy as a prognosticator of outcome following salvage radiotherapy. J Urol 2004;172: 2244–8.

[60] Stephenson AJ, Shariat SF, Zelefsky MJ, et al. Salvage radiotherapy for recurrent prostate cancer after radical prostatectomy. JAMA 2004;291: 1325–32.

[61] Touma NJ, Izawa JI, Chin JL. Current status of local salvage therapies following radiation failure for prostate cancer. J Urol 2005;173:373–9.

[62] Grado GL, Collins JM, Kriegshauser JS, et al. Salvage brachytherapy for localized prostate cancer after radiotherapy failure. Urology 1999; 53:2.

[63] Beyer DC. Permanent brachytherapy as salvage treatment for recurrent prostate cancer. Urology 1999;54:880.

[64] Chin JL, Pautler SE, Mouraviev V, et al. Results for salvage cryoablation of the prostate after radiation: identifying predictors of treatment failure and complications. J Urol 2001;165:1937–42.

[65] Ghafar MA, Johnson CW, De La Taille A, et al. Salvage cryotherapy using an argon based system for locally recurrent prostate cancer after radiation therapy: the Columbia experience. J Urol 2001;166: 1333–8.

[66] Izawa JI, Madsen LT, Scott SM, et al. Salvage cryotherapy for recurrent prostate cancer after radiotherapy: variables affecting patient outcome. J Clin Oncol 2002;20:2664–71.

[67] Han KR, Cohen JK, Miller RJ, et al. Treatment of organ confined prostate cancer with third generation cryosurgery: preliminary multicenter experience. J Urol 2003;170:1126–30.

[68] Bianco FJ, Scardino PT, Stephenson AJ, et al. Long-term oncologic results of salvage radical prostatectomy for locally recurrent prostate cancer after radiotherapy. Int J Radiat Oncol Biol Phys 2005;62: 448–53.

[69] Ward JF, Sebo TJ, Blute ML, et al. Salvage surgery for radiorecurrent prostate cancer: contemporary outcomes. J Urol 2005;173:1156–60.

[70] Stephenson AJ, Scardino PT, Bianco FJ, et al. Morbidity and functional outcomes of salvage radical prostatectomy for locally recurrent prostate cancer after radiation therapy. J Urol 2004;172: 2239–43.

[71] Moul JW, Zlotta A. Hormonal therapy options for prostate-specific antigen-only recurrence of prostate cancer after previous local therapy. BJU Int 2005;95: 285–90.

[72] Andriole G, Lieber M, Smith J, et al. Treatment with finasteride following radical prostatectomy for prostate cancer. Urology 1995;45:491–7.

[73] The Medical Research Council Prostate Cancer Working Party Investigators Group. Immediate versus deferred treatment for advanced prostatic cancer: initial results of the Medical Research Council trial. Br J Urol 1997;79:235–46.

[74] Messing EM, Manola J, Sarosdy M, et al. Immediate hormonal therapy compared with observation after radical prostatectomy and pelvic lumphadenectomy in men with node-positive prostate cancer. N Engl J Med 1999;341:1781–8.

[75] Moul JW, Wu H, Sun L, et al. Early versus delayed hormonal therapy for prostate specific antigen only recurrence of prostate cancer after radical prostatectomy. J Urol 2004;171:1141–7.

[76] D'Amico AV, Cote K, Loffredo M, et al. Determinants of prostate cancer-specific survival after radiation therapy for patients with clinically localized prostate cancer. J Clin Oncol 2002;20:4567–73.

[77] Pinover WH, Horwitz EM, Hanlon A, et al. Validation of a treatment policy for patients with prostate specific antigen failure after three-dimensional conformal prostate radiation therapy. Cancer 2003;97: 1127–33.

UROLOGIC
CLINICS
of North America

Urol Clin N Am 33 (2006) 161–166

Combined Androgen Blockade: An Update

Laurence Klotz, MD

Division of Urology, Sunnybrook and Women's College Health Sciences Centre, University of Toronto,
2075 Bayview Avenue #MG408, Toronto, Ontario M4N 3M5, Canada

Combined androgen blockade (CAB) was first described in 1979 [1]. At that time, the concept was that, in men treated with castration, the presence of adrenal androgens was responsible for continued androgenic stimulation of prostate cancer, which resulted in androgen independent progression. Over the last 25 years, an unprecedented number of clinical trials have addressed CAB versus monotherapy, and a substantial body of basic research has improved our understanding of the interactions between the anti-androgens, the androgen receptor, and androgen response elements in the genome. In this article, recent data bearing on the role of combined therapy that uses non-steroidal anti-androgens, in conjunction with androgen deprivation therapy, are reviewed. In particular, this article reviews the effect of the different non-steroidals in blocking androgen-independent activation of the androgen receptor in the androgen-depleted environment, and the potential benefit of bicalutamide in comparison to the first generation of anti-androgens (flutamide and nilutamide).

Rationale for combined therapy

Androgen-dependent cells are dependent on activation of the androgen receptor (AR) for cell growth. Under normal circumstances, androgens (especially dihydrotestosterone [DHT]) bind to the ligand binding domain of the AR. The AR, in dimeric form, is then transduced into the nucleus, where it binds to androgen response elements (AREs) in the nucleus. Nuclear co-activators and co-suppressors also bind to this complex, modulating the degree of transcription and cellular activation.

In prostate cancer, many alterations to this system occur as the disease progresses from hormone dependent to hormone independent. Two key changes include marked upregulation of the AR, which confers exquisite sensitivity to extremely small amounts of androgen; and mutation of the AR, which results in loss of specificity for androgens. Mutated ARs may be activated by non-androgen steroid hormones or by other molecules (including anti-androgens), or may be autonomously activated.

Non-steroidal anti-androgens act in two ways. It is well established that they act through competition with the testosterone metabolite dihydrotestosterone and other androgens for ligand binding sites on the androgen receptor. All three non-steroidal anti-androgens do this relatively effectively. Differences do exist: bicalutamide has a fourfold greater affinity for the AR than flutamide and nilutamide. However, it is unclear how significant this difference is at pharmacologic levels of the drugs.

The testes produce 95% of serum testosterone and the adrenal glands produce the remaining androgens [2]. After castration (whether surgical or medical), the adrenal glands continue to produce the androgens, androsterone (AS) and dehydroepiandrosterone (DHEA). DHEA is produced in 3–4 times greater amounts than testosterone, but its potency as an androgen is about 8%–10% of testosterone. The adrenal androgens are converted to testosterone in the peripheral tissues and in the prostate. These androgens may

Dr. Klotz has received honoraria from Astra Zeneca and Sanofi-Ave.

E-mail address: Laurence.klotz@sw.ca

stimulate AR activation in the castrated patient, and anti-androgens play a role in inhibiting this phenomenon.

Their blockade of androgen receptor activation by non-steroidal growth factors, cytokines, and other non-ligand-dependent activators is less well recognized [3]. They also interact with nuclear co-activators and co-suppressors of the AR. In this regard, there are significant differences between the three non-steroidal anti-androgens. In fact, the term anti-androgen is a misnomer, and may be responsible for a misperception regarding this class of drugs. The drugs actually act as androgen receptor antagonists, in that they inhibit AR activation by both androgens and non-androgenic molecules.

Molecules that activate the AR in the absence of androgens include: cytokines such as interleukin-6 and interleukin 10, growth factors such as IGF and epidermal growth factor, and signal transduction factors such as protein kinase A. These factors are capable of activating normal androgen receptors [4].

Pre-clinical data have demonstrated differences between anti-androgens in the degree to which this inhibition of androgen-independent activation occurs. Consistently, bicalutamide is a more potent blocker of this phenomenon. In addition, bicalutamide interacts more potently with nuclear co-activators and co-suppressors. Bicalutamide compared with hydroxyflutamide is a much more powerful inhibitor of the co-activator steroid receptor co-activator-1 (SRC-1), and a more potent activator of the co-suppressor nuclear receptor co-repressor (N-CoR) [5]. The net effect of bicalutamide is to dramatically reduce the cellular activation induced by the androgen receptor. The effect of flutamide in this system is much more muted.

In the presence of androgen-receptor upregulation, or mutation, the androgen receptor may become "promiscuous" and be activated by a much wider variety of ligands, cytokines, and other molecules. The non-steroidal anti-androgens differ in the degree to which they block androgen-independent activation. Flutamide was shown to activate cells with specific single-point mutations of promiscuous androgen receptors identified from patients who have androgen insensitivity syndrome [6]. Similarly, nilutamide caused transcription of a mutant androgen receptor extracted from a human metastatic cancer and with a point mutation in the same codon as the mutation in the androgen-independent cell line

LNCaP (human prostate adenocarcinoma cell line), while bicalutamide maintained antagonistic action [3]. However, in a novel cell subline, LNCaP-abl, which has a hypersensitive proliferative response to androgen, bicalutamide showed agonistic effects on androgen-receptor transactivation activity and was unable to block androgen effects [7]. Flutamide also exerted stimulatory effects on androgen receptor activity that was 2–4 times greater in LNCaP-abl cells than in LNCaP cells. For bicalutamide, the induction of reporter gene activity was lower than that seen with flutamide. The stimulatory effects of bicalutamide on androgen receptor activity were two times greater in LNCaP-abl cells than in LNCaP cells.

These studies emphasize the important biological differences between the non-steroidal anti-androgens in the androgen-depleted environment and suggest that bicalutamide may be superior to flutamide and nilutamide in delaying androgen-independent progression. Other key differences between the non-steroidal anti-androgens are their androgen receptor binding affinities and potencies, clinical efficacies, and tolerability profiles.

In vitro studies show that the binding affinity of bicalutamide for the human and rat prostate androgen receptor is 2–4 times greater than that of flutamide and twice that of nilutamide. Moreover, bicalutamide showed greater potency than flutamide in reducing intact rat ventral prostate and seminal vesicle weights [8].

The non-steroidal anti-androgens also have different tolerability profiles. Flutamide is associated with diarrhea [9,10] and liver toxicity. High rates of visual disturbances and alcohol intolerance have been reported with nilutamide. Bicalutamide is better tolerated in this regard. In a trial by Schellhammer and colleagues [11] the incidence of diarrhea was statistically significantly lower with bicalutamide plus an luteinizing hormone-releasing hormone (LHRH) agonist than with flutamide plus an LHRH agonist (12% versus 26%; $P < .001$). In that study, haematuria was the only adverse event to occur significantly more frequently with bicalutamide plus agonist than with flutamide plus agonist (12% versus 6%; $P = .007$); in most cases this was mild to moderate, unrelated to treatment (96%), and did not lead to treatment withdrawal. Overall, the incidence of withdrawal from therapy because of an adverse event was lower with bicalutamide plus agonist (10%) than with flutamide plus agonist (16%). Evidence for the effectiveness of combined therapy compared with castration alone comes from individual trials, meta-analyses of trial results, and, in the case of combined therapy using bicalutamide, from the latest analysis of historical trial data.

Individual trials

Crawford and colleagues [11] reported the first large controlled trial (603 men) to show an advantage of combined therapy over castration alone for treating metastatic prostate cancer. There were significant improvements in progression-free (median 16.5 versus13.9 months; $P = .039$) and overall (median 35.6 versus 28.3 months; $P = .035$) survival with leuprolide plus flutamide compared with leuprolide plus placebo.

This led to a confirmatory trial, the largest randomized trial of combined therapy versus monotherapy conducted to date. It studied bilateral orchidectomy plus either flutamide or placebo in 1387 patients with metastatic prostate cancer [9]. There was a trend for improved survival (a survival benefit of 10%) with combined therapy over castration alone, but this was not statistically significant (hazard rate [HR] for risk of death with flutamide versus placebo, 0.91; 90% CI 0.81–1.01; $P = .14$). A key point is that the trial was powered to detect the 25% difference that had been observed in the study by Crawford and coworkers [11]. At progression, the treatment arm was unblinded and patients who had been on placebo could then receive open-label flutamide; therefore, the trial actually compared initial with delayed combined therapy. One can speculate that the failure of the flutamide arm to achieve a statistically significant improvement may have been caused by lack of power. To demonstrate a 10% difference in mortality at 5 years, the trial would have required 3000 patients.

To date, over 31 randomized, long-term (treatment for > 1 year) trials in > 8000 men with advanced prostate cancer have investigated the effectiveness and tolerability of combined therapy, with variable results [12]. Differences between therapies are unlikely to be detected during the early follow-up, because most deaths within 1–1.5 years from diagnosis of advanced cancer are likely to be from causes other than cancer. This significantly reduces the power to detect differences in any analysis with a relatively short follow-up.

Combined therapy versus castration only

In an attempt to better understand this large volume of trial data there have been several meta-analyses [12–17]. The benefits and limitations of the various studies which compare combined therapy with castration alone were reviewed previously [14]. The most complete assessment of evidence is the meta-analysis published in 2000 by the Prostate Cancer Trialists' Collaborative Group (PCTCG), which assessed data from 27 trials (including 8275 patients) and incorporated individual patient data [13].

The PCTCG meta-analysis found an overall trend for improved survival in patients treated with combined therapy compared with castration alone, although this was not statistically significant (HR 0.958; standard error of the mean [SEM] 0.026; $P = .11$, H_2); the survival differences were not apparent before 2 years of follow-up. When steroidal and non-steroidal anti-androgens were disaggregated, combined therapy with the non-steroidal anti-androgens flutamide and nilutamide was associated with a statistically significant 8% decrease in the risk of death over castration alone (95% CI 3%–13%; $P = .005$, two-sided); this translated into a 2.9% absolute improvement in 5-year survival. However, combined therapy with the steroidal antiandrogen cyproterone acetate (CPA) was associated with a statistically significant 13% increase in the risk of death compared with castration alone (95% CI 0–27; $P = .04$, H_2), and this equated to a 2.8% reduction in 5-year survival.

In the PCTCG meta-analysis the results were independent of patient age, disease stage, or whether surgical or medical castration was used. Although the results of the trials differed, such variation could be expected by chance (the test of treatment-by-trial interaction was not significant, $P > 0.10$). Importantly, this suggests that the 8% mortality reduction seen with the non-steroidals was not simply flare blockade, since the same benefit was seen in the orchiectomy trials.

All of the PCTCG trials were performed before the recognition of the anti-androgen withdrawal phenomenon. Patients were maintained on anti-androgen until death. Insofar as anti-androgens may be agonistic as AR mutations accumulate, it is possible that this reduced the observed survival benefit of CAB when it is discontinued once disease progression occurs. However, one large retrospective study compared survival between responders and non-responders to anti-androgen withdrawal, and found no difference (median survival 13 and 12 months respectively) [18].

Bicalutamide combined therapy versus castration only

Because bicalutamide was not available when most combined versus monotherapy studies were conducted, no data on this agent were available for inclusion in the meta-analysis discussed above. There is no direct comparison of combined therapy using bicalutamide to castration alone. A double-blind, randomized trial is currently ongoing in Japan. The trial uses bicalutamide 80 mg (the registered dose in Japan) combined with an LHRH agonist versus an agonist plus placebo in 205 men who have advanced prostate cancer. Preliminary data at a median follow-up of 15 months indicate that combined therapy with bicalutamide has significant benefits over LHRH agonist monotherapy: there was an improvement in prostate-specific antigen (PSA) normalization rate (79.4% versus 38.6%; $P < .001$); reduction of the risk of treatment failure (median time to failure 22.1 months versus 15.6 months; $P = .038$) and progression (median time not reached; $P = .015$); and improvement in quality of life ($P < .001$). There were too few events to assess overall survival [19].

In a randomized, double-blind direct comparison trial in 813 men who have metastatic prostate cancer [20], there was a trend to improved overall survival with bicalutamide plus an LHRH agonist than with flutamide plus an LHRH agonist (median survival 180 weeks versus 148 weeks), although the difference did not achieve statistical significance (HR, 0.87; 95% CI 0.72–1.05; $P = .15$). This is the only trial comparing two non-steroidal anti-androgens as components of combined therapy.

At the time this trial was designed, a direct comparison of combined therapy using bicalutamide with castration alone was considered unethical, as combined therapy was considered standard care and superior to monotherapy. To estimate the benefit of bicalutamide in combined therapy Klotz and colleagues [21] used data from the Schellhammer trial [20] in conjunction with the PCTCG meta-analysis data for flutamide plus castration versus castration alone (HR 0.92; 95% CI 0.86–0.98) to calculate an estimate of the likely benefit of bicalutamide combined therapy versus castration alone.

Conventional wisdom dictates that data from different trials should not be directly compared. In fact, a methodologically validated technique has evolved to integrate the results of trials that share a common arm (in this case, flutamide as maximal androgen blockade) but differ in the alternate arm. Typically, this is used when a placebo arm may no longer be feasible or ethical. There are many disease states where the standard of care is a specific drug therapy, and a placebo-controlled trial to evaluate the benefit of a new drug is no longer ethical. Stringent criteria regarding comparability of the patient populations must be met. The PCTCG trials and the Schellhammer trial, both of which enrolled D2 (stage IV cancer with distant metastases) patients from the pre-PSA era, appear to meet these criteria. Rothmann and coworkers [22] applied the method to estimate the effect of capecitabine relative to 5-fluorouracil alone for metastatic colorectal cancer, by combining the results from a trial comparing capecitabine with 5-fluorouracil plus leucovorin, and a meta-analysis of trials comparing 5-fluorouracil plus leucovorin to 5-fluorouracil alone. Fisher and colleagues [23] described a similar application to estimate the effect of clopidogrel relative to placebo in patients who have myocardial infarction, ischemic stroke, or symptomatic peripheral arterial disease. Results from an active-controlled trial comparing clopidogrel with aspirin were used with data from 40 trials of aspirin versus placebo to obtain an estimate of the effect of clopidogrel versus placebo.

Using these methods, the HR for combined therapy using bicalutamide versus castration alone was estimated by taking the product of the HR for bicalutamide combined therapy versus flutamide combined therapy with the HR for flutamide combined therapy versus castration alone.

On applying this analysis, the balance of evidence suggests that there is a high probability that bicalutamide as part of combined therapy provides a survival advantage over castration alone. The HR is 0.80, which indicates a 20% reduction in the risk of death, and with a 95% CI of 0.66–0.98, this benefit could range from an absolute benefit of 2% to 34%. These confidence intervals are calculated from the combined standard error measurement (SEM), which was larger than the SEM from either the Schellhammer or the PCTCG meta-analysis, and reflects a greater uncertainty when results are combined. When estimating the effect of bicalutamide, it was assumed that the effect of flutamide in the trials in the PCTCG meta-analysis was of a similar magnitude to that in the study population of Schellhammer and coworkers. This would require that there are no important prognostic factors that were represented differently between the study populations (such as the extent of metastatic disease). It also would require that patients in the trials that were included in the PCTCG meta-analysis were managed similarly to those in the comparative trial of bicalutamide and flutamide. The limitation of combining data across studies is that it is impossible to completely verify the above assumptions. However, the statistical consistency of the effect of flutamide in the PCTCG analysis provides some reassurance of the validity of the assumptions.

Cost

Although combined therapy increases the cost of treating advanced prostate cancer, the evidence suggests that this cost is reasonable when compared with the cost of many other widely used cancer therapies. A recent US cost-effectiveness analysis of bicalutamide used as CAB concluded that at 5 years, the incremental cost-effectiveness ratio (ICER) for CAB, when compared with LH-RHa monotherapy, was $33,677 per quality-adjusted life-year [24]. At 10 years, the ICER for CAB was $20,053 (well within the accepted cost-effectiveness threshold). If quality adjustment was not included, the ICER for CAB was even more favorable ($20,489 at 5 years and $13,313 at 10 years). This model used the survival benefit derived from the PCTCG meta-analysis. If the survival benefit suggested by the re-analysis above is used as the basis for this estimate, the cost is substantially less.

A similar analysis was performed by a Canadian group. Canadian drug costs and a 4–7-month survival benefit with combined therapy in advanced prostate cancer were assumed to estimate the cost of combined therapy with bicalutamide per month of survival benefit, which was calculated as Can $437–$1107 [25]. The estimates of cost per month of survival gained are higher with other cancer therapies. For example, for metastatic colorectal cancer, irinotecan added to 5-fluorouracil and leucovorin provides a 2–3-month survival benefit and the cost is calculated to be Can $11,214 per month of survival gained.

Who should be treated with this approach? Recent data indicate that many men with

biochemical failure do not require early hormonal therapy, and are at low risk for a cancer death. PSA doubling time has been suggested as a useful measure to identify patients who are at risk. For patients who have metastatic disease, or PSA failure with a short doubling time (< 1 year), prostate cancer death is likely. In these patients, aggressive CAB therapy makes sense.

The timing of non-steroidal anti-androgen administration in combined therapy is an important consideration. Can the benefit of combined therapy be obtained by initiating antiandrogens at the time of progression? To date, no trial comparing early versus delayed combined therapy has been conducted. PSA responses to antiandrogens given at the time of biochemical progression occur in about 30% of patients, and these responses are generally of short (median 3 months) [18,26]. A reasonable inference from these data is that this is not likely to translate into a substantial survival benefit.

Summary

The use of combined therapy in prostate cancer management remains controversial. Combined therapy with non-steroidal anti-androgens offers a modest survival benefit compared with castration alone, which must be balanced against the potential for an increase in side-effects and a consequent adverse effect on the patient's quality of life. The inhibition of androgen-independent activation of the androgen receptor is an important component of the action of the non-steroidal anti-androgens, and the variability between the anti-androgens in this regard suggests that their activity is not simply a class effect. An estimate of the benefit of combined therapy with bicalutamide suggests there is a high probability that bicalutamide 50 mg as combined therapy provides a survival advantage over castration alone. The hazard rate for survival in this analysis was 0.80.

References

[1] Labrie F, Dupont A, Belanger A, et al. New hormonal therapy in prostatic carcinoma: combined treatment with an LHRH agonist and an antiandrogen. Clin Invest Med 1982;5(4):267–75.

[2] Partin AW, Rodriguez R. The molecular biology, endocrinology, and physiology of the prostate and seminal vesicles. In: Walsh P, editor. Campbell's urology. 7th edition. Philadelphia: WB Saunders; 1998. p. 1399.

[3] Kuil CW, Berrevoets CA, Mulder E. Ligand-induced conformational alterations of the androgen receptor analyzed by limited trypsinization. Studies on the mechanism of antiandrogen action. J Biol Chem 1995;270:27569–76.

[4] Culig Z. Androgen receptor cross-talk with cell signalling pathways. Growth Factors 2004;22(3):179–84.

[5] Hu X, Lazar MA. Transcriptional repression by nuclear hormone receptors. Trends Endocrinol Metab 2000;11:6–10.

[6] Gottlieb B, Vasiliou DM, Lumbroso R, et al. Analysis of exon 1 mutations in the androgen receptor gene. Hum Mutat 1999;14:527–39.

[7] Culig Z, Hoffmann J, Erdel M, et al. Switch from antagonist to agonist of the androgen receptor bicalutamide is associated with prostate tumour progression in a new model system. Br J Cancer 1999;81:242–51.

[8] Kolvenbag GJCM, Furr BJA, Blackledge GRP. Receptor affinity and potency of non-steroidal antiandrogens: translation of preclinical findings into clinical activity. Prostate Cancer PD 1998;1:307–14.

[9] Eisenberger MA, Blumenstein BA, Crawford ED, et al. Bilateral orchiectomy with or without flutamide for metastatic prostate cancer. N Engl J Med 1998;339:1036–42.

[10] McLeod DG. Tolerability of nonsteroidal antiandrogens in the treatment of advanced prostate cancer. Oncologist 1997;2:18–27.

[11] Crawford ED, Eisenberger MA, McLeod DG, et al. A controlled trial of leuprolide with and without flutamide in prostatic carcinoma. N Engl J Med 1989; 321:419–24.

[12] Samson DJ, Seidenfeld J, Schmitt B, et al. Systematic review and meta-analysis of monotherapy compared with combined androgen blockade for patients with advanced prostate carcinoma. Cancer 2002;95:361–76.

[13] Prostate Cancer Trialists' Collaborative Group. Maximum androgen blockade in advanced prostate cancer: an overview of the randomised trials. Lancet 2000;355:1491–8.

[14] Klotz L. Combined androgen blockade in prostate cancer: meta-analyses and associated issues. BJU Int 2001;87:806–13.

[15] Agency for Health Care Policy and Research. Relative effectiveness and cost-effectiveness of methods of androgen suppression in the treatment for advanced prostatic cancer. Available at: http://www.ahcpr.gov/clinic/tp/prostp.htm. Accessed 27 January 2004.

[16] Klotz LH, Newman T. Does maximal androgen blockade (MAB) improve survival? A critical appraisal of the evidence. Can J Urol 1996;3(3): 246–50.

[17] Bennett CL, Tosteson TD, Schmitt B, et al. Maximum androgen-blockade with medical or surgical castration in advanced prostate cancer: a meta-analysis of nine published randomized controlled trials and 4128 patients using flutamide. Prostate Cancer Prostatic Dis 1999;2(1):4–8.

[18] Small EJ, Srinivas S. The anti androgen withdrawal syndrome: experience in a large cohort of unselected patients with advanced prostate cancer. Cancer 2005;76:1428–34.

[19] Akaza H, Arai Y, Usami M, et al. Bicalutamide 80 mg in combination with a luteinizing hormone-releasing hormone agonist (LHRHa) versus LHRHa monotherapy as first-line treatment for advanced prostate cancer. Presented at the 39th Annual Meeting of the American Society of Clinical Oncology. Chicago, May 31–June 3, 2003.

[20] Schellhammer PF, Sharifi R, Block NL, et al. Clinical benefits of bicalutamide compared with flutamide in combined androgen blockade for patients with advanced prostatic carcinoma: final results of a multicentre, double-blind, randomized trial. Br J Urol 1997;80:278.

[21] Klotz L, Schellhammer P, Carroll K. A re-assessment of the role of combined androgen blockade for advanced prostate cancer. BJU Int 2004;93(9): 1177–82.

[22] Rothmann M, Li N, Chen G, et al. Design and analysis of non-inferiority mortality trials in oncology. Stat Med 2003;22:239–64.

[23] Fisher LD, Gent M, Buller HR. Active control trials: how would a new agent compare with placebo? A method illustrated with clopidogrel, aspirin and placebo. Am Heart J 2001;141:26–32.

[24] Penson D, Ramsay S, Veenstra D, et al. The cost effectiveness of combined androgen blockade with bicalutamide and LHRH agonist in men with metastatic prostate cancer. J Urol 2005;174(2): 547–52.

[25] Aprikian AG, Fleshner N, Langleben A, et al. An oncology perspective on the benefits and cost of combined androgen blockade in advanced prostate cancer. Can J Urol 2003;10:1986–94.

[26] Kassouf W, Tanguay S, Aprikian AG. Nilutamide as second line hormone therapy for prostate cancer after androgen ablation fails. J Urol 2003;169: 1742–4.

UROLOGIC CLINICS of North America

Urol Clin N Am 33 (2006) 167–179

Intermittent Androgen Deprivation: Clinical Experience and Practical Applications

Jonathan L. Wright, MD, MS[a], Celestia S. Higano, MD[b], Daniel W. Lin, MD[a],*

[a]Department of Urology, University of Washington, Box 356510, 1959 NE Pacific Street Seattle, WA 98195
[b]Division of Medical Oncology, Department of Medicine, University of Washington, Seattle, WA 98195

The role of androgen suppression in the management of metastatic prostate cancer has been well established since first described by Huggins and Hodges in 1941 [1]. Despite an initial response rate of approximately 85% in metastatic disease, all tumors, given time, develop androgen independence and progressive disease that results in median survival of 18 months [2]. Although hormonal therapy may improve urinary symptoms, decrease bone pain, and lower the risk of pathologic fractures and spinal cord compression, androgen suppression is associated with a number of side effects, such as loss of libido, hot flashes, gynecomastia, fatigue, cognitive dysfunction, depression, anemia, and loss of bone mineral density osteoporosis [3].

Prostate cancer is more frequently being diagnosed at an earlier age, and men are dying of prostate cancer at an older age. In addition, men are now treated with androgen deprivation for biochemical relapse, when there is no evidence of metastatic disease. As a result, the amount of time that patients are potentially subjected to androgen deprivation is increasing [2,4,5].

Intermittent androgen deprivation (IAD) has been investigated as a potential alternative to continuous androgen deprivation (CAD) in order to improve quality of life and potentially delay the progression to androgen independence. IAD is structured so that patients cycle on and off androgen deprivation therapy (ADT) by using pre-defined criteria and clinical thresholds, as

defined by serum prostate-specific antigen (PSA), for cessation or initiation of ADT. Patients continue to cycle until they become androgen independent (rising PSA despite a castrate level of testosterone). The literature is populated by multiple, largely single-institution, phase II trials that involve varied patient populations, treatment regimens, criteria for starting or stopping ADT, and definitions of failure. There are ongoing multi-institutional, randomized trials that will lend insight into the utility, efficacy, and feasibility of intermittent versus continuous ADT. This article discusses the theoretical benefits and rationale of IAD and reviews the completed and ongoing IAD trials. Finally, the controversies, practical applications, and future directions of IAD are addressed.

Rationale for intermittent androgen deprivation

The rationale for IAD is largely based on two theories that attempt to explain how prostate cancer cells become androgen independent in the setting of ADT. The first theory is based on clonal selection where, upon androgen withdrawal, there is selective survival of pre-existing, androgen-independent cells within the tumor. These clonal cells are thought to be poorly differentiated and eventually overtake the androgen-sensitive clones [6]. The second theory is based on tumor adaptation. This adaptive process may involve (1) mutations in the androgen receptor such that the receptor is transactivated in the absence of androgens, (2) increased levels of coactivators and alternative growth factor pathways (eg, HER2/NEU,

---

* Corresponding author.
E-mail address: dlin@u.washington.edu (D.W. Lin).

epidermal growth factor receptor [EGFR], and insulin-like growth factor 1 [IGF1]), or (3) adaptive upregulation of genes involved in cell survival (eg, BCL2, TRPM2, and HSP27) [7–12]. Finally, there are numerous other emerging proteins that are clearly involved in the transition from androgen dependence to independence and represent adaptive cellular responses for cell survival in the setting of androgen withdrawal [13]. It is beyond the scope of this article to review these theories in complete detail, thus, selected key pre-clinical studies and clinical rationale for IAD are presented.

Laboratory studies of intermittent androgen deprivation

Pre-clinical evidence for an adaptive progression of tumor cells to hormone independence primarily originates from experiments performed on the Shionogi mouse mammary carcinoma model [14]. The Shionogi model is an androgen-sensitive tumor that upon androgen withdrawal, similar to human prostate cancer, develops androgen independence with increased aggressiveness. By analyzing stem cells, Bruchovsky and colleagues [14] were able to demonstrate that an initially small number of androgen-dependent stem cells adapt to the altered hormone environment and eventually replicate. A later study from the same group in Vancouver found that intermittently exposing the surviving stem cells to androgens delays the development of androgen independence [15]. In this landmark study, Shionogi mice that were administered intermittent androgen suppression experienced a threefold longer time to androgen independence (150 days versus 50 days, P value unreported). Androgen independence did not develop until the fifth cycle of androgen exposure and withdrawal. Further work on the Shionogi androgen-sensitive tumor model has suggested that the loss of tumor apoptotic potential mediated through the *TRPM-2* (clusterin) gene may lead to overpopulation of tumor stem cells with androgen-independent lines [16,17].

In the human LNCaP model (an androgen-sensitive, PSA-secreting, human prostate cancer cell line developed from lymph node metastases), IAD yielded a twofold prolongation in the time to androgen independence (77 days versus 26 days, $P < .05$) [18]. However, experiments from the University of Washington that used the human LuCaP xenograft model, which was developed from human prostate cancer metastases, did not show a survival advantage with IAD [19].

Similarly, experiments that used the Dunning rat carcinoma model, an androgen sensitive cancer, found survival in those rats that received IAD was inferior to survival in rats that received CAD, although IAD did delay tumor growth [20,21].

Testosterone recovery

One of the potential advantages of IAD is the recovery of testosterone after cessation of androgen therapy and subsequent improvement in patient quality of life (QOL). Multiple studies have examined the time to recovery for patients on hormonal therapy for prostate cancer. Goldenberg and associates [22] first reported the recovery of testosterone at a mean of 8 weeks from cessation of ADT by luteinizing hormone-releasing hormone (LHRH) agonist and anti-androgen. The same group then demonstrated reversible medical castration with low-dose diethylstilbestrol diphosphate (DES; 0.1mg) and cyproterone acetate in 28 eugonadal men who had prostate cancer [23]. Testosterone normalized in all men after the cessation of therapy, although data on timing of testosterone recovery were not reported.

A number of subsequent studies have evaluated the reversibility of medical castration following LHRH agonist therapy. Higano and associates [24] were the next to report on return of testosterone. In 10 of 22 patients who had testosterone levels drawn, the median time to testosterone recovery was 12 weeks from the last injection (range 4–20 weeks). Oefelein [25] followed 13 patients who received a single, 3-month LHRH agonist as neoadjuvant therapy before local treatment. In this study, all men had normal baseline testosterone levels (2.41–8.27 ng/mL) and castrate levels (<0.2 ng/mL) persisted 6 months after injection in 10 of 13 (77%) patients. In another study, 14 men who had T3 or greater tumors and who received at least 2 years of primary LHRH therapy (mean 39 months, range 25–82 months) were monitored for testosterone recovery [26]. No significant change in serum testosterone occurred until 6 months after LHRH agonist withdrawal. At 1 year after ADT withdrawal, the median testosterone level was 111 ng/dL, significantly below the normal level (300–1000 ng/dL), and 4 men (29%) remained at castrate levels (<50 ng/dL).

Recently, two larger studies have been conducted to address the issue of testosterone recovery. In the first study, neoadjuvant LHRH therapy was given to 68 men for a variable period of time (median 9 months, range 1–58 months) [27]. The median time to testosterone normalization was 7 months. At 3, 6, and 12 months, 28%, 48%, and 74% of patients had testosterone levels in the normal range. In this study, longer duration of androgen deprivation therapy was associated with a significantly longer time to testosterone normalization. Specifically, in men who received < 24 months of ADT, serum testosterone normalized at a median of 6 months versus 24 months in men who received > 24 months of ADT ($P = .003$). Additionally, there was a trend toward longer time to normalization in patients over the age of 70 years ($P = .10$). Gulley and associates [28] monitored testosterone levels in 80 men who had biochemical failure after definitive local therapy for prostate cancer. Patients received 6 months of LHRH agonist monotherapy. The median time to testosterone normalization was 16.6 weeks. Patients who had low baseline testosterone levels ($P = .009$) and men older than 66 years ($P = .08$) had prolonged times to testosterone recovery. Gleason score at diagnosis, on study serum PSA levels, and prior definitive therapy were not associated with delay in testosterone recovery.

Several of the studies on IAD included testosterone measurements [24,29–34]. Three studies had high rates of testosterone recovery [30,33,34]. In the study by Crook and coworkers, 73% of men after the first cycle and 71% of men after the second cycle, recovered to 80% of normal testosterone levels, which was defined as return of serum testosterone to more than 80% of the lower limit of normal during the off-treatment interval [30]. The median time to recovery after the first and second cycle was 9 and 14 weeks respectively. Strum and colleagues [33] reported 48 of 52 (92%) patients experienced testosterone recovery after the first cycle with a median time to recovery of 12 weeks. Leibowitz and colleagues [34] reported that all men in their study who had normal pretreatment testosterone levels returned to normal levels after cessation of androgen deprivation therapy, although baseline testosterone levels were only available for half of the patients and exact timing of testosterone recovery was not reported.

In contrast, Bouchot and coworkers [29] reported 19% testosterone recovery after a mean off treatment time of 6.7 months. One possible explanation for this discrepancy comes from the differences in tumor stage. The studies by Crook and colleagues and Strum and colleagues were populated with only 0%–18% [30,33,34] metastatic disease patients. However, all patients had metastatic disease when they entered the Bouchot study [29]. The original report on IAD by Klotz [35] described normalization of testosterone in all 20 patients who had metastatic disease; however, the study used DES, which confounded comparisons to LHRH agonist studies [35]. Kurek and colleagues reported rising testosterone in all patients after androgen therapy was stopped but did not provide adequate data [31] and all patients in this study had non-metastatic disease at entry.

In summary, these findings suggest that testosterone recovery does occur after cessation of androgen deprivation therapy. Duration of ADT clearly affects the timing and degree of testosterone recovery. Patient factors, such as extent of disease and patient age may also affect the variable time to testosterone normalization as well as subsequent quality of life effects which are addressed in the following section.

Impact on quality of life and other toxicities

The side effects and toxicities of ADT are well established; however, during off-treatment intervals, men treated with IAD generally experience improvement in many symptoms related to ADT. Specifically, libido, hot flashes, energy level, and sense of well-being tend to improve during the off-treatment interval, coincident with a rise in serum testosterone. Few of the IAD studies have included formal QOL questionnaires, [29,31,32,36] and at present, there is no consensus on the best instrument for QOL analysis of men who have prostate cancer. Albrecht and colleagues [36] used an ad-hoc questionnaire and found negligible differences in QOL between on- and off-treatment times of men with metastatic disease. In another trial of patients who had metastatic disease, Bouchot and associates [29] used the European Organization for the Research and Treatment of Cancer Core Quality of Life Questionnaire C30 Version 2, a validated QOL questionnaire that included prostate cancer-specific questions. Patient scores reflected improvement in pain and urologic symptoms over baseline levels during ADT treatment, 53 to 78 ($P < .01$) and 71 to 82, ($P < .05$), respectively. During the off- treatment period, no new pain developed, but the urologic symptoms returned when scores fell from 82 during the first therapy period to 70 during the off-therapy period ($P < .05$). Hot flashes significantly improved during the off-treatment cycle (baseline 100, 52 during

ADT, 78 off ADT, $P < .01$); however, gynecomastia did not improve (baseline 100, 55 during ADT, 53 off ADT). In a study that included men who had untreated local disease as well as metastatic disease, Sato and colleagues [32] used the Functional Assessment of Cancer Therapy – General survey and the International Index of Erectile Function-5 questionnaire to assess QOL. Compared with pre-treatment, men scored worse in energy level (3.4 to 2.7, $P < .05$) and potency (14.7 to 2.4, $P < .01$) during ADT. During the off-treatment period, a statistical improvement was observed compared with the scores from the treatment period in energy level (2.7 to 3.6, $P < .01$), potency (2.4 to 11.4, $P < .01$), social and family well being (16.1 to 20.3, $P < .01$), and ability to enjoy life (3.1 to 3.6, $P < .05$).

IAD may have other benefits in addition to quality of life. The impact of IAD on bone mineral density at the spine and hip was studied in 19 men who had biochemical relapse [37]. After 9 months of ADT, the mean bone mineral density decreased 4.5% in the lumbar spine ($P < .001$) and 2.5% in the hip ($P < .001$), much greater than the expected 0.5%–1.0% annual loss of bone density. Importantly, after a median off-treatment period of 8 months, the mean change in bone mineral density was 1.5% ($P = .06$) in the spine and -0.01% in the hip ($P = .09$), reflecting the attenuation in the rate of bone loss with IAD, and thus, IAD appears to slow the decline in bone mineral density compared with what would be expected with continuous ADT.

Finally, IAD may have benefits in cognitive function relative to continuous ADT. In a trial of IAD in 19 men with biochemical relapse, cognitive function was evaluated before ADT, after 9 months of ADT, and again 3 months after stopping ADT. As a group, there were no significant changes in measures of verbal and special memory, executive function, or language ability. However, when compared with the baseline, the ability to mentally rotate complex three-dimensional figures significantly worsened during treatment, then returned to normal when testosterone levels rose during the off-treatment interval [38]. Almeida and associates [39] similarly studied 40 men with prostate cancer who were treated with CAB for 36 weeks, then followed for 18 weeks after treatment was discontinued. All subjects received multiple neuropsychological and clinical evaluations at baseline, during treatment, and after ADT was discontinued. After discontinuation of ADT, improvements in cognitive function were

reported on multiple levels, particularly in verbal memory. Regardless of study results, many men report "feeling back to normal" which is likely because of a complex network of changes caused by a rise in testosterone levels.

Clinical experience

The first reported experience of IAD in humans was from Klotz and associates in 1986 [35]. In this pre-PSA era report, 20 men received either DES (19) or flutamide (1) for advanced prostate cancer treatment. Hormonal therapy was stopped when metastatic bone pain resolved, obstructive symptoms resolved, or pulmonary metastases disappeared. Hormonal therapy was then reinitiated for recurrent symptoms. The median time off therapy in the first cycle was 8 months (44%), and 90% of men who were potent pretreatment, regained potency after hormonal cessation. Early in the PSA era, several small pilot studies were completed and used pre-defined criteria for stopping or restarting androgen therapy based on serum PSA levels [22,24,40,41].

The first clinical trial of IAD completed in the PSA era was reported in 1995 from the Vancouver group [22] and they have since published a number of follow-up studies [42–46]. Forty-seven men with either metastatic (51%) or locally advanced disease (49%) were followed for a mean of 125 weeks. Patients received total androgen blockade (TAB) with an LHRH agonist and an anti-androgen for a minimum of 24 weeks and until a PSA of < 4.0 ng/mL was reached, then therapy was discontinued to allow for testosterone recovery. TAB was restarted at pre-defined serum PSA levels which were determined by pre-ADT PSA levels. Thirty patients completed the first therapeutic cycle (mean total cycle duration of 73 weeks). Patients spent 43 weeks on ADT and 30 weeks (41%) off ADT. Fifteen patients completed a second treatment cycle: mean total cycle duration of 75 weeks, 45% off treatment. Mean time to achieve a nadir level of serum PSA was 20 weeks in cycle 1 and 18 weeks in cycle 2. Testosterone levels normalized within a mean of 8 weeks from cessation of ADT in each cycle and was paralleled by an improvement in well-being and recovery of sexual function in those with pretreatment potency (the quality of life assessment method was not provided). A schematic of the serum PSA and testosterone kinetics is represented in Fig. 1. Seven patients (15%) progressed to androgen independence; the median time to progression was 108

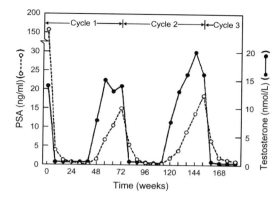

Fig. 1. Composite results of intermittent androgen suppression on 47 patients who have prostate cancer. Observations were based on 30 patients who have completed one cycle and 15 patients who have completed two cycles. The length of the first and second cycles were 73 and 75 weeks respectively. The mean treatment and no treatment intervals during the first cycle were 43 and 30 weeks; during the second cycle, 42 and 33 weeks. ○ = serum PSA; ● = serum testosterone. (*From* Goldenberg SL, Bruchovsky N, Gleave ME, et al. Intermittent androgen suppression in the treatment of prostate cancer: a preliminary report. Urology 1995;45:839–44 ; with permission.)

weeks, and the median overall survival was 166 weeks. The findings of this study fueled interest in IAD and led to a number of subsequent nonrandomized clinical studies listed in Tables 1 and 2.

Patient selection and treatment regimens in study trials

The literature on IAD includes a very heterogeneous patient population as well as varied treatment regimens, which reflects the uncertainty of appropriate timing for hormonal therapy initiation and the controversial data regarding TAB versus monotherapy as a method of androgen suppression. Studies have included patients who have biochemical failure after local definitive therapy, [30,31,47,48] patients who have only locally advanced or metastatic disease [14,32,36], or a combination of both [33,46,49–51] (Table 1). Similarly, the median baseline PSA between studies is quite variable, from < 4.5 dl/mL [48] in one study to another study where 80% of patients had an entry PSA > 80 dl/mL [36]. Most studies have primarily used total androgen blockade with both a LHRH agonist and an anti-androgen [18,24,30,31,33,46,50,52] (Table 2). Few studies have used LHRH agonists alone in all [36,51] or

some patients [29,47], and two recent studies used anti-androgen monotherapy in all [48] or most patients (59%) [49], although anti-androgen monotherapy notably does not decrease testosterone levels, which confounds comparison to other regimens.

The treatment schema for cycling on and off therapy have also varied considerably in the literature. In most reports, patients were treated initially for 6–9 months, then stopped therapy if the PSA fell below 4 ng/mL. Some series, comprised of patients primarily with biochemical recurrence or untreated local disease, used an undetectable, or near undetectable, PSA level as the indication to cycle off treatment [31,33,47–49]. Criteria for restarting ADT have generally been based on the extent of disease, whether the prostate is intact, and the initial PSA. For example, for those patients who have biochemical relapse, some regimens require re-initiation of ADT at a PSA level of 1 ng/mL in patients who have had a radical prostatectomy and 4 ng/mL in patients who were treated with radiation [24,31,45,48,49]. Other studies allow the PSA to rise to the pre-treatment baseline or a percentage of the pre-treatment baseline [24,32,45,47]. In the setting of metastatic disease, the PSA thresholds tend to be higher, and androgen blockade is restarted with a PSA of 10–20 ng/mL or symptoms [29,30,36,50,51].

The significant variance between the nonrandomized studies makes it difficult to draw firm conclusions by pooling the results on cycle duration and time off ADT (Table 3). However, some observations deserve note. First, few studies have long-term follow up on patients who complete multiple cycles of IAD. In general, regardless of treatment regimen, the total cycle length and the percentage of time off therapy for an individual patient decrease with successive cycles [46,49–52]. This may represent decreasing tumor responsiveness to androgen deprivation. Second, several authors have reported that patients who have a higher disease stage progress more quickly to androgen independence. For example, in the study by Youssef and colleagues [51], progression-free survival rates for patients who had biochemical failure, locoregional recurrence and bone metastases were 80%, 67%, and 45% respectively, $P < .02$. In the study by Albrecht and colleagues [36], patients were grouped based on extent of metastatic disease. Patients with greater metastatic burden were more likely to complete only one cycle (40% versus 20%, no P value reported). A multivariate analysis of the

Table 1
Baseline patient characteristics from IAD studies with at least 20 patients and two reported cycles

Study	Year	N	Biochemical failure	Untreated local	Local recurrence	N+	M+	Median age (yrs)	Median PSA (dl/mL)	Gleason score	Median follow-up (months)
Goldenberg [22]	1995	47	8	15	0	10	14	67.0	158.0 (mean)	NR	29
Higano [24]	1996	22	13	2	0	2	5	65.0	25.0	55% > = 7	26
Grossfeld [47]	1998	61	27	34	0	0	0	70.0	16.0	49% > = 7	30
Crooke [30]	1999	54	4	0	11	4	35		All > 10		33 (mean)
Kurek [31]	1999	44	44	0	0	0	0	TIB 70.0 RP 67.0	NR	NR	48 (mean)
Strum [33]	2000	52	19	24	0	NR	9	68.0	9.1	6.4 (median)	66
Bouchot [29]	2000	43	0	0	0	0	43	72.0	47.0	7.0 (mean)	44
De Leval [52]	2002	35	4	19	0	2	10	71.0	21.0	6.0 (median)	29
Prapotnich [50]	2003	233	90	84	0	16	43	73.0	RP 14.7 XRT 30.5 No prior 33.4	7.0 (mean)	25
Youssef [51]	2003	74	41	0	16	8	9	67.0	11.4	NR	21
Pether [46]	2003	102	38	30	0	11	23	68.5	18.5	NR	219 weeks
De la Taille [49]	2003	146	74	62	0	NR	10	72.0	69 (mean)	6.7 (mean)	46 (mean)
Albrecht [36]	2003	107	0	0	0	4	103	70.0	100% > 20 80% > 80		92 weeks
Sato [32]	2004	49	0	28	0	8	13	74.0	36.0	7.0 (median)	136 weeks (mean)
Peyromaure[a] [48]	2005	57	57	0	0	0	0	A 66.0 B 67.0	A 3.8 B 4.5	A 48% > 7 B 21% > 7	A 89 B 94
Total		1126	419	298	27	65	317				

Abbreviations: M+, metastatic disease; N+, node-positive; NR, not reported; PSA, prostate-specific antigen; RP, radical prostatectomy; XRT, radiation therapy.

[a] Patient groups: A, salvage radiotherapy; B, no salvage radiotherapy.

large series by De la Taille and colleagues [49], showed that biochemical progression-free survival rates of 93% and 52% were statistically different for patients who had localized versus metastatic disease respectively ($P = .004$). Leibowitz and Tucker [34] reported on 110 men with clinically localized prostate cancer (cT1–T3 tumors) who refused local therapy and were treated with primary "triple androgen blockade" (LHRH analog, a non-steroidal anti-androgen and finasteride) for a median of 13 months. Patients were then maintained on finasteride alone. After a median follow-up of 36 months, 77% remained off therapy at least 1 year, and no patients have restarted anti-androgen therapy. Although a PSA threshold for restarting therapy was not specified, only 8% of patients reached a PSA level > 4.0 ng/mL.

Other studies have analyzed off-treatment duration and have established prostate cancer clinico-pathologic factors and their association to progression to androgen independence in patients who receive IAD. A multivariate analysis by De la Taille and colleagues [49] reported that a Gleason score ≥ 8 ($P = .02$), off-treatment duration during the first cycle of < 1 year ($P = .04$),

and age < 70 ($P = .04$) predicted development of androgen independence and were associated with lower progression-free survival. Patients who were off treatment for > 1 year during the first cycle demonstrated a progression-free survival rate of 90% compared with 55% for patients who were off treatment in cycle one < 1 year ($P = .007$). In another study, Strum and colleagues [33] used multivariate analysis to identify predictors of prolonged time off therapy. Patients who had non-metastatic, biochemical recurrence when they entered the study ($P = .04$) and those who maintained testosterone levels < 150 ng/dL for more than 4 months off therapy ($P = .04$) experienced longer off-treatment durations. Conclusions about clinical features that predict off-treatment times are hampered by the heterogeneous patient populations and indications to cycle on or off therapy. Ongoing, large, randomized trials may shed light on these predictive factors when examined in strict clinical trial settings.

Randomized trials

The only published, randomized, controlled IAD trial in the English literature is an open-label,

Table 2
Treatment parameters from select IAD studies

Study	Year	Treatment	Indication to cycle off	Indication to cycle on	Failure definition
Goldenberg [22]	1995	LHRH/DES + AA	9 mo ADT and PSA < 4	Based on initial PSA < 10; once PSA > 2.5 10–20; once PSA 5–15 > 20; once PSA 10–20	PSA > 4 on 3 consecutive tests and castrate testosterone on TAB
Higano [24]	1996	LHRH + AA	9–12 mo ADT and PSA < 4	Based on initial PSA < 10; once PSA rises 10–100; once PSA 10–20 > 100; once PSA 20–40	PSA > 4 on 3 consecutive tests and castrate testosterone on TAB or objective evidence of progression
Grossfeld [47]	1998	LHRH (23%) LHRH + AA (77%)	Prior local treatment, PSA < 0.1 No prior treatment, PSA < 4	PSA 50% of pretreatment; PSA or > 10; or patient request	PSA rise × 2 or imaging progression on treatment
Crook [30]	1999	LHRH + AA	8 mo of ADT	PSA 10	PSA > 4 and 3 consecutive rises during TAB
Kurek [31]	1999	LHRH + AA	9 mo ADT, PSA < 0.5	pT1B, PSA > 6 post RP, PSA > 3	Not stated
Strum [33]	2000	LHRH + AA	Undetectable PSA	PSA > 5	Not stated
Bouchot [29]	2000	LHRH (25%) LHRH + AA (75%)	PSA < 4 after 6 mo of ADT	PSA > 20; or symptomatic progression	PSA > 4 at 6 mo on treatment or local failure/ mets on treatment
De Leval [52]	2002	LHRH + AA	PSA < 4 after 3–6 mo ADT	PSA > 10	PSA > 10 × 3 on TAB with castrate testosterone
Prapotnich [50]	2003	LHRH + AA	PSA < 4	PSA > 20; PSA slope > 5/mo; or symptoms	PSA fails to fall below 4 on treatment
Youssef [51]	2003	LHRH	After 6–8 mo of ADT	PSA > 10	2 consecutive PSA increases or imaging evidence of progression on treatment
Pether [46]	2003	DES/LHRH + AA	6 mo ADT, PSA < 4 at 24–32 wks	Post RP, once PSA 4–6; or based on initial PSA 20, once PSA 10–20, 10–20, once PSA 5–15	3 successive PSA rises above 4 on treatment with castrate testosterone
De la Taille [49]	2003	LHRH (29%) LHRH + AA (19%) AA (59%)	Post RP, 6 mo after undetectable PSA Post XRT, PSA < 4 No prior treatment, PSA < 1	Post RP, PSA > 4 All others, PSA > 10	PSA increase despite castrate testosterone
Albrecht [36]	2003	LHRH	80% reduction of initial PSA to a level < 20	50% rise over PSA nadir, and PSA > 20	PSA rise, clinical or radiographic progression on treatment
Sato [32]	2004	LHRH + AA	If PSA < 4 by 24–32 wks, treatment stopped at 36 wks	Based on initial PSA > 15, once PSA > 15 < 15, once PSA at baseline	3 PSA increases above level of 4 on treatment and castrate testosterone
Peyromaure [48]	2005	AA	3 mo after undetectable PSA, or higher threshold (not defined) if initial PSA > 20	PSA > 4	Persistent PSA elevation during treatment

All PSA units in ng/mL.

Abbreviations: ADT, androgen deprivation therapy; AA, antiandrogen (flutamide, nilutamide, cyproterone); LHRH, luteinizing hormone-releasing hormone; PSA, prostate-specific antigen; TAB, total androgen blockade.

Table 3
On and off-treatment cycle lengths from select IAD studies

Study	Year	Completed 1st cycle	Median 1st cycle time (months)	Median months off treatment (%)	Completed 2nd cycle	Median 2nd cycle time (months)	Median months off treatment (%)
Goldenberg [22]	1995	30	17.0	7.0 (41%)	15	17.4	7.7 (45%)
Higano [24]	1996	15	15.8	6.0 (38%)	2	21.0	10.0 (51%)
Grossfeld [47]	1998	61	17.0	9.0 (53%)	52	14.5	7.0 (48%)
Crook [30]	1999	41	15.0	8.0 (52%)	20	14.4	7.0 (48%)
Kurek [31]	1999	26	20.0	11.6 (58%)	13	17.0	8.0 (47%)
Strum [33]	2000	43	34.5	17.0 (48%)	15	31.4	14.0 (30%)
Bouchot [29]	2000	43	18.7	6.7 (36%)	35	11.9	3.8 (32%)
De Leval [52]	2002	28	12.2	8.3 (58%)	22	9.6	6.9 (61%)
Prapotnich [50]	2003	186	19.6	9.8 (68%)	92	14.3	9.7 (68%)
Youssef [51]	2003	71	17.4	9.4 (54%)	40	14.0	8.0 (57%)
Pether [46]	2003	91	22.0	11.6 (53%)	53	20.0	10.2 (51%)
De la Taille [49]	2003	117	21.6	10.5 (49%)	64	14.2	6.8 (48%)
Albrecht [36]	2003	82	8.7	3.3 (38%)	49	7.7	3.7 (49%)
Sato [32]	2004	31	19.1	10.7 (56%)	6	16.9	8.6 (51%)
Peyromaure[a] [48]	2005	A 29	14.0	8.0 (57%)	27	12.0	6.0 (50%)
		B 28	12.9	8.0 (62%)	24	14.0	8.0 (57%)

[a] Patient groups: A, salvage radiotherapy; B, no salvage radiotherapy.

non-blinded trial of 68 patients who had locally advanced, metastatic, or PSA recurrence after radical retropubic prostatectomy (RRP) [52]. Patients were randomized after 3–6 months of TAB and PSA reduction to < 4.0 ng/mL, to receive either continuous androgen deprivation or IAD. IAD patients restarted TAB after a PSA rise to > 10.0 ng/mL. Thirteen (19%) patients progressed to hormone refractory disease, 10 on CAD and 3 on IAD. Although the numbers are small, the Kaplan Meier curves were statistically different (Fig. 2; $P = .005$). On stratified analysis, the progression-free rates were higher in the IAD group versus the CAD group for those patients with a Gleason score ≥ 7 (7.1% versus 71.4%, $P = .02$) or non-metastatic disease (0.0% versus 35.8%, $P < .001$). Limitations of this study include the relatively small sample size and the heterogeneous population.

Ongoing randomized trials (Table 4)

Southwest Oncology Group

In May 1995, the Southwest Oncology Group (SWOG) activated SWOG-9346, a phase III randomized trial of intermittent versus continuous combined ADT in hormone-naïve patients who had metastatic prostate cancer. All patients receive induction with goserelin and bicalutamide. Patients are stratified according to performance status, extent of disease, and prior hormonal therapy. Those patients who have stable or declining PSA levels

after months 6 and 7 are then randomized to either continuous or intermittent androgen blockade. After 8 months of ADT, those randomized to intermittent ADT stop hormonal therapy and are followed off treatment until the PSA reaches a threshold of 20 g/mL. Formal quality of life questionnaires are collected for both study arms. This study continues to accrue subjects and has a target sample size of 1500 patients.

National Cancer Institute of Canada

The National Cancer Institute of Canada is the lead institution for CTG PR.7, a phase III randomized trial of intermittent versus continuous combined androgen deprivation therapy in patients who have biochemical recurrence after pelvic radiotherapy or radical prostatectomy followed by pelvic irradiation. Patients must have a PSA > 3 ng/mL and serum testosterone > 5 nmol/L. Randomization and treatment are similar to the previously described SWOG-9346 trial except the threshold PSA for restarting ADT is 10 ng/mL. This trial is ongoing and has a target sample size of 1340 patients. Over 800 patients have been accrued to date and this trial was expected to meet the accrual goal by the end of 2005.

Portuguese Cooperative Group

The Portuguese Cooperative Group activated SEUG-9401, a phase III randomized trial of intermittent versus continuous combined androgen deprivation therapy in hormone-naïve patients

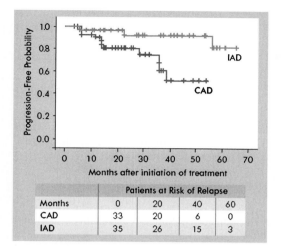

Androgen-independent biochemical progression was defined as an increasing total serum PSA level of ≥ 10 ng/mL despite continued complete androgen blockade treatment. Tick marks on the curves indicate censored patients. Patients at risk for each cohort of patients are shown below each panel. Probability of freedom from progression according to either continuous or intermittent androgen deprivation therapy for the entire cohort of patients.
Abbreviations: CAD = continuous androgen deprivation; IAD = intermittent androgen deprivation

Fig. 2. Androgen independent biochemical progression-free rates in patients with hormone naïve advanced prostate cancer. (*From* de Leval J, Boca P, Yousef E, et al. Intermittent versus continuous total androgen blockade in the treatment of patients with advanced hormone-naive prostate cancer: results of a prospective randomized multicenter trial. Clin Prostate Cancer. 2002;1:163–71; with permission.)

with newly diagnosed prostate cancer (T3 or T4 with M0 or M1 cases). All patients initially receive CPA and an LHRH agonist for 14 weeks. If the PSA falls below 4 ng/mL, patients are randomized to either continuous or intermittent ADT. Preliminary results of 605 randomized patients demonstrated that, of those who were sexually active, erectile dysfunction was less and sexual enjoyment was greater in the intermittent study arm.

Tulp Institute trial

This is an industry sponsored trial of previously untreated patients who have T2–T4 tumors with either N0, M1 or N1, M0 disease and a PSA > 10 ng/mL. Patients are induced with goserelin and nilutamide and randomized to intermittent or continuous therapy after 6 months. Patients who have M1 disease on the intermittent study arm restarted therapy when the PSA rose to 10 ng/mL; whereas, those with N1 disease did not restart until the PSA was over 20 ng/mL. The study continues to mature.

Practical applications

Although ADT is the cornerstone of advanced prostate cancer treatment, there is substantial controversy about the timing and method of androgen deprivation. IAD is predicated on the assumption that immediate ADT is superior to

Table 4
Ongoing randomized, controlled trials of IAD

Study name	Group	Entry criteria	Treatment	Status
SWOG-9346	Southwest Oncology Group	Stage IV cancer	LHRH + AA	Still accruing
NCIC CTG PR.7	National Cancer Institute of Canada	Biochemical recurrence after primary radiotherapy	LHRH + AA	Still accruing
TULP	Industry sponsored	Untreated T2-4 N0, M1 or N1, M0 cancer and PSA > 10 ng/mL	LHRH + AA	Closed (282 patients)[a]
SEUG-9401	Portuguese Cooperative Group	Untreated, locally advanced cancer	LHRH	Closed, (765 enrolled, 626 randomized)[a]
SEUG–9901	Portuguese Cooperative Group	Locally advanced or metastatic cancer	Intermittent CPA vs. continuous LHRH + CPA	NA

Abbreviations: AA, antiandrogen; CPA, cyproterone acetate; LHRH, goserelin or lupreolide; M0, no evidence of distant metastasis; M1, distant metastasis; N0, node-negative; N1, node-positive; NA, not available.

[a] Calais da Silva F, Bono A, Whelan P, et al. Intermittent androgen deprivation for locally advanced prostate cancer. Preliminary experience from an ongoing randomized controlled study of the South European urooncological group. Oncology 2003;65(Suppl 1):24–8.

delayed therapy for improved survival of patients who have advanced prostate cancer. There is growing evidence that early ADT in multiple clinical settings prolongs the time to androgen independence and improves survival [53–57].

Intermittent androgen deprivation candidates

Any patient in whom androgen deprivation therapy is being initiated could be considered for IAD. In particular, patients who do not tolerate the side effects of ADT or men concerned about potency are excellent candidates for IAD. Sexually active patients who have biochemical recurrence after primary therapy represent the most attractive patient population, if they are compliant and willing to undergo androgen deprivation. Patients who fail to reach a nadir PSA < 4 ng/mL after 6 months of ADT should probably not be offered IAD because there is a suggestion that these patients have a poor prognosis and limited response to androgen deprivation [58]. Patients should be counseled about the side effects of ADT, but should also understand that at present, although IAD may decrease the side effects and costs of ADT, data regarding the long-term efficacy for delaying progression to hormone-refractory disease and improving survival are unknown. The ongoing randomized studies will answer these important questions in the coming years.

Treatment cycle length

Treatment times in the published studies and in the ongoing randomized trials consist primarily of 6–9 months of androgen deprivation before cycling off. The biologic rationale for this treatment time is based on the goals of maximal castration effects on the tumor, yet cessation of ADT before the tumor adaptation or clonal selection. There are data to suggest that 8 months of ADT is required to reach maximal tumor regression and PSA nadir [59,60]. In a prospective, non-randomized study from the Vancouver group, 50 men received neoadjuvant androgen therapy before radical prostatectomy [60]. PSA nadir was achieved after 3 months of ADT in 22% of men, in 42% after 5 months, and in 84% after 8 months. The same group, along with the Canadian Uro-Oncology Group, then performed a randomized trial that compared PSA and pathology between 500 men who received 3 months or 8 months of neoadjuvant ADT [59]. An undetectable PSA was achieved in 43% versus 75% ($P <$ .001) of patients who received 3 versus 8 months

of ADT respectively. Prostate size, measured by transrectal ultrasound, decreased 37% after 3 months ($P <$ .001) but decreased an additional 13% after 8 months of ADT ($P <$ .03). Incidentally, positive margins were significantly lower in the 8-month group (12% versus 23%, $P =$ .01). Emerging data on molecular markers of cellular proliferation (Ki67, PCNA) and survival proteins (clusterin, BCL2) support the initial duration of ADT [61–63]. Based on these data, treatment cycles of 8–9 months are recommended.

When to restart androgen deprivation therapy

To achieve both the biological and quality-of-life benefits of IAD, the off-treatment cycle should allow adequate time for the testosterone level to rise with subsequent improvement in ADT-related symptoms. Previous studies would suggest that, in the setting of short-term (< 24 months) ADT, testosterone recovery will occur in approximately 4–6 months after withdrawal of ADT [23,25–28]. The result of testosterone recovery is an eventual rise in serum PSA, which represents the primary determinant for reinstitution of ADT. Historically, pre-determined trigger PSA levels, usually based on stage or pre-treatment baseline PSA, were used to dictate reinstitution of ADT, although the optimum PSA trigger point is unknown (Table 2). Therefore, PSA measurements are usually obtained on a frequent basis during the off-treatment period in order to restart ADT before the threshold PSA is significantly exceeded. Another indication to cycle back on to ADT is the recurrence or worsening of prostate cancer-related symptoms, although most investigators recommend the use of IAD for metastatic disease only in clinical trial settings. Until an established trigger PSA is determined from randomized studies or another, more specific, indicator is identified, individualized trigger PSAs should be used. Pre-treatment PSA, disease stage, PSA kinetics and symptoms should all be considered.

Future directions

Although the preclinical data show that IAD delays time to androgen independence and numerous phase II trials suggest potential benefit in terms of quality of life, the exact role of IAD in the treatment of prostate cancer remains unclear. Despite the fact that IAD is widely used in clinical practice, particularly for patients who experience biochemical relapse, it is still considered experimental until results from well-designed, randomized trials are available. Numerous questions remain about IAD. Is combined androgen blockade with LHRH and an anti-androgen better than LHRH analog alone? What is the optimal on-cycle and off-cycle duration in an intermittent regimen? When should ADT be re-initiated after an off-therapy cycle? What is the impact on quality of life as measured by validated instruments? What is the impact on patient survival? Despite these questions, many patients choose to be treated with IAD because of real or perceived differences in how they feel on and off ADT. Some patients may not require or benefit from additional therapy despite a rising serum PSA, and one of the current goals should be to define this cohort of patients who may be able to avoid any form of ADT. For example, the momentum of growing data, primarily from d'Amico and colleagues [64], support the use of PSA kinetics (eg, PSA velocity and PSA doubling time) to predict which patients are at high risk for progressive disease and, importantly, cancer-specific death [64–68]. With these paradigms, the clinical question would not be whether to treat with intermittent versus continuous ADT, but whether the patient would benefit from either form of ADT versus close observation alone. In the meantime, IAD will remain attractive to patients who had biochemical relapse and who are understandably concerned about the rise in their serum PSA.

The field of IAD is expanding, particularly in its application to earlier disease, such as the patient who has early biochemical recurrence after primary curative therapy. Along with the increased use of primary hormonal therapy in clinically localized prostate cancer, IAD may supplant the traditional surgical or radiotherapy options, specifically in men who have underlying co-morbidities and decreased life expectancy. Others are investigating the use of non-hormonal (eg, anti-angiogenesis inhibitor) and hormonal (eg, 5-alpha reductase inhibitors) agents during the off-treatment period, after an initial induction of ADT, as a strategy to prolong the length and number of cycles of IAD [34,69]. For example, the National Cancer Institute is studying the addition of thalidomide to IAD in patients who have biochemical relapse [69]. As the activity of other targeted agents, such as the numerous tyrosine kinase inhibitors, is better defined, these therapies will perhaps become logical additions to IAD, administered during the cycle when the agent would have its maximal effect. Until these issues are resolved, IAD remains an attractive alternative to continuous ADT for the closely monitored, compliant, and properly informed prostate cancer patient.

References

[1] Huggins C, Hodges C. Studies on prostate cancer: I. The effect of estrogen and of androgen injection on serum phosphatases in metastatic carcinoma of the prostate. Cancer Res 1941;1:293–7.

[2] Pound CR, Partin AW, Eisenberger MA, et al. Natural history of progression after PSA elevation following radical prostatectomy. JAMA 1999;281:1591–7.

[3] Higano CS. Side effects of androgen deprivation therapy: monitoring and minimizing toxicity. Urology 2003;61:32–8.

[4] Cooperberg MR, Broering JM, Litwin MS, et al. The contemporary management of prostate cancer in the United States: lessons from the cancer of the prostate strategic urologic research endeavor (CapSURE), a national disease registry. J Urol 2004;171:1393–401.

[5] Cooperberg MR, Grossfeld GD, Lubeck DP, et al. National practice patterns and time trends in androgen ablation for localized prostate cancer. J Natl Cancer Inst 2003;95:981–9.

[6] Isaacs JT, Coffey DS. Adaptation versus selection as the mechanism responsible for the relapse of prostatic cancer to androgen ablation therapy as studied in the Dunning R-3327-H adenocarcinoma. Cancer Res 1981;41:5070–5.

[7] Buchanan G, Greenberg NM, Scher HI, et al. Collocation of androgen receptor gene mutations in prostate cancer. Clin Cancer Res 2001;7:1273–81.

[8] Craft N, Shostak Y, Carey M, et al. A mechanism for hormone-independent prostate cancer through modulation of androgen receptor signaling by the HER-2/neu tyrosine kinase. Nat Med 1999;5:280–5.

[9] Feldman BJ, Feldman D. The development of androgen-independent prostate cancer. Nat Rev Cancer 2001;1:34–45.

[10] Koivisto P, Kononen J, Palmberg C, et al. Androgen receptor gene amplification: a possible molecular mechanism for androgen deprivation therapy failure in prostate cancer. Cancer Res 1997;57:314–9.

[11] Raffo AJ, Perlman H, Chen MW, et al. Overexpression of bcl-2 protects prostate cancer cells from apoptosis in vitro and confers resistance to androgen depletion in vivo. Cancer Res 1995;55:4438–45.

[12] Rocchi P, So A, Kojima S, et al. Heat shock protein 27 increases after androgen ablation and plays a cytoprotective role in hormone-refractory prostate cancer. Cancer Res 2004;64:6595–602.

[13] Nelson PS, Clegg N, Arnold H, et al. The program of androgen-responsive genes in neoplastic prostate epithelium. Proc Natl Acad Sci USA 2002;99:11890–5.

[14] Bruchovsky N, Rennie PS, Coldman AJ, et al. Effects of androgen withdrawal on the stem cell composition of the Shionogi carcinoma. Cancer Res 1990;50:2275–82.

[15] Akakura K, Bruchovsky N, Goldenberg SL, et al. Effects of intermittent androgen suppression on androgen-dependent tumors. Apoptosis and serum prostate-specific antigen. Cancer 1993;71:2782–90.

[16] Bruchovsky N, Snoek R, Rennie PS, et al. Control of tumor progression by maintenance of apoptosis. Prostate Suppl 1996;6:13–21.

[17] Akakura K, Bruchovsky N, Rennie PS, et al. Effects of intermittent androgen suppression on the stem cell composition and the expression of the TRPM-2 (clusterin) gene in the Shionogi carcinoma. J Steroid Biochem Mol Biol 1996;59:501–11.

[18] Sato N, Gleave ME, Bruchovsky N, et al. Intermittent androgen suppression delays progression to androgen-independent regulation of prostate-specific antigen gene in the LNCaP prostate tumour model. J Steroid Biochem Mol Biol 1996;58:139–46.

[19] Buhler KR, Santucci RA, Royai RA, et al. Intermittent androgen suppression in the LuCaP 23.12 prostate cancer xenograft model. Prostate 2000;43:63–70.

[20] Trachtenberg J. Experimental treatment of prostatic cancer by intermittent hormonal therapy. J Urol 1987;137:785–8.

[21] Russo P, Liguori G, Heston WD, et al. Effects of intermittent diethylstilbestrol diphosphate administration on the R3327 rat prostatic carcinoma. Cancer Res 1987;47:5967–70.

[22] Goldenberg SL, Bruchovsky N, Gleave ME, et al. Intermittent androgen suppression in the treatment of prostate cancer: a preliminary report. Urology 1995;45:839–44 [discussion: 844–5].

[23] Goldenberg SL, Bruchovsky N, Gleave ME, et al. Low-dose cyproterone acetate plus mini-dose diethylstilbestrol–a protocol for reversible medical castration. Urology 1996;47:882–4.

[24] Higano CS, Ellis W, Russell K, et al. Intermittent androgen suppression with leuprolide and flutamide for prostate cancer: a pilot study. Urology 1996;48:800–4.

[25] Oefelein MG. Time to normalization of serum testosterone after 3-month luteinizing hormone-releasing hormone agonist administered in the neoadjuvant setting: implications for dosing schedule and neoadjuvant study consideration. J Urol 1998;160:1685–8.

[26] Hall MC, Fritzsch RJ, Sagalowsky AI, et al. Prospective determination of the hormonal response after cessation of luteinizing hormone-releasing hormone agonist treatment in patients with prostate cancer. Urology 1999;53:898–902 [discussion: 902–3].

[27] Nejat RJ, Rashid HH, Bagiella E, et al. A prospective analysis of time to normalization of serum testosterone after withdrawal of androgen deprivation therapy. J Urol 2000;164:1891–4.

[28] Gulley JL, Figg WD, Steinberg SM, et al. A prospective analysis of the time to normalization of serum androgens following 6 months of androgen deprivation therapy in patients on a randomized phase III clinical trial using limited hormonal therapy. J Urol 2005;173:1567–71.

[29] Bouchot O, Lenormand L, Karam G, et al. Intermittent androgen suppression in the treatment of metastatic prostate cancer. Eur Urol 2000;38:543–9.

[30] Crook JM, Szumacher E, Malone S, et al. Intermittent androgen suppression in the management of prostate cancer. Urology 1999;53:530–4.

[31] Kurek R, Renneberg H, Lubben G, et al. Intermittent complete androgen blockade in PSA relapse after radical prostatectomy and incidental prostate cancer. Eur Urol 1999;35(Suppl 1):27–31.

[32] Sato N, Akakura K, Isaka S, et al. Intermittent androgen suppression for locally advanced and metastatic prostate cancer: preliminary report of a prospective multicenter study. Urology 2004;64:341–5.

[33] Strum SB, Scholz MC, McDermed JE. Intermittent androgen deprivation in prostate cancer patients: factors predictive of prolonged time off therapy. Oncologist 2000;5:45–52.

[34] Leibowitz RL, Tucker SJ. Treatment of localized prostate cancer with intermittent triple androgen blockade: preliminary results in 110 consecutive patients. Oncologist 2001;6:177–82.

[35] Klotz LH, Herr HW, Morse MJ, et al. Intermittent endocrine therapy for advanced prostate cancer. Cancer 1986;58:2546–50.

[36] Albrecht W, Collette L, Fava C, et al. Intermittent maximal androgen blockade in patients with metastatic prostate cancer: an EORTC feasibility study. Eur Urol 2003;44:505–11.

[37] Higano C, Shields A, Wood N, et al. Bone mineral density in patients with prostate cancer without bone metastases treated with intermittent androgen suppression. Urology 2004;64:1182–6.

[38] Cherrier MM, Rose AL, Higano C. The effects of combined androgen blockade on cognitive function during the first cycle of intermittent androgen suppression in patients with prostate cancer. J Urol 2003;170:1808–11.

[39] Almeida OP, Waterreus A, Spry N, et al. One year follow-up study of the association between chemical castration, sex hormones, beta-amyloid, memory and depression in men. Psychoneuroendocrinology 2004;29:1071–81.

[40] Horwich A, Huddart RA, Gadd J, et al. A pilot study of intermittent androgen deprivation in advanced prostate cancer. Br J Urol 1998;81:96–9.

[41] Oliver RT, Williams G, Paris AM, et al. Intermittent androgen deprivation after PSA-complete response as a strategy to reduce induction of hormone-resistant prostate cancer. Urology 1997;49:79–82.

[42] Gleave M, Goldenberg SL, Bruchovsky N, et al. Intermittent androgen suppression for prostate cancer: rationale and clinical experience. Prostate Cancer Prostatic Dis 1998;1:289–96.

[43] Goldenberg SL, Gleave ME, Taylor D, et al. Clinical experience with intermittent androgen suppression in prostate cancer: minimum of 3 years' follow-up. Mol Urol 1999;3:287–92.

[44] Hurtado-Coll A, Goldenberg SL, Gleave ME, et al. Intermittent androgen suppression in prostate cancer: the Canadian experience. Urology 2002;60: 52–6 [discussion 56].

[45] Pether M, Goldenberg SL. Intermittent androgen suppression. BJU Int 2004;93:258–61.

[46] Pether M, Goldenberg SL, Bhagirath K, et al. Intermittent androgen suppression in prostate cancer: an update of the Vancouver experience. Can J Urol 2003;10:1809–14.

[47] Grossfeld GD, Small EJ, Carroll PR. Intermittent androgen deprivation for clinically localized prostate cancer: initial experience. Urology 1998;51: 137–44.

[48] Peyromaure M, Delongchamps NB, Debre B, et al. Intermittent androgen deprivation for biologic recurrence after radical prostatectomy: long-term experience. Urology 2005;65:724–9.

[49] De La Taille A, Zerbib M, Conquy S, et al. Intermittent androgen suppression in patients with prostate cancer. BJU Int 2003;91:18–22.

[50] Prapotnich D, Fizazi K, Escudier B, et al. A 10-year clinical experience with intermittent hormonal therapy for prostate cancer. Eur Urol 2003;43:233–9 [discussion 239–40].

[51] Youssef E, Tekyi-Mensah S, Hart K, et al. Intermittent androgen deprivation for patients with recurrent/metastatic prostate cancer. Am J Clin Oncol 2003;26:e119–23.

[52] de Leval J, Boca P, Yousef E, et al. Intermittent versus continuous total androgen blockade in the treatment of patients with advanced hormone-naive prostate cancer: results of a prospective randomized multicenter trial. Clin Prostate Cancer 2002;1:163–71.

[53] The Medical Research Council Prostate Cancer Working Party Investigators Group. Immediate versus deferred treatment for advanced prostatic cancer: initial results of the Medical Research Council Trial. Br J Urol 1997;79:235–46.

[54] Bolla M, Gonzalez D, Warde P, et al. Improved survival in patients with locally advanced prostate cancer treated with radiotherapy and goserelin. N Engl J Med 1997;337:295–300.

[55] Iversen P, Johansson JE, Lodding P, et al. Bicalutamide (150 mg) versus placebo as immediate therapy alone or as adjuvant to therapy with curative intent for early nonmetastatic prostate cancer: 5.3-year median followup from the Scandinavian Prostate Cancer Group Study Number 6. J Urol 2004;172: 1871–6.

[56] Messing EM, Manola J, Sarosdy M, et al. Immediate hormonal therapy compared with observation after radical prostatectomy and pelvic lymphadenectomy in men with node-positive prostate cancer. N Engl J Med 1999;341:1781–8.

[57] Moul JW, Wu H, Sun L, et al. Early versus delayed hormonal therapy for prostate specific antigen only recurrence of prostate cancer after radical prostatectomy. J Urol 2004;171:1141–7.

[58] Miller J, Ahmann A, Drach G, et al. The clinical usefulness of serum prostate specific antigen after hormonal therapy of metastatic prostate cancer. J Urol 1992;147:956–61.

[59] Gleave ME, Goldenberg SL, Chin JL, et al. Randomized comparative study of 3 versus 8-month neoadjuvant hormonal therapy before radical prostatectomy: biochemical and pathological effects. J Urol 2001;166:500–6 [discussion 506–7].

[60] Gleave ME, Goldenberg SL, Jones EC, et al. Biochemical and pathological effects of 8 months of neoadjuvant androgen withdrawal therapy before radical prostatectomy in patients with clinically confined prostate cancer. J Urol 1996;155:213–9.

[61] July LV, Akbari M, Zellweger T, et al. Clusterin expression is significantly enhanced in prostate cancer cells following androgen withdrawal therapy. Prostate 2002;50:179–88.

[62] Paterson RF, Gleave ME, Jones EC, et al. Immunohistochemical analysis of radical prostatectomy specimens after 8 months of neoadjuvant hormonal therapy. Mol Urol 1999;3:277–86.

[63] Tsuji M, Murakami Y, Kanayama H, et al. Immunohistochemical analysis of Ki-67 antigen and Bcl-2 protein expression in prostate cancer: effect of neoadjuvant hormonal therapy. Br J Urol 1998;81: 116–21.

[64] D'Amico AV, Chen MH, Roehl KA, et al. Preoperative PSA velocity and the risk of death from prostate cancer after radical prostatectomy. N Engl J Med 2004;351:125–35.

[65] D'Amico AV, Moul JW, Carroll PR, et al. Intermediate end point for prostate cancer-specific mortality following salvage hormonal therapy for prostate-specific antigen failure. J Natl Cancer Inst 2004;96: 509–15.

[66] D'Amico AV, Moul JW, Carroll PR, et al. Surrogate end point for prostate cancer-specific mortality after radical prostatectomy or radiation therapy. J Natl Cancer Inst 2003;95:1376–83.

[67] D'Amico AV, Renshaw AA, Sussman B, et al. Pretreatment PSA velocity and risk of death from prostate cancer following external beam radiation therapy. JAMA 2005;294:440–7.

[68] Patel DA, Presti JC Jr, McNeal JE, et al. Preoperative PSA velocity is an independent prognostic factor for relapse after radical prostatectomy. J Clin Oncol 2005;23:6157–62.

[69] Arlen PM, Figg WD, Gulley J, et al. National Cancer Institute intramural approach to advanced prostate cancer. Clin Prostate Cancer 2002;1:153–62.

ELSEVIER
SAUNDERS

Urol Clin N Am 33 (2006) 181–190

**UROLOGIC
CLINICS
of North America**

Managing Complications of Androgen Deprivation Therapy for Prostate Cancer

Jeffrey M. Holzbeierlein, MD

*Department of Urology, University of Kansas Medical Center, 3901 Rainbow Blvd, Mail Stop 3016,
Kansas City, KS 66160, USA*

In 1941, Huggins and Hodges [1] became the first physicians to recognize and report that prostate cancer was androgen dependent. Their discovery resulted in a Nobel Prize. Since that time, hormonal therapy in one form or another has been used to treat prostate cancer. With the increase in the number of prostate cancer cases seen in the United States, the use of androgen deprivation therapy (ADT) as a form of treatment has continued to rise. Classically, ADT was reserved for patients who had clinically evident metastatic disease or for those who were not candidates for more definitive local therapies. With more recent data to show improved survival in patients who have limited metastatic disease and those receiving radiation for higher-stage disease, the indications for early use of ADT are expanding [2,3]. A recent report by Cooperberg and colleagues [4] documented the dramatic rise in the use of ADT from 1989 to 2001. Most dramatic was the increased use of ADT in external beam radiotherapy from 9.8% of patients to 74.6% of patients.

ADT can be accomplished in several ways. Initially, ADT was achieved through castration or by estrogen treatment. Due to the psychologic effects associated with castration and the potentially serious side effects of estrogen administration, other ways to achieve castrate states were needed. In 1985, the FDA approved the use of luteinizing hormone-releasing hormone (LHRH) analogs for the treatment of prostate cancer. Today, there are five FDA-approved LHRH agonist formulas available to treat prostate cancer: Lupron (TAP Pharmaceuticals, Lake Forest,

IL), Zoladex (Astra Zeneca Pharmaceuticals, Macclesfield, London, UK), Eligard (Atrix Laboratories, Inc., Fort Collins, CO), Viadur (Alza Corporation, Mountain View, CA), and Trelstar (Pharmacia, Peapack, NJ). With the number of patients being treated with ADT, the market for LHRH agonists has become of great interest to the pharmaceutical companies. Conservative estimates are that approximately $230 million per year are spent on LHRH agonists alone [5]. Although LHRH agonists have been the dominant form of ADT over the past decade, other nontraditional forms of chemical castration exist, such as antiandrogen monotherapy and intermittent androgen therapy. The development of these types of ADT has partly been in response to the significant side effects seen with traditional ADT. Trials to assess the efficacy of these types of treatment are ongoing. Box 1 lists the currently used forms of ADT.

With the increasing use of ADT, it is important for the urologist to recognize the potential side effects from the use of ADT and ways in which to minimize or eliminate the risks from these side effects. This article describes the potential complications of ADT and the recommendations for treatment or prevention of these complications. In addition, we examine the role of nontraditional forms of ADT and the potential benefits they offer.

Hot flashes

Hot flushes, often referred to as hot flashes, are described as a sudden intense and uncomfortable heat sensation in the face, neck, upper chest, and back. This side effect is one of the most frequent side effects of ADT, with up to 80% of the

E-mail address: jholzbeierlein@kumc.edu

Box 1. Different forms of androgen deprivation

Orchiectomy
Diethylstilbestrol
LHRH agonists
Leuprolide acetate (Lupron, Eligard)
Goserelin acetate (Zoladex)
Triptorelin pamoate (Trelstar)

LHRH antagonists
Abarelix (Planaxis)

Antiandrogens (nonsteroidal)
Flutamide (Eulexin)
Bicalutamide (Casodex)
Nilutamide (Nilandron)

Steroidal antiandrogen
Cyproterone acetate (Cyprostat)

patients describing this sensation [6–8]. Hot flashes may also be associated with nausea, flushing, or sweating, may interrupt sleep, may last for seconds or up to an hour, and may occur daily or only weekly. Triggers for hot flashes include stress, heat, sudden changes in body position, or the ingestion of hot liquids [9]. Although these attacks are not life threatening, they can be bothersome and disruptive to the patient's lifestyle. Some reports have shown that hot flashes are the most bothersome side effect of ADT, with 27% of patients in one study qualifying their hot flashes as "very distressing" [10,11]. Initially, urologists thought that with prolonged androgen deprivation hot flashes would improve or subside, but many patients continue to have hot flashes as long as they continue on ADT. It is believed that hot flashes result from the decreased feedback of testosterone to the hypothalamus, which leads to decreased endogenous peptide secretion with compensatory increased catecholamine secretion. With the thermoregulatory center for the body located in the same area, the excess catecholamines stimulate these thermal neurons, resulting in a hot flash [9,10].

Management of hot flashes

There are a number of treatments that have been used in the management of hot flashes. Many of these treatments are anecdotal and have little evidence supporting their use, and many are based on treatment strategies used for the management of hot flashes in women. Some examples of treatments include estrogen (eg, diethylstilbestrol [DES]), progestins, clonidine, phenobarbital, megestrol acetate, antidepressants, clonidine, acupuncture, soy, and vitamin E. Traditionally, one of the most commonly used medications for the treatment of hot flashes was megestrol acetate, a progestin that has been demonstrated to decrease hot flashes by up to 85% [12]. In most patients, the medication is well tolerated, but side effects can include chills (reported by 54% of patients), perceived weight gain (reported by 12% of patients), and carpal tunnel–type pain (reported by 4% of patients) [12]. Dosages are usually 20 to 40 mg/d. Dose escalation is rarely required. A case report by Sartor and colleagues [13] reported an increase in prostate-specific antigen (PSA) with the use of this medication, raising some concerns about it use; however, this is the only published report of this effect. Furthermore, this is unlikely to be a real concern because higher-dose megestrol acetate has been shown to decrease PSA [14]. The benefits of this medication include its efficacy and minimal side effects, whereas the greatest drawback of megestrol acetate is its lack of benefit on osteoporosis.

DES has been shown to be effective for the treatment of hot flashes in men on ADT [9,15]. Complete response rates of 70% and partial response rates of 20% have been reported [16]. The greatest concern about the use of DES has been its associated cardiovascular toxicity. Low doses of the medication (as low as 0.25 mg/d) that are still effective in relieving hot flashes generally avoid the cardiovascular complications associated with higher doses of estrogen (although many clinicians recommend an aspirin a day for someone on this regimen and avoid placing smokers on this regimen). Besides the cardiovascular risk, the drawbacks of using DES even at lower doses are tender gynecomastia, which causes some patients to discontinue therapy, and the difficulty in obtaining the medication. Transdermal estrogen has also been used with success at doses of 0.05 mg to 0.1 mg applied bi-weekly for 4 weeks. Overall, 83% of patients reported some improvement in their hot flashes, with major improvement seen in 67% of patients in the high-dose group and 25% in the low-dose group [15]. Side effects were limited primarily to nipple tenderness and breast enlargement. There are approximately 15 pharmacies in the United States that carry DES, although pharmacies that do compounding can produce the medication for little cost. The benefits of DES include a positive impact on osteoporosis, although it is unknown whether dosages as low as 0.25 mg/d are sufficient to prevent ADT-related osteoporosis.

One of the most popular treatments for hot flashes is antidepressants. In particular, selective serotonin reuptake inhibitors (SSRIs) have been shown to have efficacy in relieving hot flashes [17,18]. Venlafaxine hydrochloride (Effexor; Wyeth Pharmaceuticals, Collegeville, PA) and paroxetine (Paxil; Glaxo Smith Kline, Philadelphia, PA) have been shown to be effective for the treatment of hot flashes. In placebo-controlled studies of venlafaxine, the majority of patients reported a >50% decrease in hot flashes and good tolerability of the medication [17,18]. Side effects may include drowsiness, tremulousness, and dry mouth, particularly at higher doses. I typically start patients on 37.5 mg of Effexor XR, which is one of the recommended starting dosages. The drawbacks of using an SSRI are the mild side effects and the lack of effect on osteoporosis. The advantages include a generally well-tolerated, safe medication that has the additional benefit of treating depression, which is often present in patients who have cancer [17,18].

Medroxyprogesterone acetate (MPA) (Depo-Provera) was recently reported by Langenstroer and colleagues [19] to be effective in relieving hot flashes associated with ADT. In this study, patients were given 150 mg or 400 mg of intramuscular MPA for the treatment of ADT-induced hot flashes. Complete responders were defined as patients experiencing elimination of hot flashes, and partial responders were defined as patients experiencing a reduction in the number or severity of hot flashes. Up to 91% of patients in the study responded, with 48% of the patients reporting a complete response. A number of patients who stopped therapy due to resolution of hot flashes had no recurrence of their symptoms. There were no direct treatment-related side effects in this study, and there was no difference between the two dosages. Side effects that have been reported with progestin use are salt retention and exacerbation of congestive heart failure, weight gain, sexual dysfunction, and increased appetite. Advantages of this treatment for hot flashes include its relatively low side-effect profile. Drawbacks include its low availability and lack of improvement of osteoporosis; indeed, recent data concerning bone mineral density (BMD)

loss in young women using this medication for contraception has raised concerns about this treatment increasing the rate of bone loss [19].

Complementary and homeopathic treatments of the side effects of ADT are becoming increasingly popular. One such therapy is acupuncture. Hammar and colleagues [20] examined the ability of acupuncture to relieve hot flashes in men undergoing ADT. Up to 70% of patients reported decreases in hot flashes after 10 weeks of acupuncture therapy. Data on acupuncture for hot flashes in women are limited and have been somewhat controversial but generally favorable. A number of herbal preparations are available for the treatment of hot flashes, including soy, black cohosh, wild yam, dong quai, and chaste tree berry. Soy products have gained increasing interest in the treatment of hot flashes for men and women. Several commercially available products of soy have been specifically developed and marketed for this purpose. The success of soy in treating hot flashes is thought to be due to its phytoestrogenic properties. In one study conducted in women with hot flashes, soy decreased hot flashes by up to 45%, versus 30% for placebo [21]. However, a recent review of randomized controlled trials showed that only three of eight studies looking at soy for hot flashes in women have shown a benefit [22]. No randomized trials have examined the effectiveness of soy for hot flashes in men on ADT. There are other potential benefits to the use of soy in men on ADT, including possible decreases in cholesterol and PSA reduction (Jeffrey M. Holzbeierlein, MD, unpublished data, 2005). Soy beans are thought to be the best source of soy.

Vitamin E is another complementary therapy that has been postulated to be effective in reducing hot flashes, although its mechanism of action is unknown [23]. In a relatively recent placebo-controlled study on women who had hot flashes, vitamin E reduced hot flashes of up to 30% of subjects; however, 22% of subjects on placebo also experienced a decrease in symptoms [23]. Because there is some preliminary evidence to suggest a benefit of vitamin E in preventing prostate cancer, there seems to be little down side to using soy and vitamin E to relieve hot flashes.

Black cohosh has been favorably reviewed for alleviating host flashes in postmenopausal women [24]. Some recent reports demonstrate the ability of black cohosh to inhibit prostate cancer cell growth in vitro, which may be an added benefit of treating hot flashes with this preparation [25]. There have been some reports of increased liver enzymes in patients using black cohosh, but the long-term side effects remain unknown. In the authors' experience, patient acceptance of complementary therapies is generally very high, and although success may be associated with a large placebo effect, complementary therapies may be useful in some patients.

Although clonidine was initially thought to provide relief from hot flashes, a placebo-controlled randomized trial failed to demonstrate the efficacy of this medication [26]. Gabapentin has recently been touted as useful in relieving hot flashes associated with ADT, although this success has been limited to case reports [27,28]. Cyproterone acetate, a steroidal antiandrogen, which is a synthetic derivative of hydroxyprogesterone, has also been shown to be effective in reducing hot flashes by up to 80% and has been used in Europe for years, but this agent is not available in the United States [29]. Furthermore, its use has been associated with an increased cardiovascular risk, and it has no benefit for osteoporosis.

In summary, MPA, megestrol acetate, and the SSRIs are probably the best tolerated and most effective medications for the treatment of hot flashes. Although DES may be one of the most beneficial due to its positive effects on osteoporosis, concerns about its cardiovascular toxicity have tempered enthusiasm for its use. The complementary medicine approaches are favored by many patients as "natural" treatments, but the lack of well-organized, double-blind, placebo-controlled studies makes it difficult to determine their true efficacy. A summary of the treatments for hot flashes can be found in Table 1.

Osteoporosis

Osteoporosis in men on ADT remains an unrecognized and undertreated complication of androgen deprivation. This is of particular concern, considering that 33% of all hip fractures occur in men, and men have a greater mortality after hip fracture than women [30]. Stepan and colleagues [31] were the first to recognize the effects of androgen deprivation on BMD when they reported a decrease in the bone mineral content of subjects who had undergone orchiectomy for sexual delinquency. A more contemporary study examining the incidence of fracture rates in older men who underwent orchiectomy (the vast majority for prostate cancer) demonstrated a 2.5-times increased risk of fracture in the orchiectomy group [32]. The majority of fractures occurred in the hip, spine, and distal forearm, sites traditionally associated with osteoporosis. Because most patients receive their ADT through LHRH agonists, it was important to study these drugs specifically. Stoch and colleagues [33] evaluated 60 men with prostate cancer, 19 of whom received LHRH agonist therapy and 41 who did not receive ADT. Patients had their BMD measured by dual-energy x-ray absorptiometry. Bone turnover was measured using the urinary bone resorption marker N-telopeptide and the serum markers of bone formation, bone-specific alkaline phosphatase and osteocalcin. BMD values, as measured by dual-energy x-ray absorptiometry scan of multiple areas, were statistically significantly lower in the patients receiving LHRH agonists versus the untreated men with prostate

Table 1
Treatments for ADT-induced hot flashes

Agent	Dose	Reported efficacy	Side effects
Megestrol acetate	20–40 mg/d	85%	Weight gain, chills, carpal tunnel, fluid retention
SSRIs	Various	50–60%	Dry mouth, constipation, tremulousness
DES	0.25–1 mg/d	75%	Tender gynecomastia, cardiovascular toxicity
Medroxyprogesterone acetate	150 mg IM/wk	91% PR, 48% CR	Weight gain, fluid retention, CHF
Clonidine	0.1 mg/d[a]	20–30%	Rare dizziness, syncope
Soy	25–75 mg/d	10–40%	None reported
Vitamin E	400–800 IU/d	10–30%	Increased bleeding risk
Acupuncture	Weekly	Up to 70%	None reported
Gabapentin	300 mg/d	Anecdotal	Sleepiness, fatigue, dizziness
Cyproterone acetate	50 mg/d	80%	Breast tenderness, dyspnea, nausea, fatigue

Abbreviations: DES, diethylstilbestrol; SSRI, selective serotonin reuptake inhibitor.
[a] Not significantly better than placebo.

cancer. Furthermore, biochemical markers of bone turnover were significantly altered compared with untreated patients. This study confirmed that LHRH agonist use, similar to orchiectomy, results in significant BMD loss and demonstrates that the changes in the bone are not due to prostate cancer alone. A recent study demonstrated that men receiving androgen deprivation were almost 1.5 times more likely to sustain a fracture in the first year of ADT and 1.7 times more likely to require hospitalization for that fracture [34]. The authors estimate that over 3000 fractures per year can be attributed to the use of ADT. Just as alarming are recent data that showed that patients begin having effects on BMD with LHRH agonist use in as little as 9 months of therapy and as quickly as 6 months after orchiectomy [35]. It seems that the majority of the bone loss occurs within the first year and then continues at a slower pace.

The mechanism of bone loss due to androgen deprivation is not well understood. Androgen receptors have been identified on osteoblasts. However, antiandrogen monotherapy using non-steroidal antiandrogens has been shown in a cross-sectional study to have lower levels of urinary excretion of N-telopeptide and serum osteocalcin than in men treated with gonadotropin-releasing hormone agonists [36]. Therefore, the hypothesis is that, despite the blockade of androgen receptors, the presence of testosterone may be important. Androgens have been shown to mediate osteoblast proliferation and differentiation, increase bone matrix production, and increase osteocalcin secretion [37]. In addition, testosterone has been shown to stimulate growth factors such as trans-forming growth factor-β and insulin-like growth factor-1, which may be important in osteoblast proliferation [37]. The importance of the presence of testosterone may be in its peripheral conversion to estrogen. This is supported by data from Smith and colleagues [38], who reported on significant osteoporosis in a man who had normal androgen levels but had a mutation in the estrogen-receptor gene. Another study showed a significant reduction in estradiol levels in men treated with leupro-lide, further supporting the idea that estrogen is critical in the prevention of osteoporosis in men [39].

Treatment of osteoporosis

The first step in the prevention of osteoporosis associated with ADT is the recognition that it is likely to occur and instituting steps to prevent bone loss. Lifestyle modification, including smoking cessation, moderating alcohol and caffeine consumption, and regular weight-bearing exercise, are critical first steps. Seeman and colleagues [40] demonstrated that smoking and excessive alcohol consumption were independent risk factors for osteoporosis in men underscoring the need for these lifestyle modifications. Another preventive step is beginning calcium and vitamin D supplementation. A recent study demonstrated a significant vitamin D deficiency and inadequate calcium intake in men who had prostate cancer [41,42], Therefore, it is recommended that all men beginning ADT should be encouraged to maintain calcium intake at 1000 mg/d and supplemental vitamin D at 400 IU/d [41,42]. The importance of exercise in men who have ADT cannot be overemphasized. Multiple studies in men and women have shown the beneficial effect of exercise on BMD. Furthermore, a recent study showed that resistance exercise in men on ADT improved quality of life (QOL) and decreased fatigue [43].

Another option for the prevention and treatment of osteoporosis is the bisphosphonate class of medicines. These medications inhibit osteoclasts, which are involved in resorption of bone. The three main bisphosphonates are alendronate (Fosamax; Merck), pamidronate (Aredia; Novartis Pharmaceuticals), and zoledronate (Zometa; Novartis Pharmaceuticals). Of these medications, alendronate is the only oral medication. Orwoll and colleagues [42] demonstrated the effectiveness of alendronate on BMD in men who had prostate cancer and osteoporosis. In this study, a mean increase in BMD of the lumbar spine and femoral neck were observed. Many of the men in this study had normal or near-normal serum testosterone concentrations; therefore, the efficacy of this drug in hypogonadal men is unknown. Alendronate has recently become the first drug approved by the FDA for the treatment of male osteoporosis. The drawback of using an oral bisphosphonate is that it requires the medication to be taken on an empty stomach with the patient sitting in an upright position for at least 30 minutes. This is because foods and other medications can alter its absorption, and laying down increases the risk of erosive esophagitis. Pamidronate and zoledronate are intravenously administered medicines. Pamidronate at doses of 60 mg intravenously every 12 weeks has been shown to prevent BMD loss in patients on LHRH agonist therapy, although it is not FDA approved for this indication [44]. Furthermore, it has not been shown to prevent or reduce the number of skeletal-related events in men who have metastatic prostate cancer. Zoledronate, the most potent of the three bisphosphonates, has 100 to 850 times the potency of pamidronate in animal studies. It has been shown to decrease fracture rates in men who have hormone refractory prostate cancer and bone metastases [45]. Recently, a randomized, controlled trial using zoledronate to prevent bone loss in men who had prostate cancer but no metastases on LHRH agonist therapy reported favorable results. Zoledronate has received FDA approval for this indication [46]. In the men receiving zoledronate, an increase in BMD of 5.6% in the lumbar spine was seen versus a decrease of 2.2% in those on placebo. Mean BMD was also increased in the femoral neck and hip in the zoledronic acid group. Important in the use of any of the bisphosphonates is the concomitant administration of vitamin D (400 IU/d) and calcium (1200–1500 mg/d). Without adequate levels of vitamin D and calcium, the bisphosphonates are ineffective. The most common side effects of the bisphosphonates include fever, anemia, nausea, constipation, esophagitis, and hypophosphatemia [47,48]. The gastrointestinal side effects of the oral bisphosphonates can be severe; there have been reports of epigastric pain, severe esophagitis, and gastroesophageal ulceration [49]. The intravenous formulations are more associated with flu-like symptoms and reactions at the injection site. Detrimental effects on renal function with the use of zoledronate have been a concern but seem to be confined to the 8-mg dose, shorter infusion times, and smaller infusion volumes [46]. A more recently reported potential adverse effect of zoledronic acid is osteonecrosis of the jaw [50]. A review of the studies on bisphosphonates can be found in Table 2. There are several new bisphosphonates on the market that may be valuable in preventing ADT-induced osteoporosis, and clinical trials are underway evaluating a monoclonal antibody directed against osteoclasts for the prevention of osteoporosis.

Body mass and lipid changes

Along with the changes in BMD are changes in the patient's body mass and composition. Most men on ADT have an increase in their weight secondary to increased body fat [51]. Higano and colleagues [52] examined combined androgen blockade and its effect on weight. In this study, the median increase in weight was 6 kg. A similar study by Smith and colleagues [53] examined the effect of using LHRH agonists alone and found a median increase of 2.3 kg in patients' weight. In addition, from intermittent ADT studies it seems that the weight gained from ADT is not easily lost even after discontinuation of therapy [52]. Higano and colleagues [52] performed a study looking at fat distribution, body mass, and muscle mass in men after 48 weeks on ADT. In 32 out of 40 men, weight increased by 2.4%, fat body mass increased by 9.4%, and lean body mass decreased by 2.7%. Also documented in this study were an increase in cholesterol by 9% and an increase in triglycerides by 26.5%. The cause of these changes is thought to be due to changes in insulin levels associated with ADT, although an increase in sedentary activity secondary to fatigue is a common complaint of patients. A list of the metabolic changes associated with ADT is presented in Box 2. These changes may have significant implications for cardiovascular health in patients on ADT. An exercise regimen is critical in these patients because exercise has been shown to help improve fatigue and overall QOL and is helpful in managing weight gain and decreasing insulin resistance [43]. Recent data implicating a lower rate of prostate cancer in men taking statin drugs may support the aggressive use of statins in managing the increase in cholesterol seen with ADT [54].

Anemia

Fatigue is a relatively common complaint of patients on ADT, which may have its basis in anemia in some patients. The anemia seen in

Table 2
Bisphosphonate studies

Author	Drug/dose	No. of patients	Endpoints
Orwoll et al. [42]	Alendronate 10 mg po	241 men with osteoporosis	Increased BMD
Smith et al. [44]	Pamidronate 60 mg IV	47 men on ADT	BMD no change from baseline
Smith et al. [46]	Zoledronate 4 mg IV	106 men on ADT, no mets	Increased BMD

> **Box 2. Metabolic changes seen with androgen deprivation therapy**
>
> Decreased hemoglobin
> Increased uric acid
> Increased BUN
> Increased total cholesterol
> Increased fasting blood sugar
> Increased weight
> Increased inorganic phosphorus
> Increased calcium

patients on ADT is usually a normocytic, normochromic anemia thought to be due to the lack of testosterone and 5-beta dihydrotestosterone stimulation of erythroid precursors and a decrease in erythropoietin production [55]. Strum and colleagues [55] examined the incidence and severity of anemia in patients on complete androgen blockade. They found that up to 90% of patients experienced at least a 10% drop in their hemoglobin, and 13% had a decrease in their hemoglobin of 25% or more. A decrease in the hemoglobin was noted as quickly as 1 month after the initiation of ADT, although the nadir hemoglobin was not reached until 5.6 months after starting ADT. Symptoms directly related to anemia occurred in 13% of patients. Anemia was worse in patients on complete androgen blockade rather than LHRH agonist therapy alone, and when an antiandrogen was added to a patient on LHRH agonist therapy, a further drop in their hemoglobin was seen. The authors found that the anemia was typically easily corrected with the subcutaneous administration of recombinant human erythropoietin. Previous reports suggested that the anemia seen with ADT reversed fairly rapidly with discontinuation of therapy; however, a more recent report showed that resolution of anemia in patients receiving long-term ADT often took > 1 year [55]. Antiandrogen monotherapy also seems to be associated with anemia, although the mechanism of this effect is not clear [55]. Some clinicians have recommended following hemoglobin levels every 2 to 3 months in patients on ADT and more closely if patients are symptomatic.

Sexual dysfunction

A decrease in libido often followed by a decrease in sexual function is a well-recognized side effect of ADT. Because testosterone plays

a significant role in the maintenance of libido and sexual function, these are common changes with ADT that usually occur within the first year of therapy and often within several months of the initiation of ADT. The lack of testosterone may have a direct effect on the cavernosal nerves involved in erections [56]. Baba and colleagues [56] performed a study of orchidectomized rats and demonstrated a decrease in the number of NAPDH diaphorase-stained fibers in the rat corpus cavernosum and dorsal nerve as compared with control animals. This suggests that testosterone has peripheral effects, in addition to central effects, that are important in erectile function. Most standard treatments for erectile dysfunction, such as oral agents, vacuum erection devices, intracorporal injection therapy, or placement of a penile prosthesis, are good options. Other forms of ADT, specifically antiandrogen monotherapy and intermittent androgen deprivation, have also been shown to be associated with significantly improved sexual function.

Cognitive dysfunction

Recent research has examined the effect of ADT on memory and cognitive function [57]. In a study by Salminen and colleagues [58], the decline in testosterone in patients on ADT was associated with a decline in visuomotor skills and reaction times and impaired recognition of letters. Delayed recall of objects was improved. In another study of hypogonadal male geriatric patients not known to have prostate cancer, testosterone replacement improved spatial ability, verbal memory, and fluency [59]. These findings have significant implications for the effects of ADT on cognitive function. Although no specific treatment for this decline in cognitive dysfunction has been recommended, it has been suggested that the fall in estradiol levels associated with the decline in testosterone is responsible for many of the cognitive changes; therefore, estrogen replacement may be beneficial [60].

Intermittent androgen ablation

The use of intermittent rather than continuous androgen deprivation remains a controversial topic within urology. It is unknown whether this provides the same, better, or worse survival as continuous androgen deprivation. Several studies in prostate cancer cell lines and in mouse models suggest that intermittent androgen ablation delays the time to the development of hormone refractory disease; however, this has not been substantiated in humans [61,62]. QOL is improved on intermittent androgen ablation as opposed to continuous therapy [63]. Many of the side effects of androgen deprivation can be avoided or reversed with the "holiday" periods of intermittent therapy. For example, patients report improved sexual function, fewer hot flashes, and an improved sense of well-being [63]. Furthermore, bone loss associated with ADT seems to slow or stop during the off-treatment periods [64]. A trial by the Southwest Oncology Group seeking to determine if intermittent androgen deprivation has equivalent survival rates in men with metastatic prostate cancer is underway. If this trial demonstrates noninferiority, then patients who have metastatic prostate cancer may have significant improvements in their QOL on intermittent androgen deprivation without compromising efficacy.

Antiandrogen monotherapy

Another nontraditional option for androgen deprivation is the use of antiandrogen monotherapy. Typically, bicalutamide (Casodex; Astra-Zeneca) at 150 mg/d, flutamide (Eulexin; Scherring-Plough) at 250 mg three times a day, or nilutamide (Nilandron; Aventis) 100 mg three times a day are the recommended medications and dosages for this therapy. For metastatic disease, this therapy has been shown to be inferior to castration or LHRH agonist therapy [65]. However, in the PSA-only setting without evidence of metastatic disease, no difference in survival has been seen [66]. In terms of QOL, because testosterone is preserved, patients report statistically significant improvements in sexual interest and physical capacity [66]. Furthermore, the use of antiandrogen monotherapy largely avoids hot flashes and osteoporosis, although anemia remains a side effect. Despite these advantages, antiandrogen monotherapy has not been approved by the FDA for this use and has not gained widespread acceptance, perhaps in part due to the significant costs to the patient.

Summary

Although androgen deprivation, or hormonal therapy, is not chemotherapy in the traditional sense, the side effects of ADT should not be underestimated. Some side effects, such as

osteoporosis and anemia, can be severe and can cause significant medical problems and therefore require more aggressive intervention, whereas others, although not life threatening, have a significant impact on QOL. As evidence mounts for a survival benefit for prostate cancer patients with early ADT, there will be an increased need to recognize, prevent, and treat the side effects of ADT. Some modifications, such as exercise, diet, and vitamin supplementation, are simple and may have great benefit. The incidence and scope of the side effects of ADT, such as the effects on cognitive function, are not completely understood, but an increasing number of studies seem to be focusing on these issues. With intermittent androgen ablation or antiandrogen monotherapy, many of these side effects may be reversible or preventable. Proper counseling of patients beginning ADT is necessary in helping patients recognize and report side effects of their treatment.

References

[1] Huggins C, Hodges C. Studies on prostate cancer. I. The effect of castration, of estrogen and of androgen injection on serum phosphatases in metastatic carcinoma of the prostate. Cancer Res 1941;1:293–7.
[2] Messing EM, Manola J, Sarosdy M, et al. Immediate hormonal therapy compared with observation after radical prostatectomy and pelvic lymphadenectomy in men with node-positive prostate cancer. N Engl J Med 1999;341:1781–8.
[3] Bolla M, Gonzalez D, Warde P, et al. Improved survival in patients with locally advanced prostate cancer treated with radiotherapy and goserelin. N Engl J Med 1997;337:295–300.
[4] Cooperberg MR, Gorssfeld GD, Lubeck DP, et al. national practice patterns and time trends in androgen ablation for localized prostate cancer. J Natl Cancer Inst 2003;95:981–9.
[5] Bonzani RA, Stricker HJ, Peabody JO, et al. Cost comparison of orchiectomy and leuprolide in metastatic prostate cancer. J Urol 1998;160:2446–9.
[6] Schow DA, Renfer LG, Rozenski TA, et al. Prevalence of hot flashes during and after neoadjuvant hormonal therapy for localized prostate cancer. South Med J 1998;91:855–7.
[7] Charig CR. Flushing: long term side effect of orchiectomy in treatment of prostatic carcinoma. Urology 1989;33:175–8.
[8] Karling P, Hammar M, Varenhorst E. Prevalence and duration of hot flashes after surgical or medical castration in men with prostatic carcinoma. J Urol 1994;152:1170–3.
[9] Smith JA. Management of hot flushes due to endocrine therapy for prostate carcinoma. Oncology 1996;10:1319–22.

[10] Smith JA. A prospective comparison of treatments for symptomatic hot flashes following endocrine treatment for carcinoma of the prostate. J Urol 1994;152:132–4.

[11] Frodin T, Aluval G, Varenhorst E. Measurement of skin blood-flow and water evaporation as a means of objectively assessing hot flashes after orchidectomy in patients with prostatic cancer. Prostate 1985;7: 203–8.

[12] Loprinzi CL, Michalak JL, Quella SK, et al. Megestrol acetate for the prevention of hot flashes. N Engl J Med 1994;331:347–52.

[13] Sartor O, Eastham JA. Progressive prostate cancer associated with the use of megestrol acetate administered for control of hot flashes. South Med J 1998; 92:415–6.

[14] Dawson NA, Conaway M, Halabi S, et al. A randomized study comparing standard versus moderately high dose megestrol acetate for patients with advanced prostate carcinoma: cancer and leukemia group B study 9181. Cancer 2000;88:825–34.

[15] Gerber GS, Zagaja GP, Ray PS, et al. Transdermal estrogen in the treatment of hot flashes in men with prostate cancer. Urol 2000;55:97–101.

[16] Miller JI, Ahmann FR. Treatment of castration induced menopausal symptoms with low dose diethylstilbestrol in men with advanced prostate cancer. Urology 1992;40:499–502.

[17] Loprinzi CL, Pisansky TM, Fonseca R, et al. Pilot evaluation of venlaflaxine hydrochloride for the therapy of hot flashes in cancer survivor. J Clin Oncol 1998;16:2377–81.

[18] Quella SK, Loprinzi CL, Sloan J, et al. Pilot evaluation of venlafaxine for the treatment of hot flashes in men undergoing androgen ablation therapy for prostate cancer. J Urol 1999;162:98–102.

[19] Langenstroer P, Karmer B, Cutting B, et al. Parenteral medroxyprogesterone for the management of lutenizing hormone releasing hormone induced hot flashes in men with advanced prostate cancer. J Urol 2005;174:642–5.

[20] Hammar M, Grisk J, Grimes O, et al. Accupuncture treatment of vasomotor symptom sin men with prostatic carcinoma: a pilot study. J Urol 1999;161:853–6.

[21] Albertazzi P, Parsini F, Bonaccorsi G, et al. The effect of dietary soy supplementation on hot flashes. Obstet Gynecol 1998;91:6–11.

[22] Kronenberg F, Fugh-Berman A. Complementary and alternative medicine for menopausal symptoms: a review of randomized, controlled trials. Ann Intern Med 2002;137:805.

[23] Barton DL, Loprinzi CL, Quella SK, et al. Prospective evaluation of vitamin E for hot flashes in breast cancer survivors. J Clin Oncol 1998;16:495–500.

[24] Fugate SE, Church CO. Nonestrogen treatment modalities for vasomotor symptoms associated with menopause. Ann Pharmacother 2004;38:1482–99.

[25] Jarry H, Thelen P, Chirstoffel V, et al. Cimicifuga racemosa extract BNO 1055 inhibits proliferation of the human prostate cancer cell line LNCaP. Phytomedicine 2005;12:178–82.

[26] Parra RO, Gregory JL. Treatment of post-orchiectomy hot flashes with trasndermal administration of clonidine. J Urol 1990;142:753–4.

[27] Stearns V. Management of hot flashes in breast cancer survivors and men with prostate cancer. Curr Oncol Rep 2004;6:285–90.

[28] Jeffery SM, Pepe JJ, Pupovich LM, et al. Gabapentin for hot flashes in prostate cancer. Ann Pharmacother 2002;36:433–6.

[29] Cervenakov I, Kopecny M, Jancar M, et al. "Hot flush", an unpleasant symptom accompanying antiandrogen therapy of prostatic cancer and its treatment by cyproterone acetate. Int Urol Nephrol 2000;32:72–9.

[30] Morote J, Martinez E, Trilla E, et al. Influence of the type and length of continuous androgen suppression in the development of osteoporosis in patients with prostate cancer [abstract]. J Urol 2003;169(Suppl):931.

[31] Stepan JJ, Lachman M, Zvioina J, et al. Castrated men exhibit bone loss effect of calcitonin treatment on biochemical indices of bone remodeling. J Clin Endocrin Metab 1989;69:523–7.

[32] Melton JL, Alothman KI, Khosla S, et al. Fracture risk following bilateral orchiectomy. J Urol 2003; 169:1747–50.

[33] Stoch SA, Parker RA, Chen L, et al. Bone loss in men with prostate cancer treated with gonadotropin releasing hormone agonists. J Clin Endocrinol Metab 2001;86:27–37.

[34] Shahinian VB, Kuo YF, Freeman JL, et al. Risk of fracture after androgen deprivation for prostate cancer. N Engl J Med 2005;352:152–64.

[35] Agarwal MM, Khandelwal N, Mandal AK, et al. Factors affecting bone mineral density in patients with prostate carcinoma before and after orchidectomy. Cancer 2005;103:2042–52.

[36] Smith MR, Fallon MA, Goode MJ. Cross sectional study of bone turnover during bicalutamide monotherapy for prostate cancer. Urology 2003;61: 127–31.

[37] Wiren K, Orwoll E. Androgens and bone: basic aspects. In: Orwoll E, editor. Osteoporosis in men. San Diego (CA): Academic Press; 1989. p. 211–74.

[38] Smith EB, Boyd J, Frank GR, et al. Estrogen resistance caused by a mutation in the estrogen receptor gene in a man. N Engl J Med 1994;331:1056–61.

[39] Smith MR, McGovern FJ, Fallon MA, et al. Low bone mineral density in hormone naive men with prostate carcinoma. Cancer 2001;91:2238–45.

[40] Seeman E, Melton LJ, O'Fallon WM, et al. Risk factors for spinal osteoporosis in men. Am J Med 1983; 75:977–83.

[41] Bilezikian JP. Osteoporosis in men. J Clin Edocrinol Metab 1999;84:3431–4.

[42] Orwoll E, Ettinger M, Weiss S, et al. Aledronate for the treatment of osteoporosis in men. N Engl J Med 2000;343:604–10.

[43] Segal RJ, Reid RD, Courneya KS, et al. Resistance exercise in men receiving androgen deprivation therapy for prostate cancer. J Clin Oncol 2003;21:1653–9.

[44] Smith MR, McGovern FJ, Zietman AL, et al. Pamidronate to prevent bone loss during androgen deprivation therapy for prostate cancer. N Engl J Med 2001;345:948–55.

[45] Lipton A, Small E, Saad F, et al. The new bisphosphonate Zometa (zolendronic acid) decreases skeletal complications in both osteolytic and osteoblastic lesions: a comparison to pamidronate. Cancer Invest 2002;20(Suppl 2):45–54.

[46] Smith MR, Eastham JA, Gleason DM, et al. Randomized controlled trial of zolendronic acid to prevent bone loss in men receiving androgen deprivation therapy for nonmetastatic prostate cancer. J Urol 2003;169:2008–12.

[47] Major PP, Lipton A, Berenson J, et al. Oral bisphosphonates: a review of clinical use in patients with bone metastases. Cancer 2000;61:6–14.

[48] Cheer SM, Noble S. Zoledronic acid. Drugs 2001;61: 799–805.

[49] Body JJ. Dosing regimens and main adverse events of bisphosphonates. Semin Oncol 2001;4(Suppl 1):49–53.

[50] Vannucchi AM, Ficarra G, Antonioli E, et al. Osteonecrosis of the jaw associated with zoledronate therapy in a patient with multiple myeloma. Br J Haematol 2005;128:738.

[51] Tayek JA, Herber D, Byerly LO, et al. Nutritional and metabolic effects of gonadotropin releasing hormone agonist treatment for prostate cancer. Metabolism 1990;39:1314–9.

[52] Higano CS, Ellis W, Russell K, et al. Intermittent androgen suppression with leuprolide and flutamide for prostate cancer: a pilot study. Urology 1996;48: 800–4.

[53] Smith MR, Finklestein JS, McGovern FJ, et al. Changes in body composition during androgen deprivation therapy for prostate cancer. J Clin Endocinol Metab 2002;87:599–602.

[54] Shannon J, Tewoderos S, Garzotto M, et al. Statins and prostate cancer risk: a case controlled study. Am J Epidemiol 2005;162:318–25.

[55] Strum SB, McDermed JE, Scholz MC, et al. Anaemia associated with androgen deprivation in patients with prostate cancer receiving combined hormone blockade. Br J Urol 1997;79:933–41.

[56] Baba K, Yajima M, Carrier S, et al. effect of testosterone on the number of NADPH diaphorase stained fibers in the rat corpus cavernosum and dorsal nerve. Urology 2000;56:533–8.

[57] Green HJ, Pakenham KI, Headley BC, et al. Altered cognitive function in men treated for prostate cancer with luteinizing hormone releasing hormone analogues and cyproterone acetate: a randomized controlled trial. Br J Urol 2002;90:427–32.

[58] Salminen EK, Portin RI, Koskinen A, et al. Associations between serum testosterone fall and cognitive function in prostate cancer patients. Clin Cancer Res 2004;10:7575–82.

[59] Tan RS. Andropause and testosterone supplementation for cognitive loss. J Androl 2002;23:45–6.

[60] Salminen EK, Portin RI, Koskinen AI, et al. Estradiol and cognition during androgen deprivation in men with prostate carcinoma. Cancer 2005;103: 1381–7.

[61] Akakura K, Bruchosvsky N, Goldberg SL, et al. Effects of intermittent androgen suppression on androgen-dependent tumors: apoptosis and serum prostate-specific antigen. Cancer 1993;71:2782–90.

[62] Sato N, Gleave ME, Bruchosvsky N, et al. Intermittent androgen suppression delays progression to androgen independent regulation of prostate specific antigen gene in the LNCaP prostate tumor model. J Steroid Biochem Mol Biol 1996;58:139–46.

[63] Grossfeld GD, Small EJ, Lubeck DP, et al. Androgen deprivation therapy for patients with clinically localized (stages T1 to T3) prostate cancer and for patients with biochemical recurrence after radical prostatectomy. Urology 2001;58:56–64.

[64] Jiang PY, Higano S. the dynamics of bone mineral density during intermittent androgen suppression in prostate cancer patients without bone metastases. Proc Am Soc Clin Oncol 2002; [abstract 789a].

[65] Tyrrell CJ, Kaisary AV, Iversen P, et al. A randomized comparison of 'Casodex'(bicalutamide) 150mg monotherapy versus castration in the treatment of metastatic and locally advanced prostate cancer. Eur Urol 1998;33:447–56.

[66] Iversen P, Tyrrell CJ, Kaiary AV, et al. Bicalutamide monotherapy compared with castration in patients with non-metastatic locally advanced prostate cancer: 6.3 years of follow-up. J Urol 2000;164: 1979–82.

ELSEVIER
SAUNDERS

Urol Clin N Am 33 (2006) 191–199

UROLOGIC
CLINICS
of North America

The Role of Bisphosphonates in Preventing Skeletal Complications of Hormonal Therapy

Scott M. Gilbert, MD[a], James M. McKiernan, MD[b],*

[a]*Department of Urology, University of Michigan, 3875 Taubman Center,
1500 East Medical Center Drive, Ann Arbor, MI 49109, USA*
[b]*Department of Urology, Columbia University College of Physicians & Surgeons,
161 Fort Washington Avenue, New York, NY 10032, USA*

Prostate cancer is the most common solid-organ malignancy diagnosed in men and is the second leading cause of cancer death in the United States. In 2005, an estimated 232,090 incident cases were diagnosed, and greater than 30,000 men died from prostate cancer [1]. The prevalence is approximately 1.6 million cases, and the estimated life-time risk of developing prostate cancer is 16% for the average American man [2]. Advanced cases of prostate cancer are associated with bone metastases in 65% to 75% of cases, and approximately 80% to 90% of men who die of prostate cancer develop bony metastases during the course of their disease [3]. Bony disease places the patient at risk for skeletal morbidity, including pathologic fracture. Furthermore, androgen deprivation therapy (ADT), a common therapy used in managing advanced and metastatic prostate cancer, can hasten bone mineral density (BMD) loss in this population of men. Exposure to ADT is not limited to patients who have advanced disease. Increasing numbers of patients who have localized prostate cancer and those who have rising prostate-specific antigen levels after radical prostatectomy are being managed with adjuvant ADT, even though no survival benefit has been demonstrated [4,5]. Recent data suggest that treatment of prostate cancer with ADT is associated with a significant risk of osteoporosis.

ADT-associated osteoporosis

It is estimated that 2 million men are affected by osteoporosis in the United States [6]. Although men experience a gradual age-related loss of BMD of 7% to 12% per decade beginning at age 30, primary male osteoporosis is not common [7]. Most men who have clinically significant osteoporosis are older than 70 years of age and have risk factors that contribute to decreased bone mineralization, such as hypogonadism, thyroid and parathyroid disorders, glucocorticoid excess, alcoholism, osteomalacia, and malignancy [8].

The relationship between decreased BMD and ADT is well established [9,10]. Androgen suppression reduces BMD approximately 3% to 7% per year [11]. Recent reports have demonstrated that men who have prostate cancer receiving ADT have BMD measurements from 6.5% to 17.3% lower than BMD measurements of men not treated with ADT [12]. One study reported that spinal and femoral BMD were 1.7% and 5.2% less after 2 years and 14% and 28% less after 10 years of ADT, respectively, compared with age-matched control subjects [13].

Although treatment with ADT is linked to decreased BMD, there is evidence that men who have hormone-naive prostate cancer have higher-than-expected rates of osteoporosis. Several studies have reported osteopenia and osteoporosis in men who have prostate cancer before initiation of ADT. Wei and colleagues [14] found that five of eight patients (63%) who had hormone-naive prostate cancer had osteopenia or osteoporosis. In a larger study, Smith and colleagues [15]

* Corresponding author.

E-mail address: jmm23@columbia.edu
(J.M. McKiernan).

identified 14 of 41 (34%) prostate cancer patients without exposure to ADT who had dual-energy x-ray absorptiometry (DEXA) criteria for osteopenia or osteoporosis. Using quantitative CT scan, which is a more sensitive test, 39 of 41 (95%) of these men met criteria for significant loss in BMD. Conde and colleagues [16] reported a high prevalence of osteopenia and osteoporosis in 34 men who had nonmetastatic, hormone-naive prostate cancer. Twenty-five (73.5%) men were diagnosed with osteopenia (55.9%) or osteoporosis (17.6%) at baseline using DEXA. Advanced age, lower body mass index, and elevated prostate-specific antigen levels correlated significantly with decreased BMD.

BMD is the most important predictor of osteoporotic fractures in healthy men and women [17–19]. Although the relationship between decreased ADT-associated BMD and risk of osteoporotic fracture in men who have prostate cancer has not been addressed in a prospective clinical trial, several retrospective studies and a recent population-based analysis support a close relationship. Townsend and colleagues [20] studied 224 men receiving luteinizing hormone-releasing agonist for prostate cancer retrospectively and reported an overall fracture rate of 9% and a 5% incidence of osteoporotic fractures. These rates are more than three times the incidence of fractures expected in normal men of similar age. Two retrospective studies have examined fracture rates in men who have prostate cancer treated with surgical castration and reported a marked increase in the cumulative fracture rate in men undergoing orchiectomy [21,22].

Other studies have noted a relationship between increased risk of fracture and ADT. One study reported a 6% fracture rate in men treated with ADT for >6 months [23]. Another study of 181 men who had prostate cancer reported that those treated with ADT were at a fivefold increased risk for skeletal fractures compared with reported rates in age-matched control subjects. The 5- and 10-year fracture rates were 13% and 33%, respectively. Duration of androgen ablation, race, and body mass index <25 kg/m^2 were significantly associated with risk of fracture [24]. In a retrospective analysis of 87 men who had prostate cancer treated with ADT, Diamond and colleagues [25] reported that 44% of patients were found to have radiographic evidence of spinal fracture, of which 13% were symptomatic and clinically significant. An additional study found that 35% of men initiating ADT for

prostate cancer sustained a fracture over a 7-year period [26].

A recent analysis of the National Cancer Institute sponsored Surveillance, Epidemiology and End Results program found a significant difference in fracture rate between men who had prostate cancer receiving and not receiving ADT [27]. The study reported a 19.4% fracture rate in men who had prostate cancer treated with ADT compared with a 12.6% rate in prostate cancer patients not receiving ADT ($P < .001$). The risk of fracture increased with number of doses of gonadotropin-releasing hormone agonist administered during the first year after diagnosis, and ADT was an independent predictor of fracture in multivariate analysis (Fig. 1).

Fractures are associated with substantial morbidity and mortality, particularly in men. Men who experience hip fractures suffer greater impairment and have a higher rate of fracture-related mortality than women [28]. In addition, men have a greater probability of being undertreated after a fracture [29]. Approximately 20% to 30% of hip fractures occur in men, and 50% to 60% of men die within 1 year of the fracture [30,31]. Atraumatic hip fractures in men are associated with a 32% excess mortality in the year after the fracture [32], and the estimated 5-year mortality rate after hip or spine fracture is 20% greater

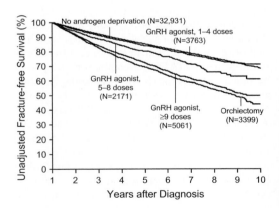

Fig. 1. Unadjusted fracture-free survival among patients who have prostate cancer, according to ADT. The survival curves start at 12 months after diagnosis, and androgen deprivation was initiated within 6 months of diagnosis. The number of doses is the number administered within 12 months of diagnosis. GnRH, gonadotropin-releasing hormone. *From* Shahinian VB, Kuo YF, Freeman JL, et al. Risk of fracture after androgen deprivation for prostate cancer. N Engl J Med 2005; 352:159; with permission.

than expected [30]. The detrimental association between fracture and mortality extends to men who have prostate cancer. Oefelein and colleagues [33] identified a negative association between skeletal fracture and overall survival in 195 prostate cancer patients treated with chronic ADT.

Preventative treatment

Patients at risk for osteoporosis should be counseled on adequate daily calcium and vitamin D supplementation to minimize bone demineralization. Although these measures reduce bone loss and decrease fracture risk in elderly men and women [34], the benefit may be reduced in men treated with ADT. In two randomized clinical trials, calcium (500 mg) and vitamin D (400 IU) supplementation did not prevent significant decreases in BMD in control subjects beginning ADT [35,36]. Weight-bearing exercise is known to increase BMD in healthy older men and women [37] and should be recommended in prostate cancer patients initiating ADT. Estrogen therapy has been studied in men undergoing ADT, and although BMD is maintained with estrogen therapy, cardiovascular and thromboembolic complications are a concern [38]. Recent studies report reduced risk using low-dose estrogen therapy. Some studies suggest that low doses of estrogen can reduce rapid bone turnover and resorption [39] and improve BMD [40]. Ockrim and colleagues [40] used transdermal estradiol therapy in 20 prostate cancer patients in conjunction with ADT and reported effective testosterone suppression and tumor response without significant cardiovascular toxicity. The authors also reported diminished andropause symptoms, improved quality of life, and increased BMD. Calcitonin has also been evaluated in ADT-associated osteoporosis, but results have been disappointing thus far [41].

Bisphosphonates are pyrophosphate analogs that decrease bone resorption, primarily through direct inhibition of osteoclast activity and proliferation. Proposed mechanisms of action include inhibition of osteoclastogenesis and induction of osteoclast apoptosis [42]. The efficacy of oral bisphosphate therapy for primary male osteoporosis has been established with several randomized clinical trials. Orwoll and colleagues [43] investigated the efficacy of oral alendronate in men who had primary osteoporosis. Alendronate (10 mg/d) administered with vitamin D and calcium resulted in significant increases in BMD at the lumbar spine, femoral neck, trochanter, hip, and total body

compared with patients treated with vitamin D, calcium, and placebo. Vertebral fractures were also significantly reduced; 1% of patients in the alendronate group suffered a vertebral fracture compared with 7% in the placebo group. Gonnelli and colleagues [44] reported similar results and showed that bisphosphonate therapy continued to increase BMD each year with therapy. Alendronate is FDA approved for treatment of primary male osteoporosis, and risedronate is approved for use in men who have glucocorticoid-induced osteoporosis.

Bisphosphonate therapy in advanced and metastatic prostate cancer

The efficacy of bisphosphonate therapy in preventing androgen deprivation-associated osteoporosis in men who have advanced, nonmetastatic prostate cancer has been examined in four clinical trials involving three agents (Table 1). Smith and colleagues [35] studied the effect of intravenous pamidronate in men who had locally advanced, lymph node–positive, or recurrent prostate cancer. Study participants were without evidence of bone metastases and had not received ADT before study enrollment. The treatment group received pamidronate, vitamin D, and calcium concomitantly with leuprolide androgen deprivation. A placebo was substituted for pamidronate in the control group. BMD was maintained at the lumbar spine, trochanter, femoral neck, and total hip sites at 24 and 48 weeks in the pamidronate group. The control group experienced BMD losses at all sites except for the femoral neck. In men treated with leuprolide alone, the mean BMD decreased by 3.3% in the lumbar spine, 2.1% in the trochanter, and 1.8% in the total hip at 48 weeks. Additionally, quantitative CT scan assessment of the lumbar spine revealed an 8.5% loss of trabecular bone at 48 weeks in the control group. Trabecular bone in the lumbar spine did not change significantly in the pamidronate group throughout the study period (2.0% decrease from baseline, $P = .32$). The absolute difference in change in trabecular BMD was 6.5% between the two groups ($P = .02$) (Fig. 2). Biochemical markers of bone metabolism were also assessed and showed increased levels in patients not receiving pamidronate.

More recently, Smith and colleagues [36] reported the results of a multicenter prospective clinical trial designed to assess that effect of the bisphosphate zoledronic acid on BMD in 106

Table 1
Summary of clinical trials evaluating the efficiency of bisphosphonates in men who have prostate cancer treated with ADT

Study	Patients	Bisphosphonate therapy	ADT	BMD	Biochemical markers	Fracture[a]	Toxicity
Smith et al. [35]	47 men Advance or recurrent CaP No metastases	Pamidronate 60 mg IV q12 wk 48-wk duration	GnRH agonist Leuprolide	Treatment group No significant change Control group ↓ 3.3% lumbar spine ↓ 1.8% total hip	Control group ↑ DPD and NTP relative to treatment group	Not assessed	Treatment group 5 (24%) serious 3 (14%) acute-phase reaction Control group 3 (14%) serious
Smith et al. [36]	106 men Advanced CaP No metastases	Zoledronic acid 4 mg iv q3 mo 1-yr duration	GnRH agonist ± antiandrogen or orchiectomy	Treatment group ↑ 5.6% lumbar spine ↑ 1.1% total hip Control group ↓ 2.2% lumbar spine ↓ 2.8% total hip	Not measured	Treatment group 5 fractures Control group 3 fractures	Treatment group 24% severe 2 withdrawals Control group 39% severe 3 withdrawals
Morabito et al. [47]	48 men Advanced CaP No metastases T score <−2.5 SD	Neridronate 25 mg im q1 mo 1-yr duration	GnRH agonist triptoreline	Treatment group No significant change	Treatment group No change	Not assessed	Treatment group Transient acute-phase reaction in 3/24 (12.5%) patients after first dose
Magno et al. [48]	60 men Advanced CaP No metastases T score <−2.5 SD	Neridronate 25 mg im q1 mo 1-yr duration	Triptoreline and bicalutamide (50 mg) Bicalutamide (150 mg)	Control group ↓ 4.9% lumbar spine ↓ 1.9% total hip Treatment groups ↑ 2.5% at lumbar spine and ↑ 1.6% at total hip w/AA Control groups ↓ 4.9% at lumbar spine w/MAB	Control group 72.8% ↑ DPD 26.6% ↑ BALP Treatment groups ↓ DPD w/AA No change w/MAB Control groups ↑ DPD w/MAB No change w/AA	Not assessed	Treatment group Transient acute-phase reaction in 3/30 (10%) patients after first dose

Abbreviations: AA, antiandrogen therapy; BALP, bone alkaline phosphatase; CaP, prostate cancer; DPD, deoxypyridinoline; MAB, maximum androgen blockade; NTP, N-telopeptide; Rx bisphosphonate treatment.
[a] Trial was not designed to assess fractures. Fractures were nonclinical, asymptomatic and defined as new-incident cases or worsening of preexisting vertebral fractures.

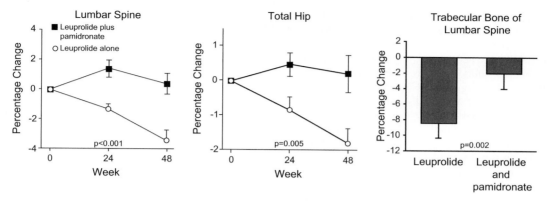

Fig. 2. Mean changes from baseline in BMD in men who have prostate cancer treated with leuprolide alone or leuprolide and pamidronate at the lumbar spine, total hip, and trabecular bone of lumbar spine. *Adapted from* Smith MR, McGovern FJ, Zietman AL, et al. Pamidronate to prevent bone loss during androgen-deprivation therapy for prostate cancer. N Engl J Med 2001;345:951; with permission.

men who had advanced nonmetastatic prostate cancer treated with ADT. A total of 47 men in the zoledronic acid group and 42 men in the placebo group received all five does of study medication. The authors reported that the mean BMD of the lumbar spine increased by 5.6% in men receiving zoledronic acid and decreased by 2.2% in men randomized to placebo treatment, resulting in a difference of 7.8% in mean percent change at 1 year ($P < .001$). The mean BMD of the femoral neck, trochanter, and total hip increased in the zoledronic acid group and decreased in the placebo group (Fig. 3). Although no patient suffered from a clinical (symptomatic) fracture, there were five radiographically diagnosed new or worsening vertebral fractures in the zoledronic acid group and three in the placebo group. Although these results are encouraging, one important study limitation is that site-specific fracture rates were not measured. In fact, no clinical trial has examined whether preventing BMD loss in this population translates into reduced fracture rate, and this remains an important question that should be addressed.

A recent trial evaluated the ability neridronate, a bisphosphonate used in the management of Paget disease [45] and malignant hypercalcemia [46], to prevent bone loss in prostate cancer patients treated with ADT. Morabito and colleagues [47] randomized 48 men who had prostate cancer and osteoporosis (T score < -2.5 SD) equally to intramuscular neridronate (25 mg) in addition to calcium (400 mg) and cholecalciferol (400 IU) supplements (treatment group) or calcium (400 mg) and cholecalciferon (400 IU) without neridronate therapy (control group). All patients

received ADT with triptorelin depot. Bone turnover was assessed with urine markers (deoxypyridinoline [DPD] and bone alkaline phosphatase [BALP]), and bone loss was evaluated with DEXA scan. DPD and BALP levels were significantly elevated in the control group, corresponding to increase bone turnover rates. DPD levels

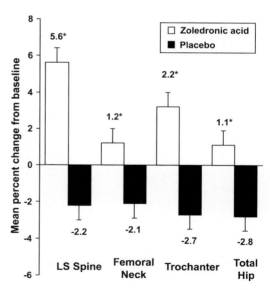

Fig. 3. Least square mean percent change from baseline in BMD at the lumbar spine, femoral neck, trochanter, and total hip. *$P < .001$ (ANOVA) for comparison between zoledronic acid and placebo. *From* Smith MR, Eastham J, Gleason DM, et al. Randomized controlled trial of zoledronic acid to prevent bone loss in men receiving androgen deprivation therapy for nonmetastatic prostate cancer. J Urol 2003;169:2011; with permission.

increased 72.8% above baseline, and BALP levels were elevated 26.6% above baseline in patients not receiving bisphosphonate therapy. Urine markers were not significantly changed in the neridronate group (−9.87% DPD and −13.30% BALP at 12 months) (Fig. 4). At 12 months, BMD decreased significantly in the control group at the lumbar spine (0.738 g/cm^2 at baseline versus 0.702 g/cm^2 at 12 months) and total hip (0.804 g/cm^2 at baseline versus 0.789 g/cm^2 at 12 months). Patients receiving neridronate did not experience any significant change in BMD and showed slight increases in bone mineralization at all assessed sites. Fracture rates were not mentioned in the study; however, the side effect profile of neridronate was limited to an acute-phase reaction in three patients (12.5%).

A more recent study from the same group assessed the efficacy of bisphosphonate therapy in patients treated with maximum androgen blockade (triptorelin + bicalutamide) and with antiandrogen therapy (bicalutamide) alone [48]. Sixty patients who had advanced prostate cancer and osteoporosis were randomized to ADT strategy with or without neridronate therapy (total of four groups). Patients treated with neridronate and maximum androgen blockade did not experience significant changes in BMD at the lumbar spine or total hip. Those treated with maximum androgen blockage without adjuvant bisphosphonate therapy experienced significant bone loss at both sites. A slight, nonsignificant decrease in

BMD was seen in patients treated with bicalutamide alone (without neridronate), and patients who received both bicalutamide and neridronate experienced a significant increase in BMD. These results indicate a difference in bone loss in patients treated with maximum androgen blockage compared with androgen receptor antagonist therapy alone. Patients treated with bicalutamide seem to have an attenuated decrease in BMD compared with those exposed to gonadotropin-releasing hormone (GnRH) agonists, and adjuvant bisphosphonate therapy increased bone mineralization in the former population.

Although bisphosphonate therapy has been shown to reduce the risk of fracture and the need for palliative radiotherapy in metastatic breast cancer [49] and multiple myeloma [50], the role of bisphosphonates in metastatic prostate cancer is not well established [51] and is currently under study [52,53]. The benefit of bisphosphonates on BMD in this group of patients seems to be maintained. In an early study, etidronate was shown to reverse bone loss in men who had metastatic prostate cancer treated with combined androgen blockade [54]. Another study from the same group evaluated the efficacy of a single infusion of intravenous pamidronate on BMD in a small group of men who had metastatic prostate cancer [55]. Diamond and colleagues [55] studied 21 men who had metastatic prostate cancer and bone metastases treated with combined androgen blockade and reported significant decreases in

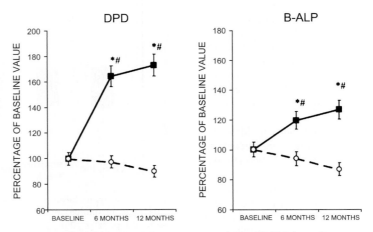

Fig. 4. Changes in urinary excretion of DPD and serum concentrations of BALP in patients treated with (open circle) and without (closed boxes) neridronate. Values are expressed as the mean ± SD percentages of baseline values. *$P < .05$ for comparisons from baseline; #$P < .05$ for comparisons between groups. *From* Morabito N, Gaudio A, Lasco A, et al. Neridronate prevents bone loss in patients receiving androgen deprivation therapy for prostate cancer. J Bone Miner Res 2004;19:1768; with permission.

serum bone Gla-protein concentrations (16.8%) and urinary excretion of DPD (18.5%) after bisphosphonate therapy. Treatment with intravenous pamidronate resulted in BMD increases of 7.8% in the lumbar spine assessed by quantitative CT and 2% in the total femoral neck assessed by DEXA. Conversely, treatment with placebo was associated with 5.7% and 2.3% decreases in BMD in the lumbar spine and total femoral neck, respectively. The differences in BMD between the treatment and placebo groups were statistically significant ($P = .0007$).

Adverse effects of bisphosphonate therapy

Although generally well tolerated, bisphosphonate therapy is associated with attendant side effects. The most common side effects associated with oral bisphosponates are mild nausea and abdominal pain. Intravenous administration is associated with a self-limited, acute-phase reaction. Typically, symptoms can be reduced with intravenous hydration. Side effects and adverse reactions of specific agents have resulted in participant withdrawal from clinical trials. In the pamidronate trial published in the *New England Journal of Medicine*, Smith and colleagues [35] reported serious adverse reactions in a total of eight study participants—three (14%) in the group treated with ADT and five (24%) in the combination ADT and bisphosphonate group. Two patients treated with pamidronate withdrew from the study secondary to adverse reactions, and an additional three patients (14%) experienced transient arthralgias and fevers consistent with the acute-phase reaction associated with intravenous bisphosphonate administration. In the zoledronic acid trial published 2 years later in the *Journal of Urology*, severe adverse reactions were reported in 24% of patients in the treatment group and in 39% of patients in the placebo group. There were five withdrawals secondary to adverse events—two from the zoledronic acid group and three from the placebo group [36]. Ten to twelve percent of men treated with intramuscular neridronate experience a transient acute-phase reaction [47,48]. Patients and clinicians should be aware of the side-effect profiles of these medications before initiation of therapy.

Summary

ADT is associated with decreased BMD and increased fracture rates in men who have prostate cancer. Men suffer excess morbidity and mortality after clinically significant fractures and may be at risk for undertreatment. Moreover, fracture is associated with decreased overall survival in men who have prostate cancer. Bisphosphonates inhibit osteoclast activity and have been shown to be beneficial in multiple myeloma and in patients who have lytic bone lesions secondary to breast cancer. Several randomized clinical trials have assessed the efficacy of bisphosphonate therapy in patients who have advanced and metastatic prostate cancer. The current evidence suggests that bisphosphonates reduce bone turnover and increase or maintain BMD in patients treated with ADT. Fracture rates have not been formally studied with randomized clinical trials; however, the stabilization of BMD theoretically should decrease the risk of fracture in this population of men. Despite these findings, bisphosphonate therapy has not become standard clinical practice in managing these men. In fact, a recent review of 184 patients who had prostate cancer treated with ADT for >1 year revealed that only 8.7% were evaluated with DEXA scan, and only 5.4% were treated with bisphosphonates [56]. Although further research and formal recommendations are needed, patients placed on androgen deprivation should be counseled regarding preventative measures, and BMD measurement should be strongly considered. Administration of bisphosphonate therapy should be instituted in cases with clinical evidence of decreased BMD or fracture.

References

[1] Jemal A, Murray T, Ward E, et al. Cancer statistics. CA Cancer J Clin 2005;2005(55):10–30.
[2] Jemel A, Murray T, Samuels A, et al. Cancer statistics. CA Cancer J Clin 2003;2003(53):5–26.
[3] Carlin BI, Andriole GL. The natural history, skeletal complications, and management of bone metastases in patients with prostate carcinoma. Cancer 2000; 88(Suppl):2989–94.
[4] Cooperberg MR, Grossfeld GD, Lubeck DP, et al. National practice patterns and time trends in androgen ablation for localized prostate cancer. J Natl Cancer Inst 2003;95:981–9.
[5] Meng MV, Grossfeld GD, Sadetsky N, et al. Contemporary patterns of androgen deprivation therapy use for newly diagnosed prostate cancer. Urology 2002;60(Suppl 1):7–12.
[6] Lindsay R, Cosman F. Osteoporosis. In: Braunwald E, Fauci AS, Kasper DL, et al, editors. Harrison's principles of internal medicine. 15th edition. New York: McGraw-Hill; 2001. p. 2226–37.

[7] Siddiqui NA, Shetty KR. Osteoporosis in older men: discovering when and how to treat it. Geriatrics 1994;54:20–37.

[8] Kelepouris N, Harper KD, Gannon FM. Severe osteoporosis in men. Ann Intern Med 1995;123:452–60.

[9] Mittan D, Lee S, Miller E, et al. Bone loss following hypogonadism in men with prostate cancer treated with GnRH analogs. J Clin Endocrinol Metab 2002;87:3656–61.

[10] Daniell HW, Dunn SR, Ferguson DW, et al. Progressive osteoporosis during androgen deprivation therapy for prostate cancer. J Urol 2000;163:181–6.

[11] Oefelein MG, Resnick MI. The impact of osteoporosis in men treated for prostate cancer. Urol Clin North Am 2004;31:313–9.

[12] Diamond TH, Higano CS, Smith MR, et al. Osteoporosis in men with prostate carcinoma receiving androgen-deprivation therapy: recommendations for diagnosis and therapies. Cancer 2004;100:892–9.

[13] Kiratli B, Srinivas S, Perkash I, et al. Progressive decrease in bone density over 10 years of androgen deprivation therapy in patients with prostate cancer. Urology 2001;57:127–32.

[14] Wei JT, Gross M, Jaffe CA, et al. Androgen deprivation therapy for prostate cancer results in significant loss of bone density. Urology 1999;54:607–11.

[15] Smith MR, McGovern FJ, Fallon MA, et al. Low bone mineral density in hormone-naïve men with prostate carcinoma. Cancer 2001;91:2238–45.

[16] Conde FA, Sarna L, Oka RK, et al. Age, body mass index, and serum prostate-serum antigen correlate with bone loss in men with prostate cancer not receiving androgen deprivation therapy. Urology 2004;64:335–40.

[17] Burger H, de Laet CE, van Daele PL, et al. Risk factors for increased bone loss in an elderly population: the Rotterdam study. Am J Epidemiol 1998;147:871–9.

[18] Nguyen TV, Eisman JA, Kelly PJ, et al. Risk factors for osteoporotic fractures in elderly men. Am J Epidemiol 1996;144:255–63.

[19] Melton LJ III, Atkinson EJ, O'Fallon WM, et al. Long-term fracture prediction by bone mineral assessed at different skeletal sites. J Bone Miner Res 1993;8:1227–33.

[20] Townsend SF, Sanders WH, Northway RO, et al. Bone fractures associated with luteinizing hormone-releasing hormone agonists used in the treatment of prostate adenocarcinoma. Cancer 1997;79:545–50.

[21] Daniell HW. Osteoporosis after orchiectomy for prostate cancer. J Urol 1997;157:439–44.

[22] Melton LJ, Alothman KI, Khosla S, et al. Fracture risk following bilateral orchiectomy. J Urol 2003;169:1747–50.

[23] Hatano T, Oishi Y, Furuta A, et al. Incidence of bone fracture in patients receiving luteinizing hormone-releasing agonists for prostate cancer. BJU Int 2000;86:449–52.

[24] Oefelein MG, Ricchuiti V, Conrad W, et al. Skeletal fracture associated with androgen suppression induced osteoporosis: the clinical incidence and risk factors for patients with prostate cancer. J Urol 2001;166:1724–8.

[25] Diamond TH, Bucci J, Kersley JH, et al. Osteoporosis and spinal fractures in men with prostate cancer: risk factors and effects of androgen deprivation therapy. Urology 2004;172:529–32.

[26] Krupski TL, Smith MR, Lee WC, et al. Natural history of bone complications in men with prostate cancer initiating androgen deprivation therapy. Cancer 2004;101:541–9.

[27] Shahinian VB, Kuo YF, Freeman JL, et al. Risk of fracture after androgen deprivation for prostate cancer. N Engl J Med 2005;352:154–64.

[28] Stock H, Schneider A, Strauss E. Osteoporosis: a disease in men. Clin Orthop 2004;425:143–51.

[29] Kiebzak GM, Beinart GA, Perser K, et al. Undertreatment of osteoporosis in men with hip fracture. Arch Intern Med 2002;162:2217–22.

[30] Diamond TH, Thornley SW, Sekel R, et al. Hip fractures in elderly men: prognostic factors and outcomes. Med J 1997;167:412–5.

[31] De Laet CE, Pois HA. Fractures in the elderly: epidemiology and demography. Best Pract Res Clin Endocrinol Metab 2000;14:171–9.

[32] NIH Consensus Development Panel on Osteoporosis Prevention, Diagnosis, and Therapy. Osteoporosis prevention, diagnosis, and therapy. JAMA 2001;285:785–95.

[33] Oefelein MG, Ricchiuti V, Conrad W, et al. Skeletal fractures negatively correlate with overall survival in men with prostate cancer. J Urol 2002;168:1005–7.

[34] Dawson-Hughes B, Harris SS, Krall EA, et al. Effect of calcium and vitamin D supplementation on bone density in men and women 65 years of age and older. N Engl J Med 1997;337:670–6.

[35] Smith MR, McGovern FJ, Zietman AL, et al. Pamidronate to prevent bone loss during androgen-deprivation therapy for prostate cancer. N Engl J Med 2001;345:948–55.

[36] Smith MR, Eastham J, Gleason DM, et al. Randomized controlled trial of zoledronic acid to prevent bone loss in men receiving androgen deprivation therapy for nonmetastatic prostate cancer. J Urol 2003;169:2008–12.

[37] Vincent KR, Braith RW. Resistance exercise and bone turnover in elderly men and women. Med Sci Sport Exerc 2002;34:17–23.

[38] Eriksson S, Eriksson A, Stege R, et al. Bone mineral density in patients with prostate cancer treated with orchidectomy and with estrogens. Calcif Tissue Int 1995;57:97–9.

[39] Scherr D, Pitts WR, Vaughan ED. Diethylstilbestrol revisited: androgen deprivation, osteoporosis and prostate cancer. J Urol 2002;167:535–8.

[40] Ockrim JL, Lalani EN, Laniado ME, et al. Transdermal estradiol therapy for advanced prostate

cancer: forward to the past? J Urol 2003;169: 1735–7.

[41] Stepan JJ, Iachman M, Zverina J, et al. Castrated men exhibit bone loss: effect of calcitonin treatment on biochemical indices of bone remodeling. J Clin Endocrinol Metab 1989;69:523–7.

[42] Russell RG, Croucher PI, Rogers MJ. Bisphosphonates: pharmacology, mechanism of action and clinical use. Osteoporos Int 1999;9(Suppl 2):S66–80.

[43] Orwoll E, Ettinger M, Weiss S, et al. Alendronate for the treatment of osteoporosis in men. N Engl J Med 2000;343:604–10.

[44] Gonnelli S, Cepollaro C, Montagnani A, et al. Alendronate treatment in men with primary osteoporosis: a three-year longitudinal study. Calcif Tissue Int 2003;73:133–9.

[45] Filipponi P, Cristallini S, Policani G, et al. Paget's disease of bone: benefits of neridronate as a first treatment and in cases of relapse after clodronate. Bone 1998;23:543–8.

[46] O'Rourke NP, McCloskey EV, Rosini S, et al. Treatment of malignant hypercalcemia with aminohexane bisphosphonate (neridronate). Br J Cancer 1994;69:914–7.

[47] Morabito N, Gaudio A, Lasco A, et al. Neridronate prevents bone loss in patients receiving androgen deprivation therapy for prostate cancer. J Bone Miner Res 2004;19:1766–70.

[48] Magno C, Anastasi G, Morabito N, et al. Preventing bone loss during androgen deprivation therapy for prostate cancer: early experience with neridronate. Eur Urol 2005;47:575–81.

[49] Hortobagyi GN, Theriault RL, Porter L, et al. Efficacy of pamidronate in reducing skeletal complications in patients with breast cancer and lytic bone metastases. Protocol 19 Aredia Breast Cancer Study Group. N Engl J Med 1996;335: 1785–91.

[50] Berenson JR, Lichtenstein A, Porter L, et al. Efficacy of pamidronate in reducing skeletal events in patients with advanced multiple myeloma. Myeloma Aredia Study Group. N Engl J Med 1996; 334:488–93.

[51] Ross JR, Saunders Y, Edmonds PM, et al. Systemic review of role of bisphosphonates on skeletal morbidity in metastatic cancer. BMJ 2003;327:469–75.

[52] Saad F, Gleason DM, Murray R, et al. A randomized, placebo-controlled trial of zoledronic acid in patients with hormone-refractory metastatic prostate carcinoma. J Natl Cancer Inst 2002;94: 1458–68.

[53] Saad F, Gleason DM, Murray R, et al. Long-term efficacy of zoledronic acid for the prevention of skeletal complications in patients with metastatic hormone-refractory prostate cancer. J Natl Cancer Inst 2004;96:879–82.

[54] Diamond T, Campbell J, Bryant C, et al. The effect of combined androgen blockade on bone turnover and bone mineral densities in men treated for prostate carcinoma: longitudinal evaluation and response to intermittent cyclic etidronate therapy. Cancer 1998;83:1561–6.

[55] Diamond TH, Winters J, Smith A, et al. The antiosteoporotic efficacy of intravenous pamidronate in men with prostate carcinoma receiving combined androgen blockade. Cancer 2001;92:1444–50.

[56] Tanvetyanon T. Physician practice of bone mineral density testing and drug prescribing to prevent or treat osteoporosis during androgen deprivation therapy. Cancer 2005;103:237–41.

Mechanisms Leading to the Development of Hormone-Resistant Prostate Cancer

Susan Kasper, PhD*, Michael S. Cookson, MD

Department of Urologic Surgery, A-1302 MC, Vanderbilt University Medical Center, Nashville, TN 37232-2765, USA

It has been appreciated for more than 60 years that prostate cancer cells are responsive to androgen deprivation therapy (ADT). In 1941, Huggins and Hodges [1] observed the beneficial effects of hormonal therapy on prostate cancer cells, and the importance of this contribution was later recognized by the awarding of a Nobel Prize. In addition to surgical castration, there are various methods used to achieve castrate levels of testosterone. Medical castration can be achieved with the use of estrogens, gonadotropin-releasing hormone (GnRH) agonists, and antagonists [2]. In addition, agents that block the androgen receptor (androgen receptor antagonists) and medications that affect androgen synthesis may be used alone or in combination to block the effects of androgens. The majority of ADT is administered injection using GnRH agonists, and it is recommended that this therapy be continued even after the tumors progress to hormone refractory cancer status [3]. This article provides an overview of ADT in advanced prostate cancer (PCa) and discusses the potential mechanisms by which hormonal resistance to therapy develops.

ADT

ADT remains the cornerstone of treatment in the management of patients who have advanced

Supported by the National Institute of Diabetes & Digestive & Kidney Diseases (R01 DK60957, R01 DK059142) and the Frances Preston Laboratories of the T.J. Martell Foundation (S.K.).

* Corresponding author.

E-mail address: susan.kasper@vanderbilt.edu (S. Kasper).

prostate cancer. This includes patients who have locally advanced disease and metastases at the time of presentation and high-risk patients who relapse after initial therapy. Early detection, including the widespread use of prostate-specific antigen (PSA), has significantly reduced the number of men who have advanced or metastatic disease at the time of presentation, and data are emerging that show that deaths from prostate cancer are on the decline [4,5]. Despite these encouraging statistics, it has been estimated that up to 40% of men with clinically localized disease suffer recurrence after initial therapy with curative intent. PSA recurrence is conservatively estimated to affect about 50,000 men each year, having become the most common presentation of advanced prostate cancer [6]. The majority of these men will undergo treatment with ADT earlier in their disease course than historically administered, placing them at risk for the development of androgen-independent progression even before evidence of radiographic progression.

Several studies, historical and contemporary, have validated the efficacy of ADT in patients who have advanced and metastatic disease. In the 1960s, the Veterans Administration Cooperative Study Group conducted the first large, randomized study investigating the efficacy of ADT in men who had advanced prostate cancer [7]. A reexamination of the data demonstrated a survival advantage for men who had locally advanced and metastatic prostate cancer treated with 1 mg/d of diethylstilbestrol as compared with patients treated with placebo, low (0.2 mg), or high (5 mg) diethylstilbestrol [8]. A more contemporary study conducted by the Medical Research Council further validated the use of ADT in men who have locally advanced and metastatic prostate cancer [9]. There were also reductions in the complications of prostate cancer, including reduced skeletal metastases, pathologic fractures, spinal cord compression, and ureteral obstruction, in favor of immediate therapy. This study has been criticized because many patients on the observation arm received no hormonal therapy despite progression of disease and death from prostate cancer [9].

The use of ADT among patients having failed initial therapy is common, often occurring when biochemical relapse is the only evidence of recurrent disease. In a retrospective, observational, multicenter database analysis of patients treated with early versus delayed ADT for PSA recurrence after prior radical prostatectomy, early treatment was an independent predictor of delayed clinical metastases only for high-risk patients [10]. In addition to its use in metastatic and recurrent prostate cancer, ADT is often instituted much earlier in the disease process. Support for this is inferred from a randomized study of 98 men who had positive lymph nodes at the time of radical prostatectomy. This study compared immediate ADT with observation until time of progression and demonstrated a significant overall and PCa-specific survival advantage in favor of immediate treatment [11]. At a median follow-up of 10 years, approximately two thirds of the patients who received ADT were alive, compared with 49% of those on observation. The cause-specific survival was 87.2% in patients receiving early ADT versus 56.9% in the delayed-treatment group [12].

The use of ADT in combination with primary treatment based on high-risk features at the time of diagnosis has emerged as the standard of care. Several randomized studies have demonstrated an overall survival benefit when comparing radiation therapy alone with radiation therapy plus ADT in men who have locally advanced tumors [13,14]. D'Amico and colleagues [15] recently reported results of a randomized trial of 3-dimensional conformal radiation therapy with or without 6 months of ADT therapy in 206 patients who had prostate cancer. All of these patients had a Gleason score of at least 7, evidence of extraprostatic disease, or a PSA of 10 ng/mL or higher. After a median follow-up of 4.5 years, patients randomized to receive combination therapy had a significantly higher survival ($P = .04$) and lower prostate cancer–specific mortality ($P = .02$). Kaplan-Meier estimates of 5-year survival rates were 88% in the combination therapy versus 78% (95% confidence interval, 68–88) in the radiation-alone group. Rates of survival-free of salvage ADT at 5 years were 82% in the radiation therapy plus ADT group versus 57% in the radiation alone group. These data support the early use of hormonal therapy in combination with radiation therapy among high-risk patients.

In summary, ADT is an effective form of palliation among men who have metastatic disease and has significantly improved survival when used in combination with radiation therapy for high-risk patients who have local or regional disease. Increasingly, ADT is being initiated earlier in the disease process in an attempt to delay or prevent the progression of disease and complications thereof. Yet, most of these tumors progress to androgen independence and become refractory to androgen ablation [16]. At that point, the options are limited and up until recently were palliative in nature. Recently, two randomized phase III studies demonstrated for the first time improvements in survival using chemotherapy, offering hope for the future to patients who have hormone refractory disease [17]. A better understanding of the mechanisms through which these tumors survive in the absence of androgens is a first step toward targeting therapies aimed at reducing deaths from this disease.

Potential mechanisms for promoting hormonal resistance

Reactivation of the androgen receptor

The observation that advanced PCa progresses to androgen independence and becomes refractory to ADT has sparked interest in the role of androgens in PCa development and progression. Androgens exert most of their biologic activities through binding to androgen receptor (AR). During ADT, subcellular localization of AR seems to be nuclear, suggesting that the AR signaling pathway can be activated when serum androgen levels are greatly reduced [18]. Nuclear AR was observed in COS cells after treatment with hydroxyflutamide, implying that nuclear localization should also be observed in patients undergoing antiandrogen therapy [19]. In a microarray study comparing gene expression profiles of hormone-naive PCa with primary PCa after short-term ADT and with androgen-resistant metastatic tumor samples, Holzbeierlein and colleagues [20] demonstrated that many genes altered expression in response to 3 months of ADT, including known targets of

AR, such as PSA (kallikrein [KLK]-3) and KLK2. Gene expression profiles of androgen-resistant metastatic tumors were similar to that of hormone-naive lesions but were distinct from that of primary tumors after short-term ADT. These data suggest that AR signaling has been reactivated in androgen-resistant tumors. Several mechanisms by which AR may be activated during the development of hormone-refractory prostate cancer (HRPC) include AR gene amplification, altered AR phosphorylation, AR mutations, androgen-independent activation of AR through other signaling pathways and altered activity of AR co-regulators. Any combination of these mechanisms could occur during HRPC development.

AR gene amplification and increased AR levels

It is postulated that 20% to 30% of recurrent HRPC samples exhibit AR gene amplification [21,22]. In a cohort of 51 patients, Edwards and colleagues [23] correlated AR gene amplification with AR protein expression in 102 matched hormone-sensitive and HRPC specimens. AR gene amplification occurred in 20% of hormone-resistant tumors (compared with 2% of hormone-sensitive tumors) and increased AR expression correlated with AR gene amplification in 80% of HRPC. PSA levels were significantly lower in hormone-resistant tumors compared with matched hormone-sensitive tumors. Increased AR expression without AR amplification occurred in 35% of cases [23], suggesting that alternative mechanisms (eg, AR phosphorylation) promoted hormone resistance [24]. Thus, AR amplification with increased AR expression correlates at best with a subset of prostate cancer cases.

Increased AR gene expression and protein levels were generated in a transgenic mouse model by targeting the murine AR gene under control of the rat probasin promoter to the prostatic epithelium to assess the direct effects of AR overexpression on prostate cancer development [25]. Transgenic mice older than 1 year developed focal areas of intraepithelial neoplasia (PIN) resembling human high-grade PIN, indicating that AR overexpression during prostate development induced PIN formation but was insufficient to induce adenocarcinoma or metastasis [25]. In contrast, overexpression of AR in the LAPC4 prostate cancer cell and xenograft models converted prostate cancer growth from androgen-sensitive to hormone refractory disease [26]. Thus, the effectiveness of

increased AR expression to promote recurrent disease likely depends not only on AR expression levels but also on the status of the prostate cancer cell.

Protein stability or AR phosphorylation are alternative mechanisms by which circulating AR levels or activity may increase. In recurrent CWR22 tumors and cell lines derived from recurrent prostate tumors, AR stability increased two to four times that observed in androgen-sensitive CWR22 tumors, and AR stabilization correlated with increased proliferation induced by very low androgen levels [27]. AR is stabilized and protected against proteolytic degradation when phosphorylated at serines 80, 93, and 641 and transcriptionally activated when the receptor is phosphorylated at serines 213, 506, and 650 [24]. AR phosphorylation by mitogen-activated protein kinase and Akt sensitizes AR to low circulating levels of dihydrotestosterone (DHT), estrogens, or antiandrogens [24].

AR mutations

Mutations facilitate the reactivation of AR signaling by other steroid hormones and growth factors. This was initially demonstrated in LNCaP cells where a threonine to alanine substitution at residue 877 (T877A) in AR resulted in the transactivation of an androgen-regulated reporter gene in response to progesterone, 17β-estradiol, or hydroxyflutamide [28]. The histidine to tyrosine substitution at residue 874 (H874Y) appearing in CWR22 epithelial tumors was more responsive to estradiol, progesterone, hydroxyflutamide, and the adrenal androgen dehydroepiandrosterone than wild-type AR [29]. The T877A mutation was detected in 5 of 16 patients who received combined ADT with the AR antagonist flutamide compared with 1 of 17 patients treated with ADT alone, suggesting that AR mutations could occur in response to selective pressure from flutamide treatment [30]. In a trial for antiandrogen withdrawal, 184 bone marrow biopsies were obtained. Of these, 48 had detectable PCa [31]. AR sequence analysis detected single-point mutations (residues 877, 879, 741, or 756) in 5 of the 48 samples, and frequency of AR mutations was similar regardless of long-term exposure to bicalutamide or flutamide [31]. An AR substitution mutation of glutamic acid to glycine at residue 231 (E231G) promoted development of PIN, adenocarcinoma, and metastases in transgenic mice overexpressing this mutant AR [32].

A comprehensive list of AR mutations in prostate cancer and androgen insensitivity syndromes can be found in the updated AR mutation database [33]. Approximately 85 AR mutations have been found in PCa tissue, with most being single-base substitutions due to somatic rather than germline mutations. Somatic mutations in PCa colocalize to six targeted areas: two in the N terminal (residues 54–92 and 253–282) and four in the ligand binding domain (residues 654–689, 688–721, 723–738, and 867–917) [34]. Many of these mutations have not been functionally evaluated in the laboratory, and therefore their role in AR activation in response to different agonists or in providing a growth advantage during HRPC development remains to be elucidated.

Altered activity of AR co-regulators

Increased activation of the AR promoter may occur through altered activity of AR co-regulators. Expression of transcriptional intermediary factor 2 (TIF2) and steroid receptor coactivator 1 increased in recurrent CWR22 tumors [35]. AR transactivation in response to TIF2 overexpression resulted in hypersensitivity to androstenedione, estradiol, and progesterone and to dihydrotestosterone treatment [35]. Bicalutamide functioned as an agonist in LAPC4 cells overexpressing AR through the differential recruitment of polymerase II, steroid receptor coactivator 1, and nuclear receptor corepressor to the PSA gene promoter [26].

ARA70 was the first AR coactivator discovered. In transient transfection studies, ARA70 increased AR stability and enhanced AR activation by hydroxyflutamide, cyproterone acetate, and bicalutamide [36,37]. The coactivator ARA55 increased AR-regulated transcriptional activity in the presence of 17β-estradiol and hydroxyflutamide [38]. Other co-regulators in the AR signaling pathway include CBP, Tip60, ARA55, ARA54, gelsolin, Stat3, and RAC3 [39–41].

The coactivator p300 induced PSA promoter activity in LNCaP cells maintained in long-term culture in the presence of interleukin-6, a cytokine important in late-stage PCa [42]. Furthermore, the PSA promoter became more responsive to p300 than to androgens, and this increased activity was, in part, independent of AR [42]. Thus, p300 may regulate androgen-dependent genes in the absence or low levels of AR during late-stage PCa.

Foxa1 and Foxa2 are proteins that belong to the forkhead box a (Foxa) superfamily of transcription factors that play a central role in intestinal and hepatic gene regulation [43]. Mirosevich and colleagues [43] demonstrated that although LNCaP and PC-3 cells expressed Foxa1, Foxa2 expression was only observed in PC-3 cells. Furthermore, Foxa2 positively regulated the androgen-dependent PSA promoter in an androgen- and AR-independent manner. Foxa1 protein was expressed in human prostate carcinomas irrespective or Gleason grade, whereas Foxa2 was detected only in neuroendocrine small-cell carcinomas and high Gleason grade adenocarcinomas [43]. Thus, Foxa2 regulation of gene expression seems to correlate with PCa progression to androgen independence.

In summary, modulation of the combination of coactivators and corepressors with AR upregulate AR expression and activity in PCa and that these changes often enhance the agonistic effects of AR antagonists. The list of identified AR coregulators has continued to increase [44,45], but their role in recurrent PCa has not been fully investigated.

Ligand-independent activation of AR

Studies have shown that nonsteroid receptor signaling pathways can be activated in an androgen-depleted environment. Overexpression or amplification of the HER2/neu gene were observed in a subset of PCa patients [46] and elevated serum levels of the HER2/neu extracellular domain occurred in patients that failed therapy [47]. In the absence of DHT, HER2/neu overexpression could rescue LNCaP cells from growth inhibition induced by androgen deprivation in vitro and shortened the latency of LNCaP/HER2 tumor formation in castrated SCID mice in vivo [46]. PSA secretion increased 6 to 7 fold in LNCaP/HER2 cells compared with the LNCaP parental cell line. In LAPC-4 cells, which express wild-type human AR, HER2/neu activated the PSA enhancer/promoter 15 fold in the absence of androgen treatment [46]. Thus, HER2/neu could substitute for androgens and promote prostate cancer cell growth. Furthermore, Casodex could not block HER2/neu-activated AR signal transduction, indicating that this pathway was independent of the ligand-binding domain [46]. Yeh and colleagues [48] reported that HER2/neu increased PSA expression through the MAP kinase pathway and that addition of MAP-kinase inhibitors suppressed AR transactivation. AR activation occurred through phosphorylation of the N-terminal, confirming that HER2/neu-induced

AR signaling was independent of the ligand binding domain. Thus, HER2/neu signaling may be an important mechanism in the development of androgen-independent prostate cancer.

The phosphoinositide 3-kinase-Akt pathway has also been implicated in the ligand-independent activation of AR. HER2/neu can activate Akt, resulting in an Akt:AR interaction, phosphorylation of AR serine residues 213 and 791 and cell survival and growth upon androgen withdrawal [49]. In vivo, overexpression of a constitutively active Akt increased tumor growth in the LNCaP xenograft model [50].

Growth factors such as insulin-like growth factor 1 (IGF-1), epidermal growth factor, and keratinocyte growth factor can activate AR-mediated PSA gene transcription, and this activation can be blocked by Casodex [51]. Thus, IGF-1 activity seems to be dependent on the ligand-binding domain of AR. Chan and colleagues [52] found that men with increased IGF-1 plasma levels had a relative risk of 4.3 fold of developing prostate cancer compared to men with normal IGF-1 serum levels. It is unclear whether these effects occur through the direct interaction with AR or through another mechanism.

Primary and metastatic prostatic adenocarcinomas contain a subpopulation of neuroendocrine (NE) cells, which are not eliminated by ADT [53]. Although >50% of all malignant prostatic tumors contain NE-like cells and metastatic PCa with NE differentiation indicates poorer prognosis [54], the function of NE secretory peptides and amines is not clear [55]. Jin and colleagues [52] investigated the role of NE cells on PCa growth by implanting NE-10 xenografts (established from a NE prostate carcinoma) into one flank and LNCaP xenografts into the opposing flank of nude mice. In intact mice, NE-10 tumors increased serum PSA levels, AR expression, and xenograft tumor volume [53]. Serum PSA levels, LNCaP AR expression levels, cell proliferation, and tumor volume remained elevated in castrated mice bearing NE-10 and LNCaP xenografts compared with castrated mice bearing only LNCaP xenografts [53]. Xenograft This study suggests that NE cells secrete factors that promote tumor cell survival and proliferation and AR signaling during androgen deprivation.

Cancer stem cells

Cancer stem cells arise from a multipotent stem cell that undergoes self-renewal and accumulates genetic alterations during its long lifespan (Fig. 1) [56]. Thus, cancer cell fate is determined by a combination of genetic mutations or altered gene expression that occur during tumor development. Another view is that during the continuum of cell determination and differentiation, maturation arrest of stem cell differentiation influences the development of malignant potential [57]. For example, in normal development, prostate epithelial cells invade the mesenchymal pad during branching morphogenesis. A transformed prostate epithelial cell from this stage may intrinsically be more invasive or have more motility than a differentiated prostate epithelial cell harboring the same mutation. Thus, a combination of the particular cell stage in which these mutations occur along with the specific mutations may account for the multifocal nature of prostate cancer.

Prostatic stem cells are thought to reside in the basal cell compartment [58]. The most compelling evidence is derived from the mouse castration model where withdrawal of androgens results in apoptosis in approximately 90% of epithelial cells, leaving the basal cell layer intact [59]. Androgen replacement induces these pluripotent cells to amplify and undergo differentiation to repopulate the prostate with basal, luminal, and NE epithelial cells [59,60]. NE cells are thought to arise from a common epithelial precursor, although there is some evidence that they may be derived from the neural crest during embryogenesis [61].

The role of basal cells in prostate development was recently analyzed in prostates that did not express the basal cell marker p63. Because p63-null mice were postnatally lethal, urogenital sinus of p63($-/-$) mouse embryos were rescued by grafting them under the renal capsule of adult male nude mice [62]. They developed into prostate containing luminal and neuroendocrine but not basal epithelial cells [62]. This study suggests that p63 is essential for the differentiation of basal cells but that it (and therefore basal cells) is not required for differentiation into luminal or neuroendocrine epithelial cells. Whether all cells within the basal compartment of the prostate are p63+ remains to be determined.

Numerous studies have attempted to identify or isolate prostate stem cells from human pathologic samples. The absence of the cell cycle inhibitor p27^{kip1} in transient amplifying prostate cells suggests that they arose from a p27^{kip1}-negative basal cell [59]. Decreased p27^{kip1} expression has been detected in high-grade PIN, invasive primary, and pelvic lymph node specimens [59]. Prostate

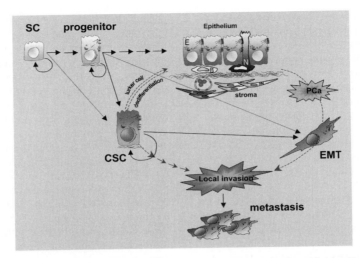

Fig. 1. Development of hormone-resistant PCa through stem cell or EMT mechanisms. Stem cells (SC) are a good candidate for the origin of cancer stem cells (CSC). Because stem cells have a long life and a large replicative potential, any mutation(s) accumulating in this cell population are passed on to the transient amplifying cells. Unlike terminal differentiation observed in normal cells, a mutant clone continues to expand and develop into a tumor. Another source of PCa stem cells are the progenitor or transient amplifying cells, which form the intermediate between the stem cell and the terminally differentiated cell. These cells may represent the androgen-independent lurker cell [18], which is thought to reside in the prostate. Clonal expansion of a number of mutant stem/progenitor cells, possibly selected for by therapy, could account for the multifocal nature of PCa. An alternative mechanism of tumor development involves normal prostate epithelial cells that have undergone dedifferentiation in response to loss of heterozygosity or mutation. These genomic changes promote increased survival and proliferation. As tumors cells become more neoplastic, EMT increases cell motility at the leading edge of the tumor, resulting in local invasiveness and metastasis. B, basal cell; E, epithelial cell; F, fibroblast; N, neuroendocrine cell; SM, smooth muscle cell.

progenitor cells seem to express basal and luminal epithelial cell markers, including cytokeratins CK5, CK14, CK8, CK18, CK19, and p63 and GSTpi [63]. Another study proposed that at 17 weeks of gestation, the keratin phenotype of basally located cells were CK5 and CK14 positive but CK18 negative [64]. Further studies are required to positively identify the prostate stem cell.

Cell surface molecules and colony formation assays have been used to identify prostate stem cells in culture. Collins and colleagues [65] isolated basal cells from primary human prostate cell cultures using antibodies to the basal cell surface marker CD44. Within this population, only cells expressing α2-integrin generated prostate-like glands expressing PSA and prostatic acid phosphatase in the xenograft model [65]. Although proliferative basal cells expressing α2-integrin could be separated by a rapid rate of adherence to type I collagen, they could not be differentiated based on whether they formed type I and type II colonies [65]. In a similar study, Hudson and colleagues [66] could not correlate β1- or α6-integrin expression with colony type, suggesting that stem cells are likely not clustered together but distributed among the basal cell population. In three-dimensional culture on Matrigel, cells formed structures reminiscent of prostate epithelium, suggesting that these could be the progeny of stem cells [66].

A number of proteins, such as CD133, CD44, c-kit, and NANOG, have been identified as putative stem cell markers [56]. In prostate, putative prostate cancer stem cells were identified as rare isolated cells that expressed breast cancer resistant protein but not AR, p63, synaptophysin, or smooth muscle α-actin [67]. These breast cancer resistant protein–positive AR⁻ cells actively excluded androgens in culture and seemed to undergo clonal expansion in the xenograft model postcastration. Thus, survival and expansion of an androgen-resistant cancer stem cell could result in the recurrence of hormone refractory disease.

Epithelial-mesenchymal transition

Through epigenetic changes and genetic alterations, cancer cells acquire limitless proliferative potential, becoming self-sufficient in proliferation signals and insensitive to growth inhibitory signals and apoptosis. They also undergo epithelial-mesenchymal transition (EMT), whereby they loose polarity and transform into a migratory mesenchymal phenotype. This process occurs at the invasion front of a metastasizing primary tumor [68] and can be activated by oncogenes, specific growth factors, or extracellular matrix components binding their cellular receptors [68–70].

EMT is characterized by decreased E-cadherin expression, increased expression of mesenchymal markers (eg, vimentin) and spindle-shaped morphology [69]. E-cadherin induces the formation of cell–cell contacts by clustering into small junctional complexes, which develop into adherens junctions and promote the formation of desmosomes [71]. Disruption of the E-cadherin–catenin complex results in downregulation of E-cadherin expression, transcriptional downregulation of cell–cell adhesion components, progressive destabilization of cell–cell adhesion structures, and degradation of cell/cell adhesion [72]. Perl and colleagues [73] demonstrated that loss of E-cadherin correlated with the transition of well-differentiated adenoma to invasive carcinoma in the Rip1Tag2 transgenic model for pancreatic β-cell carcinogenesis. Repression of E-cadherin expression by transcriptional regulators such as Snail, Smad-interacting protein 1, and Twist have emerged as critical steps in influencing EMT. TWIST is a key factor in the development of breast cancer metastasis by promoting EMT, and *TWIST* gene amplification is associated with the acquisition of resistance to the anticancer drug Taxol [74]. TWIST is also overexpressed in approximately 90% of prostate cancers, and increasing TWIST protein levels correlate with increasing Gleason grade [74]. Ectopic TWIST expression in LNCaP cells resulted in protection against Taxol-induced apoptosis [74]. In the androgen-independent prostate cancer cell lines DU-145 and PC-3, downregulation of TWIST expression through small interfering RNA inhibited EMT and promoted E-cadherin expression and suppression of invasion and migration [74]. These studies imply that therapies effectively reducing TWIST expression could promote a less invasive, epithelial cell phenotype that would be sensitive to second-line interventions such as Taxol.

PSA is a serine protease secreted by normal and tumor prostate epithelial cells and is used as the serum biomarker for PCa. Veveris-Lowe and colleagues [75] demonstrated that in PC-3 cells,

overexpression of exogenous PSA promoted EMT as seen by the transition to a more mesenchymal cell morphology, decreased E-cadherin expression, and increased vimentin expression. Similar results were seen when KLK4 was overexpressed in PC-3 cells. Although these kallikreins increased cell motility, they did not promote invasion in a Matrigel invasion assay [75], suggesting other events were required before metastasis occured. Other molecular mechanisms that govern EMT in tumor progression include the receptor tyrosine receptor kinase/Ras-, TGF-β, Wnt-, Notch-, Hedgehog-, and NF-κB–dependent pathways [68–70]. Increasing evidence suggests that EMT plays a key role in the acquisition of cell motility, which promotes local invasion at the leading tumor edge and metastasis. Factors that control the EMT process could become targets for developing more effective cancer therapies that prevent the development of metastatic potential.

Summary

Advanced and metastatic prostate cancer remains a potentially lethal tumor, and although ADT remains the most effective, treatment the limitations of its efficacy have been realized for more than a half a century. Patients who progress to androgen independence die of their disease. It is through an enhanced understanding of mechanisms involving AR activation and comprehension of processes such as the emergence of cancer stem cells or EMT cells that new therapies can developed to combat this challenging disease. Given the multiple pathways in which hormone refractory prostate cancer develops, it is conceivable that true progress in terms of improved survival will rely on a combination of treatments designed to address the various avenues of androgen resistance.

References

[1] Huggins C, Hodges CV. The effect of castration, of estrogen and of androgen injection on serum phosphatases in metastatic carcinoma of the prostate. Cancer Res 1941;1:293–7.

[2] Sharifi N, Gulley JL, Dahut WL. Androgen deprivation therapy for prostate cancer. JAMA 2005;294:238–44.

[3] Chang SS, Benson MC, Campbell SC, et al. Society of Urologic Oncology position statement: redefining the management of hormone-refractory prostate carcinoma. Cancer 2005;103:11–21.

[4] Crawford ED. Epidemiology of prostate cancer. Urology 2003;62(Suppl 1):3–12.

[5] Jemal A, Murray T, Ward E, et al. Cancer statistics, 2005. CA Cancer J Clin 2005;55:10–30.

[6] Ward JF, Moul JW. Treating the biochemical recurrence of prostate cancer after definitive primary therapy. Clin Prostate Cancer 2005;4:38–44.

[7] The Veterans Administration Co-operative Urological Research Group. Treatment and survival of patients with cancer of the prostate. Surg Gynecol Obstet 1967;124:1011–7.

[8] Byar DP. Proceedings: The Veterans Administration Cooperative Urological Research Group's studies of cancer of the prostate. Cancer 1973;32:1126–30.

[9] The Medical Research Council Prostate Cancer Working Party Investigators Group. Immediate versus deferred treatment for advanced prostatic cancer: initial results of the Medical Research Council Trial. Br J Urol 1997;79:235–46.

[10] Moul JW, Wu H, Sun L, et al. Early versus delayed hormonal therapy for prostate specific antigen only recurrence of prostate cancer after radical prostatectomy. J Urol 2004;171:1141–7.

[11] Messing EM, Manola J, Sarosdy M, et al. Immediate hormonal therapy compared with observation after radical prostatectomy and pelvic lymphadenectomy in men with node-positive prostate cancer. N Engl J Med 1999;341:1781–8.

[12] Messing EM. Re: disease progression and survival of patients with positive lymph nodes after radical prostatectomy. Is there a chance of cure? J Urol 2003;170:1955–6.

[13] Bolla M, Collette L, Blank L, et al. Long-term results with immediate androgen suppression and external irradiation in patients with locally advanced prostate cancer (an EORTC study): a phase III randomised trial. Lancet 2002;360:103–6.

[14] Pilepich MV, Caplan R, Byhardt RW, et al. Phase III trial of androgen suppression using goserelin in unfavorable-prognosis carcinoma of the prostate treated with definitive radiotherapy: report of Radiation Therapy Oncology Group Protocol 85-31. J Clin Oncol 1997;15:1013–21.

[15] D'Amico AV, Manola J, Loffredo M, et al. 6-month androgen suppression plus radiation therapy vs radiation therapy alone for patients with clinically localized prostate cancer: a randomized controlled trial. JAMA 2004;292:821–7.

[16] Debes JD, Tindall DJ. Mechanisms of androgen-refractory prostate cancer. N Engl J Med 2004;351: 1488–90.

[17] Petrylak DP. The current role of chemotherapy in metastatic hormone-refractory prostate cancer. Urology 2005;65(Suppl):3–7.

[18] Feldman BJ, Feldman D. The development of androgen-independent prostate cancer. Nat Rev Cancer 2001;1:34–45.

[19] Kemppainen JA, Lane MV, Sar M, et al. Androgen receptor phosphorylation, turnover, nuclear transport,

and transcriptional activation. Specificity for steroids and antihormones. J Biol Chem 1992;267:968–74.

[20] Holzbeierlein J, Lal P, LaTulippe E, et al. Gene expression analysis of human prostate carcinoma during hormonal therapy identifies androgen-responsive genes and mechanisms of therapy resistance. Am J Pathol 2004;164:217–27.

[21] Koivisto P, Kononen J, Palmberg C, et al. Androgen receptor gene amplification: a possible molecular mechanism for androgen deprivation therapy failure in prostate cancer. Cancer Res 1997;57:314–9.

[22] Linja MJ, Savinainen KJ, Saramaki OR, et al. Amplification and overexpression of androgen receptor gene in hormone-refractory prostate cancer. Cancer Res 2001;61:3550–5.

[23] Edwards J, Krishna NS, Grigor KM, et al. Androgen receptor gene amplification and protein expression in hormone refractory prostate cancer. Br J Cancer 2003;89:552–6.

[24] Edwards J, Bartlett JM. The androgen receptor and signal-transduction pathways in hormone-refractory prostate cancer. Part 1: modifications to the androgen receptor. BJU Int 2005;95:1320–6.

[25] Stanbrough M, Leav I, Kwan PW, et al. Prostatic intraepithelial neoplasia in mice expressing an androgen receptor transgene in prostate epithelium. Proc Natl Acad Sci USA 2001;98:10823–8.

[26] Chen CD, Welsbie DS, Tran C, et al. Molecular determinants of resistance to antiandrogen therapy. Nat Med 2004;10:33–9.

[27] Gregory CW, Johnson RT Jr, Mohler JL, et al. Androgen receptor stabilization in recurrent prostate cancer is associated with hypersensitivity to low androgen. Cancer Res 2001;61:2892–8.

[28] Veldscholte J, Ris-Stalpers C, Kuiper GG, et al. A mutation in the ligand binding domain of the androgen receptor of human LNCaP cells affects steroid binding characteristics and response to anti-androgens. Biochem Biophys Res Commun 1990;173:534–40.

[29] Tan J, Sharief Y, Hamil KG, et al. Dehydroepiandrosterone activates mutant androgen receptors expressed in the androgen-dependent human prostate cancer xenograft CWR22 and LNCaP cells. Mol Endocrinol 1997;11:450–9.

[30] Taplin ME, Bubley GJ, Ko YJ, et al. Selection for androgen receptor mutations in prostate cancers treated with androgen antagonist. Cancer Res 1999;59:2511–5.

[31] Taplin ME, Rajeshkumar B, Halabi S, et al. Androgen receptor mutations in androgen-independent prostate cancer: Cancer and Leukemia Group B Study 9663. J Clin Oncol 2003;21:2673–8.

[32] Han G, Buchanan G, Ittmann M, et al. Mutation of the androgen receptor causes oncogenic transformation of the prostate. Proc Natl Acad Sci USA 2005; 102:1151–6.

[33] Gottlieb B, Beitel LK, Wu JH, et al. The androgen receptor gene mutations database (ARDB): 2004 update. Hum Mutat 2004;23:527–33.

[34] Buchanan G, Greenberg NM, Scher HI, et al. Collocation of androgen receptor gene mutations in prostate cancer. Clin Cancer Res 2001;7:1273–81.

[35] Gregory CW, He B, Johnson RT, et al. A mechanism for androgen receptor-mediated prostate cancer recurrence after androgen deprivation therapy. Cancer Res 2001;61:4315–9.

[36] Yeh S, Chang C. Cloning and characterization of a specific coactivator, ARA70, for the androgen receptor in human prostate cells. Proc Natl Acad Sci USA 1996;93:5517–21.

[37] Miyamoto H, Yeh S, Wilding G, et al. Promotion of agonist activity of antiandrogens by the androgen receptor coactivator, ARA70, in human prostate cancer DU145 cells. Proc Natl Acad Sci USA 1998;95:7379–84.

[38] Fujimoto N, Yeh S, Kang HY, et al. Cloning and characterization of androgen receptor coactivator, ARA55, in human prostate. J Biol Chem 1999;274:8316–21.

[39] Culig Z, Comuzzi B, Steiner H, et al. Expression and function of androgen receptor coactivators in prostate cancer. J Steroid Biochem Mol Biol 2004;92:265–71.

[40] Culig Z, Steiner H, Bartsch G, et al. Mechanisms of endocrine therapy-responsive and -unresponsive prostate tumours. Endocr Relat Cancer 2005;12:229–44.

[41] Edwards J, Bartlett JM. The androgen receptor and signal-transduction pathways in hormone-refractory prostate cancer. Part 2: androgen-receptor cofactors and bypass pathways. BJU Int 2005;95:1327–35.

[42] Debes JD, Comuzzi B, Schmidt LJ, et al. p300 regulates androgen receptor-independent expression of prostate-specific antigen in prostate cancer cells treated chronically with interleukin-6. Cancer Res 2005;65:5965–73.

[43] Mirosevich J, Gao N, Gupta A, et al. The expression and role of Foxa proteins in prostate cancer. Prostate 2005; In press.

[44] Heinlein CA, Chang C. Androgen receptor in prostate cancer. Endocr Rev 2004;25:276–308.

[45] Wang L, Hsu CL, Chang C. Androgen receptor corepressors: an overview. Prostate 2005;63:117–30.

[46] Craft N, Shostak Y, Carey M, et al. A mechanism for hormone-independent prostate cancer through modulation of androgen receptor signaling by the HER-2/neu tyrosine kinase. Nat Med 1999;5:280–5.

[47] Arai Y, Yoshiki T, Yoshida O. c-erbB-2 oncoprotein: a potential biomarker of advanced prostate cancer. Prostate 1997;30:195–201.

[48] Yeh S, Lin HK, Kang HY, et al. From HER2/Neu signal cascade to androgen receptor and its coactivators: a novel pathway by induction of androgen target genes through MAP kinase in prostate cancer cells. Proc Natl Acad Sci USA 1999;96:5458–63.

[49] Wen Y, Hu MC, Makino K, et al. HER-2/neu promotes androgen-independent survival and growth of prostate cancer cells through the Akt pathway. Cancer Res 2000;60:6841–5.

[50] Graff JR, Konicek BW, McNulty AM, et al. Increased AKT activity contributes to prostate cancer progression by dramatically accelerating prostate tumor growth and diminishing p27Kip1 expression. J Biol Chem 2000;275:24500–5.

[51] Culig Z, Hobisch A, Cronauer MV, et al. Androgen receptor activation in prostatic tumor cell lines by insulin-like growth factor-I, keratinocyte growth factor, and epidermal growth factor. Cancer Res 1994;54:5474–8.

[52] Chan JM, Stampfer MJ, Giovannucci E, et al. Plasma insulin-like growth factor-I and prostate cancer risk: a prospective study. Science 1998;279:563–6.

[53] Jin RJ, Wang Y, Masumori N, et al. NE-10 neuroendocrine cancer promotes the LNCaP xenograft growth in castrated mice. Cancer Res 2004;64:5489–95.

[54] Cussenot O, Villette JM, Cochand-Priollet B, et al. Evaluation and clinical value of neuroendocrine differentiation in human prostatic tumors. Prostate Suppl 1998;8:43–51.

[55] Vashchenko N, Abrahamsson PA. Neuroendocrine differentiation in prostate cancer: implications for new treatment modalities. Eur Urol 2005;47:147–55.

[56] Reya T, Morrison SJ, Clarke MF, et al. Stem cells, cancer, and cancer stem cells. Nature 2001;414:105–11.

[57] Sell S, Pierce GB. Maturation arrest of stem cell differentiation is a common pathway for the cellular origin of teratocarcinomas and epithelial cancers. Lab Invest 1994;70:6–22.

[58] Isaacs JT, Coffey DS. Etiology and disease process of benign prostatic hyperplasia. Prostate Suppl 1989;2:33–50.

[59] De Marzo AM, Meeker AK, Epstein JI, et al. Prostate stem cell compartments: expression of the cell cycle inhibitor p27Kip1 in normal, hyperplastic, and neoplastic cells. Am J Pathol 1998;153:911–9.

[60] Rumpold H, Heinrich E, Untergasser G, et al. Neuroendocrine differentiation of human prostatic primary epithelial cells in vitro. Prostate 2002;53:101–8.

[61] Aumuller G, Leonhardt M, Janssen M, et al. Neurogenic origin of human prostate endocrine cells. Urology 1999;53:1041–8.

[62] Kurita T, Medina RT, Mills AA, et al. Role of p63 and basal cells in the prostate. Development 2004;131:4955–64.

[63] Wang Y, Hayward S, Cao M, et al. Cell differentiation lineage in the prostate. Differentiation 2001;68:270–9.

[64] Xue Y, Smedts F, Debruyne FM, et al. Identification of intermediate cell types by keratin expression in the developing human prostate. Prostate 1998;34:292–301.

[65] Collins AT, Habib FK, Maitland NJ, et al. Identification and isolation of human prostate epithelial

stem cells based on alpha(2)beta(1)-integrin expression. J Cell Sci 2001;114:3865–72.

[66] Hudson DL, O'Hare M, Watt FM, et al. Proliferative heterogeneity in the human prostate: evidence for epithelial stem cells. Lab Invest 2000;80:1243–50.

[67] Huss WJ, Gray DR, Greenberg NM, et al. Breast cancer resistance protein-mediated efflux of androgen in putative benign and malignant prostate stem cells. Cancer Res 2005;65:6640–50.

[68] Thiery JP. Epithelial-mesenchymal transitions in tumour progression. Nat Rev Cancer 2002;2:442–54.

[69] Grunert S, Jechlinger M, Beug H. Diverse cellular and molecular mechanisms contribute to epithelial plasticity and metastasis. Nat Rev Mol Cell Biol 2003;4:657–65.

[70] Gotzmann J, Mikula M, Eger A, et al. Molecular aspects of epithelial cell plasticity: implications for local tumor invasion and metastasis. Mutat Res 2004; 566:9–20.

[71] Garrod D, Chidgey M, North A. Desmosomes: differentiation, development, dynamics and disease. Curr Opin Cell Biol 1996;8:670–8.

[72] Wijnhoven BP, Dinjens WN, Pignatelli M. E-cadherin-catenin cell-cell adhesion complex and human cancer. Br J Surg 2000;87:992–1005.

[73] Perl AK, Wilgenbus P, Dahl U, et al. A causal role for E-cadherin in the transition from adenoma to carcinoma. Nature 1998;392:190–3.

[74] Kwok WK, Ling MT, Lee TW, et al. Up-regulation of TWIST in prostate cancer and its implication as a therapeutic target. Cancer Res 2005;65: 5153–62.

[75] Veveris-Lowe TL, Lawrence MG, Collard RL, et al. Kallikrein 4 (hK4) and prostate-specific antigen (PSA) are associated with the loss of E-cadherin and an epithelial-mesenchymal transition (EMT)-like effect in prostate cancer cells. Endocr Relat Cancer 2005;12:631–43.

ELSEVIER
SAUNDERS

Urol Clin N Am 33 (2006) 211–217

UROLOGIC
CLINICS
of North America

Advancing Prostate Cancer: Treatment Options for the Urologist

William T. Lowrance, MD, Sam S. Chang, MD*

Department of Urologic Surgery, A1302 Medical Center North, Vanderbilt University Medical Center,
Nashville, TN 37232-2765, USA

Advancing prostate cancer often presents the practicing urologist with serious treatment dilemmas. This patient population is extremely diverse, constantly evolving, and treatment options must be tailored to each individual patient. Patients who have advancing prostate cancer include those who have a prostate specific antigen (PSA) only recurrence (biochemical recurrence) after local therapy, and patients treated with androgen ablation therapy that demonstrate a rising PSA (generally considered hormone-refractory). Hormone-refractory prostate cancer is defined by consecutive PSA elevations despite castrate levels of testosterone. The onset of hormone-refractory prostate cancer has historically had a dismal prognosis; median survival has been reported in the 2–3 year range [1]. Oefelein and coworkers [2], however, recently demonstrated that this reported range of survival was not consistent with current clinical presentations. They reported the median survival after the development of hormone-refractory disease was approximately 40 months in those patients who had evidence of skeletal metastasis and 68 months in patients who did not have skeletal metastasis.

Huggins and Hodges [3] are credited with the discovery of androgen deprivation therapy for metastatic prostate cancer in 1941. Since their sentinel work, many advances have been made in the treatment of progressive prostate cancer, yet androgen ablation therapy is at best a temporary solution for most patients. The mechanisms by which prostate cancer cells become hormone independent are the subject of intense research but are still largely unknown.

The clinician must take individual patient histories into account when determining a treatment strategy. Prior therapies, current rate of disease progression, symptoms, and evidence of clinical and radiographic metastatic disease are just a few of the issues that must be carefully considered when adopting a treatment plan. The authors have attempted to outline a logical progression of treatment choices for the practicing urologist based on a case presentation that includes hormonal manipulations, chemotherapeutic options, and adjunctive therapies.

Case presentation

A 78 year-old white male who had prostate cancer with a Gleason score of 3 + 4 underwent radical prostatectomy 9 years ago. He had a PSA-only recurrence 3 years ago and subsequently initiated luteinizing hormone releasing hormone (LHRH) analog therapy. At that time there was no evidence of metastatic disease. His PSA quickly became undetectable until recently. Six months ago, his PSA was 0.3 ng/mL and has increased to 0.6 ng/mL. The patient still has no evidence of clinical disease.

When patients with prostate cancer experience disease progression, many are treated at some point with androgen deprivation. There is some debate about the timing of androgen deprivation therapy in men with asymptomatic advancing prostate cancer. For patients who have metastatic disease, Messing and coworkers [4] support immediate androgen deprivation therapy before the patient becomes symptomatic. Most patients,

---

* Corresponding author.

E-mail address: sam.chang@vanderbilt.edu (S.S. Chang).

regardless of whether they are asymptomatic or symptomatic, will have a palliative and biochemical response to the withdrawal of androgens. The duration of the response is dependent on several factors, particularly the presence or absence of radiographically demonstrated skeletal metastatic disease. For patients who have skeletal metastasis, response to androgen deprivation is approximately 3 years [2]. Response durations average more than 5 years for patients who have limited metastatic disease or no metastatic disease [2,5,6]. Many patients who are treated with androgen deprivation are thus destined to have a limited remission.

Patients who have progressive prostate cancer after androgen deprivation therapy should, at a minimum, have testosterone levels that are castrate before they are classified as having hormone refractory disease. The most common form of androgen ablation is LHRH agonists with or without antiandrogens. Although several randomized controlled trials have shown that maximum androgen blockade (LHRH agonist combined with an antiandrogen) offers a modest survival advantage over LHRH agonist therapy alone, many physicians and patients choose only LHRH therapy because of cost, side effects, and minimal survival benefit from maximum androgen blockade [7–11]. Castrate levels of testosterone can also be achieved with bilateral simple orchiectomy. Other alternative approaches that spare castrate levels of testosterone, such as antiandrogens (steroidal or nonsteroidal) with or without 5-alpha reductase inhibitors, have increased in popularity over the years [12]. However, randomized data that show the equivalence to other methods of castration are not available.

Regardless of the method, it is recommended that serum testosterone be measured for patients who have a rising PSA while on androgen deprivation therapy. If the patient does not have a testosterone level < 50 ng/dL, the initial therapeutic approach should be targeted toward testosterone reduction or complete blockade. Prospective clinical trials have not been performed to demonstrate a clinical benefit in maintaining castration once a patient relapses; however, retrospective studies have demonstrated a probable benefit [13,14]. Most clinicians do recommend that castration be continued despite disease progression, based on evidence that administration of exogenous testosterone has been shown to worsen patient symptoms [15].

Castrate patients who have progression of prostate cancer, either by PSA rise or by clinical manifestations, are appropriate candidates for systemic therapies. For those patients who may have had only LHRH therapy, an antiandrogen should be added to the treatment regimen. For those patients treated with maximum androgen blockade with an antiandrogen and LHRH agonist, the first therapeutic maneuver can be antiandrogen withdrawal. PSA declines after such a maneuver are well recognized, and occasional radiographic responses have been noted as well. The response of antiandrogen withdrawal varies with the half-life of the antiandrogen used. Flutamide (Eulexin; half-life approximately 6 hours) withdrawal responses typically occur within 28 days; whereas, bicalutamide (Casodex; half-life approximately 6 days) withdrawal responses may take up to 8 weeks [16].

The patient's PSA is observed for several months, but unfortunately it continues to climb even after the addition of an antiandrogen and the subsequent withdrawal of the antiandrogen.

At this point, secondary hormonal manipulators can be considered, especially in asymptomatic patients, because these agents are relatively nontoxic. In general, the benefit from a second-line hormone therapy is several months, but can be longer. Potential therapeutic choices within the class of second-line hormonal therapies include less commonly used antiandrogens (eg, nilutamide), adrenal and testicular enzyme inhibitors (eg, ketoconazole), corticosteroids, and estrogens.

Patients may respond differently to various antiandrogens, and no comparative trials are available to suggest that one might be better than another. Responses are clearly possible for patients who have failed one antiandrogen and are then treated with another [17,18]. However, relief of symptoms with antiandrogens used in the second-line setting has been uncommon. In the original leuprolide +/− flutamide randomized Intergroup clinical trial, the addition of flutamide to patients who failed daily leuprolide (lupron), had no effect upon patient survival [19].

Estrogens are active in patients who have both symptomatic and asymptomatic hormone-refractory disease. Mechanisms of action are not clearly understood, and randomized trials to evaluate estrogens in the second-line setting are not available. High doses of estrogens (eg, intravenous fosfestrol) are associated with a high risk of thromboembolic events; these potentially serious adverse effects have substantially limited the use of these agents [20]. Lower doses of estrogens (eg, oral diethylstilbestrol [DES] at 1–3 mg) are clearly active and are typically well tolerated except for nipple tenderness and gynecomastia. DES at an oral dose of 3 mg/day is associated with PSA declines in approximately 42% of patients [21].

Adrenal suppressants such as ketoconazole or aminoglutethimide may have benefit in selected patients. Ketoconazole (600–1200 mg/day) plus hydrocortisone demonstrated a surprisingly high response rate in terms of PSA reduction and potential reduction of symptoms in single-institution phase II trials [22]. Wilkerson and Chodak demonstrated that an intermediate dose of ketoconazole (300 mg) combined with hydrocortisone replacement provided a significant reduction in PSA in more than 50% of their patients and toxicity was limited. However, toxicity from ketoconazole at high doses may be problematic; gastrointestinal distress, visual disturbances, fatigue, and liver function abnormalities are not uncommon. Again, a lower dose of ketoconazole has been shown to be effective and have a better side effect profile [23]. Although these agents are commonly used in patients who have prostate cancer, they do not have a US Food and Drug Administration (FDA) indication.

Although not FDA approved, glucocorticoids such as hydrocortisone, prednisone, and dexamethasone are known to be active agents in prostate cancer. Side effects are clearly dose related, but dose-response curves for the treatment of prostate cancer have not been ascertained. Palliation of symptoms and PSA declines have been described in approximately one-third of the cases treated with low-dose (10–20 mg/day) prednisone [24]. Higher PSA response rates have been described with dexamethasone, a more potent glucocorticoid [25]. Glucocorticoids have been used in a number of randomized multicenter trials and have a well-defined side effect profile, including glucose intolerance, redistribution of body fat, easy bruising, and steroid myopathies. Care should be taken before abruptly discontinuing glucocorticoids to avoid an Addisonian crisis.

Despite the addition of estrogen, the patient's PSA continues to rise and is now 5.5 ng/mL only 18 months after it first began to increase. No clinical symptoms are present.

There is considerable debate about when to order a bone scan or a computed tomography (CT) scan in patients who have advancing prostate cancer. Clearly, if a patient has symptoms such as bone pain, an imaging study may be indicated regardless of PSA value. In asymptomatic patients, the PSA level can be used as a guide for ordering imaging studies. Many studies have attempted to define the optimal PSA level for ordering radionuclide bone scans. Cher and co-workers [26] found that the chance of having a positive bone scan when the PSA was 10 ng/mL or less was approximately 1% to 2%. They concluded there was little utility in ordering bone scans until the PSA level rose above 30–40 ng/mL. Swindle and colleagues [27] take a slightly more conservative approach and conclude that bone scans should be reserved for patients who have PSA values > 10–20 ng/mL or those with a rapidly rising PSA. Recent data presented by Chodak and colleagues [28] suggest that bone scans are not indicated when the PSA level is < 5 ng/mL in asymptomatic patients who have undergone local therapy for prostate cancer.

CT sensitivity for detecting local recurrence has been shown to be as low as 36% [29]. Despite the poor sensitivity of CT in diagnosing local recurrence, it can be effective for evaluating advancing or metastatic prostate cancer. CT scan is a valuable tool for identifying areas of prostate cancer progression and makes it possible to evaluate both soft tissue and bones. There are no official guidelines that outline PSA values of when one should consider ordering a bone scan or CT scan. Again, each patient scenario must be considered on an individual basis.

This patient desires aggressive therapy and evaluation. Although he continues to be asymptomatic, he is found to have bilateral pelvic lymphadenopathy on CT scan and a small, left ischial lesion on bone scan.

Until the past decade, chemotherapy was regarded as futile in patients who had metastatic hormone-refractory prostate cancer. Recently, two prospective randomized, phase-III trials have been published that report a palliative and survival benefit of certain chemotherapy regimens in patients who have systemic symptoms and good performance status. Both SWOG 9916 and TAX 327 are landmark studies that demonstrate the effectiveness of docetaxel (taxotere) chemotherapy in treating advanced prostate cancer.

The traditional FDA approved chemotherapeutic regimen for hormone-refractory prostate cancer was a combination of mitoxantrone and prednisone. In the SWOG 9916 trial, this regimen was compared with docetaxel combined with estramustine. The TAX 327 trial compared two schedules of docetaxel and prednisone against mitoxantrone and prednisone. In 770 patients,

SWOG 9916 demonstrated a 23% improvement in median survival when every 3 week doses of docetaxel and estramustine were compared with mitoxantrone and prednisone (18 months versus 15 months; $P = .008$) [30]. In TAX 327 a survival difference was also demonstrated when comparing every 3 week docetaxel/prednisone versus mitoxantrone/prednisone (18.9 months versus 16.5 months; $P = .009$). A significant improvement in pain response and a $> 50\%$ decrease in serum PSA was also observed in TAX 327 [31]. Interestingly, there was no survival advantage with the weekly dosing of docetaxel and prednisone. These studies provide the first prospective, randomized data that demonstrate a survival benefit for patients who have metastatic hormone-refractory disease and are treated with chemotherapy. Docetaxel has now been approved by the FDA for treatment of metastatic hormone-refractory prostate cancer. Other drug combinations and schedules with docetaxel are the subject of active clinical investigation, because single agent docetaxel is not the final answer. Docetaxel may have a role in the neoadjuvant setting for locally advanced disease or possibly for treating patients who have PSA-only relapse. A small trial by Febbo and coworkers [32] showed that neoadjuvant docetaxel decreased PSA by more than 50% and also decreased tumor volume on endorectal MRI. Currently there are multiple clinical trials to examine other roles for docetaxel in the treatment of advanced prostate cancer. It is difficult to create precise and universal algorithms for the use of docetaxel because of the heterogeneous nature of prostate cancer and the lack of prospective trials in the different disease states. The optimal timing and regimen remain unknown at this time.

The patient has a PSA decline, but after six months, despite docetaxel treatment, our patient becomes symptomatic from his bone metastasis. A repeat bone scan demonstrates progression of the lesion in his left ischium.

In addition to systemic therapies, other therapeutic interventions are important for castrate patients who have progressive hormone-refractory disease, especially if they have bony metastases, local progression, or pain symptoms. These treatments include bone-targeted therapies, local control of cancer complications, and aggressive pain management.

Bone-targeted therapies can optimize outcomes for patients with bony metastases include integrating the timely use of radiotherapy, bone-seeking radiopharmaceuticals, and bisphosphonate therapy. These bone-targeted therapies attempt to improve quality of life and may slow progression of disease.

External beam radiotherapy (EBRT) is the standard for treatment of focal, painful, osseous metastases and in the treatment and prevention of spinal cord and nerve root compression. Early suspicion of possible epidural disease is important, and significant pain should trigger a neurological evaluation including an MRI scan [33]. For patients who have neurologic compromise, neurosurgical stabilization should be combined with urgent EBRT and steroidal therapy (dexamethasone 4–10 mg/qid) to optimize results. For other patients who have focal, painful, osseous metastases, a short course of EBRT is highly effective for palliation of pain; partial response rates $> 80\%$ and complete response rates of 25%–40% have been reported [34,35]. However, the optimal fractionation schedule is controversial and varies greatly between a single fraction and 10 treatments over 2 weeks [36,37].

Bisphosphonate therapy with zoledronic acid is one category of therapy for metastatic prostate cancer targeted to bone that has FDA approval. Bisphosphonates are pyrophosphate analogs that block osteoclast activity in normal and diseased bone, tilting the balance in favor of bone stabilization and recovery. A recent randomized, prospective study from Saad and colleagues [38] demonstrated a beneficial effect for zoledronic acid in patients who had hormone-refractory prostate cancer and bone metastases that were evident with radiographs. Adverse skeletal related events (eg, fracture, need for EBRT, or need for surgery) were less common in patients treated with zoledronic acid (33.3%) versus placebo (44.2%), and the time to first skeletal related event was substantially delayed in the treatment group. In addition, the progressive increase in average pain intensity that was seen in the placebo group was abrogated in patients who were in the treatment group, which suggests a palliative effect. Other measures to optimize bone health, such as supplementation with calcium (1200 mg/day) and vitamin D (400–800 IU/day) and counseling about the importance of a healthy diet, regular weight-bearing exercise, smoking cessation, and moderation of alcohol intake, should be strongly considered [39].

Bone-seeking radiopharmaceuticals, such as Strontium 89, Samarium 153 (both FDA approved), and Rhenium 188, also have a role in the management of diffuse symptomatic metastatic disease. These agents have potential for palliation at multiple sites and may delay development of the next symptomatic sites. The most commonly used agent has been Strontium 89, typically administered as a single dose of 150 MBq (4 mCi). Subjective response rates range from 35% to 89% [40–42] and the duration of response ranges from 3 to 12 months [41]. Complete resolution of painful symptoms may be seen in 10% of patients; a flare in pain has been reported in 23% of patients [42]. The combination of strontium with doxorubicin for patients with advanced androgen-independent prostate cancer who have responded to induction chemotherapy may lead to a survival benefit (27.7 months versus 16.8 months; $P = .0014$) according to one small randomized trial [43]. Samarium 153 also has been associated with pain relief in approximately two-thirds of patients in placebo-controlled, randomized trials [44,45]. There is, however, reluctance to pursue the use of bone-seeking radiopharmaceuticals because of the bone marrow suppression that can ensue.

After external beam radiation therapy our patient's bone pain improves. Unfortunately, he develops lower urinary tract symptoms and hematuria.

Patients who have advanced prostate cancer can also develop local progression that can manifest as ureteral or bowel obstruction, urinary retention, chronic irritative voiding symptoms, persistent hematuria, or troublesome proctitis. Close urologic monitoring is recommended for early recognition and treatment of these conditions, which can be associated with substantial morbidity. There are various local control measures that can substantially improve quality of life.

Medical management, such as anticholinergic therapy for voiding symptoms or steroid enemas for proctitis, is preferred, but some patients may require surgical intervention (eg, limited transurethral resection) for obstruction. The patient may even require more extensive surgery, such as urinary or bowel diversion, either by intubation (urethral, suprapubic catheter, or nephrostomy tube) or surgery (diverting colostomy or ileal conduit), to optimize quality of life. Other therapies that target localized disease in this setting are considered experimental; examples include radiofrequency ablation, cryosurgery, high intensity focused ultrasound, and chemoembolization.

Supportive and palliative-care measures are particularly important for patients who have hormone-refractory prostate cancer, especially as disease progresses and quality-of-life considerations take precedence. The presence or absence of pain should always be ascertained when the patient is evaluated; if pain is present, it should be assessed in detail. Current guidelines suggest initial management should consist of nonsteroidal anti-inflammatory drugs (NSAIDs) or acetaminophen for mild pain, or opioids for moderate to severe pain [46–48]. Use of immediate-release preparations over a period of 24–48 hours will establish the appropriate dose of slow-release medication. Conversion to morphine equivalent doses is often helpful.

After conversion to a slow-release preparation, immediate-release drugs can be used for relief of "breakthrough" pain. Patients should be instructed to document the use of breakthrough medications to adjust the slow-release preparation accordingly. Because gastrointestinal motility is slowed by opioids, a bowel regimen that consists of both a stool softener and a stimulant should be initiated simultaneously. Bulk-forming agents should be avoided in this setting because patients who do not drink enough fluid can actually become more constipated. Nausea may be temporary and should be treated with antiemetics. Metaclopramide enhances gastric motility and can alleviate nausea and vomiting. Some patients may require chronic antiemetic therapy.

When oral opioid therapy is no longer adequate, additional strategies should be considered, including NSAIDs, antidepressant or anticonvulsant drugs, and parenteral opioids. Rarely, an interventional approach such as a nerve block, chordotomy, or insertion of an epidural or intrathecal catheter is required. Other non-pharmacological approaches should also be considered. Psychological, psychosocial, and spiritual strategies should be explored where appropriate.

Most patients who have advanced hormone-refractory prostate cancer will experience pain at some time during disease progression, and the assessment and treatment of pain should be a top priority. Good pain management frequently involves a multidisciplinary team consisting of the urologist, medical and radiation oncologists, a pain specialist, a psychologist, and nurse or hospice personnel.

Summary

Since the landmark discovery by Huggins and Hodges over half a century ago, much progress has been made in regard to treating advancing prostate cancer. Our understanding of and ability to treat hormone-refractory prostate cancer is constantly evolving. There are numerous clinical trials underway to evaluate novel chemotherapeutic agents and their effectiveness against various stages of prostate cancer. Today's urologist has multiple treatment options available. The treatment strategies presented here include hormonal manipulations, chemotherapeutic options, and adjunctive therapies, and can serve as a guide when caring for this patient population. A mutlidisciplinary approach is important to maximize patient survival and quality of life. The heterogeneity of patients who have advancing prostate cancer makes their treatment especially challenging and necessitates individualized care.

References

[1] Eisenberger MA, Carducci MA. Chemotherapy for hormone-resistant prostate cancer. Campbell's Urology, vol. 4. 8th edition. Philadelphia: Saunders; 2002.

[2] Oefelein MG, Agarwal PK, Resnick MI. Survival of patients with hormone refractory prostate cancer in the prostate specific antigen era. J Urol 2004;171(4): 1525–8.

[3] Huggins C, Hodges C. Studies on prostate cancer. I: The effect of castration of estrogen and androgen injection on serum phosphatases in metastatic carcinoma of the prostate. Cancer Res 1941;1:293.

[4] Messing E. The timing of hormone therapy for men with asymptomatic advanced prostate cancer. Urol Oncol 2003;21(4):245–54.

[5] Oefelein MG, Ricchiuti VS, Conrad PW, et al. Clinical predictors of androgen-independent prostate cancer and survival in the prostate-specific antigen era. Urology 2002;60(1):120–4.

[6] Crawford ED, Allen JA. Treatment of newly diagnosed state D2 prostate cancer with leuprolide and flutamide or leuprolide alone, phase III, intergroup study 0036. J Steroid Biochem Mol Biol 1990; 37(6):961–3.

[7] Maximum androgen blockade in advanced prostate cancer: an overview of the randomised trials. Prostate Cancer Trialists' Collaborative Group. Lancet 2000;355(9214):1491–8.

[8] Eisenberger MA, Blumenstein BA, Crawford ED, et al. Bilateral orchiectomy with or without flutamide for metastatic prostate cancer. N Engl J Med 1998;339(15):1036–42.

[9] Smith JA, Chang SS, Keane TE, et al. Androgen deprivation: research, results, and reimbrusement. Contemporary Urology 2005; June.

[10] Aprikian AG, Fleshner N, Langleben A, et al. An oncology perspective on the benefits and cost of combined androgen blockade in advanced prostate cancer. Can J Urol 2003;10(5):1986–94.

[11] Amling CL. Advanced prostate cancer treatment guidelines: a United States perspective. BJU Int 2004; 94(Suppl 3):7–8.

[12] Fleshner NE, Trachtenberg J. Combination finasteride and flutamide in advanced carcinoma of the prostate: effective therapy with minimal side effects. J Urol 1995;154(5):1642–5 [discussion 1645–46].

[13] Pienta KJ, Redman B, Hussain M, et al. Phase II evaluation of oral estramustine and oral etoposide in hormone-refractory adenocarcinoma of the prostate. J Clin Oncol 1994;12(10):2005–12.

[14] Taylor CD, Elson P, Trump DL. Importance of continued testicular suppression in hormone-refractory prostate cancer. J Clin Oncol 1993;11(11): 2167–72.

[15] Fowler JE, Whitmore WF. The response of metastatic adenocarcinoma of the prostate to exogenous testosterone. J Urol 1981;126:372–5.

[16] Schellhammer PF, Venner P, Haas GP, et al. Prostate specific antigen decreases after withdrawal of antiandrogen therapy with bicalutamide or flutamide in patients receiving combined androgen blockade. J Urol 1997;157(5):1731–5.

[17] Sartor O, Eastham JA. Progressive prostate cancer associated with use of megestrol acetate administered for control of hot flashes. South Med J 1999; 92(4):415–6.

[18] Scher HI, Liebertz C, Kelly WK, et al. Bicalutamide for advanced prostate cancer: the natural versus treated history of disease. J Clin Oncol 1997;15(8): 2928–38.

[19] Crawford ED, Eisenberger MA, McLeod DG, et al. A controlled trial of leuprolide with and without flutamide in prostatic carcinoma. N Engl J Med 1989; 321(7):419–24.

[20] Ferro MA, Gillatt D, Symes MO, et al. High-dose intravenous estrogen therapy in advanced prostatic carcinoma. Use of serum prostate-specific antigen to monitor response. Urology 1989;34(3):134–8.

[21] Smith DC, Redman BG, Flaherty LE, et al. A phase II trial of oral diethylstilbesterol as a second-line hormonal agent in advanced prostate cancer. Urology 1998;52(2):257–60.

[22] Small EJ, Baron AD, Fippin L, et al. Ketoconazole retains activity in advanced prostate cancer patients with progression despite flutamide withdrawal. J Urol 1997;157(4):1204–7.

[23] Wilkinson S, Chodak G. An evaluation of intermediate-dose ketoconazole in hormone refractory prostate cancer. Eur Urol 2004;45(5):581–4 [discussion 585].

[24] Tannock I, Gospodarowicz M, Meakin W, et al. Treatment of metastatic prostatic cancer with low-dose prednisone: evaluation of pain and quality of life as pragmatic indices of response. J Clin Oncol 1989;7(5):590–7.

[25] Nishimura K, Nonomura N, Yasunaga Y, et al. Low doses of oral dexamethasone for hormone-refractory prostate carcinoma. Cancer 2000;89(12):2570–6.

[26] Cher ML, Bianco FJ Jr, Lam JS, et al. Limited role of radionuclide bone scintigraphy in patients with prostate specific antigen elevations after radical prostatectomy. J Urol 1998;160(4):1387–91.

[27] Swindle PW, Kattan MW, Scardino PT. Markers and meaning of primary treatment failure. Urol Clin North Am 2003;30(2):377–401.

[28] Chodak GW, Iverson P, McLeod DG, et al. Prostate-specific antigen levels as a predictor of positive bone scans during follow-up after standard care for prostate cancer: data from the bicalutamide early prostate cancer program. Poster presented at the annual meeting of the American Urological Association, San Antonio, Texas; May 21–26, 2005.

[29] Kramer S, Gorich J, Gottfried HW, et al. Sensitivity of computed tomography in detecting local recurrence of prostatic carcinoma following radical prostatectomy. Br J Radiol 1997;70(838):995–9.

[30] Petrylak DP, Tangen C, Hussain M, et al. SWOG 99–16: Randomized phase III trial of docetaxel (D)/estramustine (E) versus mitoxantrone (M)/prednisone (P) in men with androgen-independent prostate cancer (AIPCA). Proc Am Soc Clin Oncol 2004;23:2 [plenary presentation #3].

[31] Eisenberger MA, De Wit R, Berry W, et al. A multicenter phase III comparison of docetaxel (D) + prednisone (P) and mitoxantrone (MTZ) + P in patients with hormone-refractory prostate cancer (HRPC). Proc Am Soc Clin Oncol 2004;23:2 [plenary presentation #4].

[32] Febbo PG, Richie JP, George DJ, et al. Neoadjuvant docetaxel before radical prostatectomy in patients with high-risk localized prostate cancer. Clin Cancer Res 2005;11(14):5233–40.

[33] Chang SS, Benson MC, Campbell SC, et al. Society of Urologic Oncology position statement: redefining the management of hormone-refractory prostate carcinoma. Cancer 2005;103(1):11–21.

[34] Gaze MN, Kelly CG, Kerr GR, et al. Pain relief and quality of life following radiotherapy for bone metastases: a randomised trial of two fractionation schedules. Radiother Oncol 1997;45(2):109–16.

[35] Nielson OS, Bentzen SM, Sandberg E, et al. Randomized trial of single dose versus fractionated palliative radiotherapy of bone metastases. Radiother Oncol 1998;47:233–40.

[36] Ben-Josef E, Shamsa F, Williams AO, et al. Radiotherapeutic management of osseous metastases: a survey of current patterns of care. Int J Radiat Oncol Biol Phys 1998;40(4):915–21.

[37] Chow E, Danjoux C, Wong R, et al. Palliation of bone metastases: a survey of patterns of practice among Canadian radiation oncologists. Radiother Oncol 2000;56(3):305–14.

[38] Saad F, Gleason DM, Murray R, et al. A randomized, placebo-controlled trial of zoledronic acid in patients with hormone-refractory metastatic prostate carcinoma. J Natl Cancer Inst 2002;94(19):1458–68.

[39] Ross RW, Small EJ. Osteoporosis in men treated with androgen deprivation therapy for prostate cancer. J Urol 2002;167(5):1952–6.

[40] Oosterhof GO, Roberts JT, de Reijke TM, et al. Strontium(89) chloride versus palliative local field radiotherapy in patients with hormonal escaped prostate cancer: a phase III study of the European Organisation for Research and Treatment of Cancer, Genitourinary Group. Eur Urol 2003;44(5):519–26.

[41] Pons F, Herranz R, Garcia A, et al. Strontium-89 for palliation of pain from bone metastases in patients with prostate and breast cancer. Eur J Nucl Med 1997;24(10):1210–4.

[42] Kraeber-Bodere F, Campion L, Rousseau C, et al. Treatment of bone metastases of prostate cancer with strontium-89 chloride: efficacy in relation to the degree of bone involvement. Eur J Nucl Med 2000;27(10):1487–93.

[43] Tu SM, Millikan RE, Mengistu B, et al. Bone-targeted therapy for advanced androgen-independent carcinoma of the prostate: a randomised phase II trial. Lancet 2001;357(9253):336–41.

[44] Serafini AN, Houston SJ, Resche I, et al. Palliation of pain associated with metastatic bone cancer using samarium-153 lexidronam: a double-blind placebo-controlled clinical trial. J Clin Oncol 1998;16(4):1574–81.

[45] Sartor O, Reid RH, Hoskin PJ, et al. Samarium-153-Lexidronam complex for treatment of painful bone metastases in hormone-refractory prostate cancer. Urology 2004;63(5):940–5.

[46] Managment of cancer pain. 1994. Rockville, MD: Department of Health and Human Services, Public Health Service, Agency of Health Care Policy and Research, publication # AHCPR 94–0592.

[47] Principles of analgesic use in treatment of acute pain and cancer pain. 5th edition. Glenview (IL): American Pain Society; 2003.

[48] American Cancer Society's Guide to pain control. Powerful methods to overcome cancer pain. Atlanta (GA): American Cancer Society; 2001.

ELSEVIER
SAUNDERS

Urol Clin N Am 33 (2006) 219–226

UROLOGIC
CLINICS
of North America

Radiation Therapy and Radio-nuclides for Palliation of Bone Pain

Juanita Crook, MD, FRCPC

*Department of Radiation Oncology, University of Toronto/Princess Margaret Hospital,
610 University Avenue, Toronto, Ontario M5G 2M9, Canada*

The therapeutic goals in the management of metastatic prostate cancer are to optimize quality of life and effectively palliate pain from bone metastases. An integrated approach to pain management, and the timely use of palliative radiotherapy and radio-isotopes are key components. Pain relief should be both expedient and durable because the pain from bone metastases can markedly diminish a patient's mobility and quality of life, and is often compounded by anxiety and depression [1].

External radiotherapy

Radiotherapy is the cornerstone of the management of painful osseous metastases and the treatment and prevention of spinal cord and nerve root compression. Bone metastases are associated with a significant increase in morbidity, largely caused by pain, which becomes refractory to analgesia. Androgen ablation is the initial treatment of choice but most patients become hormone refractory within 2–3 years. A short course of external beam radiotherapy is very effective in pain palliation: response rates are more than 80% and complete response rates are 15%–40% [1–3]. The response is quicker and more durable than that from any of the systemic therapies [4]. The median onset of pain relief is 3 weeks [5] and the duration is 13–24 weeks [1,5]. Despite the fact that palliation represents almost 50% of the practice of radiotherapy [4], and the palliation of bone

pain is the most common palliative referral, the optimal fractionation schedule remains controversial and varies from one health care system to another. Several randomized trials (Table 1) have addressed this issue and have failed to show a dose-response effect. A single fraction of 6–10 Gy appears to be as effective as a more prolonged fractionation scheme such as 20 Gy in 5 fractions, 30 Gy in 10 fractions, or 40.5 in 15 fractions [1,3,5–8]. A meta-analysis of 3260 patients randomized in seven studies did not detect a difference in complete and overall pain relief between single and multi-fraction regimens, or evidence for a dose response in the various multi-fraction schedules [9].

Endpoints

One of the problems with assessing the published literature on efficacy of palliative treatment is the lack of uniformity in assessment of response. Patient self-assessment of pain score and requirements for analgesics are common to all, but pain assessment scales vary and the need for narcotic analgesics may be altered by pain other than at the index site. Response may be defined as an improvement in the pain score of at least one increment in a 5-point scale of none, mild, moderate, severe, or intractable [1,3], or an improvement of 2 points on an 11-point scale [5]. Others use a 4-point scale (none, mild, moderate, or severe) [10,11], or a visual-analog scale [3,12]. A complete response may be defined as a pain score of zero regardless of analgesic intake, or may require a pain score of zero and an analgesic score

E-mail address: Juanita.crook@rmp.uhn.on.ca

Table 1
Randomized trials of various fractionation schemes

Author (year)	n	Schedules compared	% prostate	Onset & duration	Morbidity	Re-treatments
Tong et al. [11]	266 (solitary)	40.5/15/3 wks vs 20/5/1 wk	14%[a]	Onset faster for 20/5	fractures in treated site 18% vs 4%	24% for 20/5[b]
Tong et al. [11]	750 (multiple sites)	30/10/2 wks 15/5/1 wk 20/5/1 wk 25/5/1 wk	14%[a]	RR 90% Med duration 12 wks nd		23% for 15/5[b]
Blitzer [13]	759 (subset of Tong)	Per Tong	14%	ns	ns	11–16% for 40.5/15, 30/10, 20/5 & 25/5 23% for 15/5
Price et al. [10]	288	8/1/1 d vs 20/5/1 wk	10%	nd	nd	15/140 (11%) vs 4/148 (3%)
Gaze et al. [1]	280	10/1/1 d vs 22.5/5/1 wk	27%	nd duration: 13.5 vs 14 wk RR 84% vs 89% CR 15% vs 14%	nd	ns
Nielson et al. [3]	241	8/1/1 d vs 20/5/1 wk	33%	RR 80% vs 82% CR 15% each arm	nd	25/120 (21%) 8/1 vs 14/119 (12%) (20/5)
Yarnold [14]	765	8/1/1 d vs 20/5/1 wk 30/10/2 wks	34%	78% RR CR 57% vs 58%	nd	23% (8/1) vs 10% (20/5 or 30/10)
Steenland et al. [5]	1171	8/1/1 d vs 24/6/1 wk	24%	TTR 3 wks both arms TTP 20 vs 24 wks	nd	25% (8/1) vs 7% (24/6)
Hartsell et al. [8]	897	8/1/1 d vs 30/10/2 wks	50%	CR 15% (8/1) vs 18% PR 50% vs 48%	Grade 2–4 acute toxcitiy higher in 30/10 arm 17% vs 10% $P < 0.0001$	ns

Abbreviations: CR, Complete response; nd, no difference; ns, not stated; RR, response rate; TTP, time to progression; TTR, time to response.

[a] Overall % of prostate primaries in the solitary and multiple metastatic populations combined [13].

[b] 16% re-treatment rate overall.

of zero. Other important considerations are tolerance of treatment (nausea, vomiting, and fatigue), subsequent pathologic fracture or development of cord compression at the index site, or need for re-treatment at that site. Changes in systemic treatment may also confound results.

The Radiation Therapy Oncology Group (RTOG) 74-02 trial provides a dramatic example of how the method of analysis and definition of endpoint can influence results. This trial was first reported by Tong and coworkers [11] and concluded that short fractionation schedules were as effective as more protracted fractionation schemes. The data were subsequently re-analyzed

by Blitzer [13] and the opposite conclusion was reported: higher total doses from more prolonged fractionation schemes were associated with better outcome. Blitzer combined the solitary and multiple metastases populations that had been analyzed separately in the original report, and analyzed them together, but excluded 45% of the 266 patients randomized in the solitary metastasis, often because the lesions weren't truly solitary, and 18% of the patients randomized to the multiple metastases group. The remaining 759 (only 75% of the original study) were analyzed with an emphasis on "complete combined pain relief" (ie, zero pain score and zero analgesic intake). With this endpoint, the most prolonged fractionation scheme showed a significant advantage ($P = .003$). However, the endpoints discussed in the original publication by Tong and colleagues [11], such as frequency, promptness, and duration of pain relief were not discussed. A short course of radiotherapy that produces prompt pain relief and that can subsequently be maintained with lesser doses of analgesics may be more beneficial to a patient who has a limited life span than the commitment to a 3 or 4 week course of therapy for a marginally better result.

Similarly, the work of Arcangeli and coworkers [12] is often cited as evidence that prolonged fractionation and high total dose offer significant advantages in palliation of bone pain. They report results for 205 patients who were selected to receive either 40–46 Gy in 20–23 fractions in 5+ weeks, 30–36 Gy in 10–12 fractions in 2+ weeks, or 8–28 Gy in 1–4 consecutive fractions. Short courses were selected when there was a risk of bone fracture and longer courses when performance status was good and a longer life expectancy was anticipated. Not surprisingly, they reported fewer complete responses with a short course of radiotherapy, and longer survival with a protracted course, clearly a reflection of the different patient populations selected for each treatment type.

Acute tolerance

The literature fails to demonstrate any difference in acute tolerance of single fractions versus the various more prolonged one-, two- or three-week fractionation schemes. Nielson [3] (n = 241) compared a single 8 Gy to 20 Gy in 5 fractions over 1 week and reported no difference in acute toxicity between the two arms; 65% of patients reported no adverse effects. Steenland [5] (n = 1171) compared a single 8 Gy to 24 Gy in 6 fractions and similarly found no difference in acute nausea, vomiting, or fatigue between the two arms. The only serious adverse effects were one case of ileus in the 24 Gy in six arms, and one case of enteritis in the single 8 Gy arm. Gaze and colleagues [1] (n = 280) randomized patients to a single 10 Gy versus 22.5 Gy in 5 fractions over one week. There was no difference between the two arms in the incidence or severity of acute toxicity; 63% of patients reported no anorexia, nausea, or vomiting. The majority (73%) reported some degree of fatigue. Ninety-five percent of patients were

followed until death and no adverse late effects were noted. When single fractions are compared with a 2 week fractionated course of 30 Gy in 10 fractions, Price [10] (n = 288) found no difference in acute tolerance, although in a recent RTOG randomized study, Hartsell and colleagues [7,8] (n = 897) reported a significantly higher incidence of grade 2–4 acute toxicity in the protracted fractionation arm (17% versus 10%; $P < .001$).

Re-treatments

It is apparent from reviewing the randomized trials that the need for re-treatment of the index site may be higher in the single fraction group [5,14]. The largest randomized trial reported is that of the Dutch Bone Metastasis Study, which randomized 1171 patients to receive either a single fraction of 8 Gy or 6 fractions of 4 Gy (24 Gy in 6). Response to treatment was seen in 71% of patients (78% for prostate primaries, with 41% complete responses); the median time to response was 3 weeks in both treatment arms. No difference was found between the two arms in quality of life, side effects, or changes in pain medication requirements [5]. However, re-treatment for repeat palliation at the same site was more common in the single fraction group (25%) than in the more protracted fractionation arm (7%, $P < .001$) and occurred earlier, at an average of 14 weeks versus 23 weeks. However, the authors noted that the treating physicians were more apt to offer re-treatment after a single fraction, because this tended to occur at a lower pain score than did re-treatments after a fractionated course. Although the frequency of re-treatment in the single fraction arm undermined some of the economic advantage of this approach, there was still an overall cost saving. For patients in a group characterized by limited life expectancy and for whom travel can be very uncomfortable, the fact that 75% can be effectively palliated with a single fraction of radiotherapy cannot be over-emphasized. A subsequently published economic analysis [15] of this trial concluded that single fraction radiotherapy provided equivalent pain relief and quality of life at a lower medical and societal cost.

Konski [16] recently analyzed the cost-effectiveness of various possible treatment scenarios for metastatic prostate cancer including supportive care and pain medication only, chemotherapy with mitoxantrone and prednisone, and multi-fraction and single fraction palliative radiotherapy.

Although multi-fraction radiotherapy had a slightly higher "quality-adjusted life (QAL) months" rating (6.25 versus 6.1), single fraction radiotherapy was the most cost-effective palliative treatment as measured in $/QAL-years: $6857 versus $36,000 for multi-fraction regimens.

Fractures and cord compression

In the RTOG randomized trial, Tong and coworkers [11] reported that for the solitary metastasis population (n = 277), subsequent fractures occurred in 18% of patients treated with 40.5 Gy in 15 fractions over 3 weeks as compared with 4% of those receiving 20 Gy in 5 fractions over 1 week. Unfortunately, this trial did not have a single fraction arm. Results of a study by Nielson and colleagues [3] support the RTOG finding. They compared a single 8 Gy versus 20 Gy in 5 fractions and found the fracture rate to be 5% in both arms of the trial. Steenland and coworkers [5] (n = 1171) randomized patients to a single 8 Gy versus 24 Gy in 6 fractions and reported the subsequent fracture rate to be 4% in the 8 Gy arm as compared with only 2% in the multi-fraction arm ($P < 0.05$).

In the trial conducted by Steenland and coworkers [5], cord compressions were seen in 2% of each study arm. Price's much smaller study [10] (n = 288) reported one cord compression in the multi-fraction regimen versus 2 in the single fraction arm.

Practice patterns

Despite the solid evidence base and obvious economic advantages of a single fraction, surveys of patterns of care from the United States [6], Canada [17], Australia, and New Zealand [18] continue to indicate that longer fractionation schemes are preferred, specifically 30 Gy in 10 fractions in the United States, and 20 Gy in 5 fractions in Canada, Australia, and New Zealand. The reasons behind this are not clear. A survey of patterns of care in the United States by Ben Josef and coworkers [6] revealed that longer fractionation schemes were preferred by an overwhelming 98% of the 817 practitioners who responded to the survey. The preferred fractionation was 30 Gy in 10 fractions over 2 weeks for 77% of practitioners; 40 Gy in 15 fractions in 3 weeks and 40 Gy in 20 fractions in 4 weeks were ranked second and third. The longer fractionation schemes were particularly popular among physicians in private practice and those in practice for more than 15 years. It was suggested by the authors that reimbursement considerations may be instrumental in the choice of fractionation. Rose and Kagan [4] published an American College of Radiology consensus statement on the radiotherapeutic palliation of bone metastases. Single fractions of 6–8 Gy were only thought to be appropriate in the case of rib metastases. However, in Canada, only 10% of 172 practitioners would prefer 30 Gy in 10 fractions over 2 weeks, and the most commonly prescribed dose was 20 Gy in 5 fractions over 1 week. Only 17% preferred a single fraction [17], although this was used more commonly for prostate primaries (31%). In the Australian and New Zealand practice survey, prescription also varied with primary tumor site, and single fractions were used for palliation of bone pain in 42% of lung, 28% of prostate, and only 15% of breast primaries [18]. All three of these national surveys were performed before the publication of the Dutch bone metastases trial [5] (n = 1171) and the recent RTOG 97-14 trial [7, 8]. The influence of these trials on practice patterns has yet to be evaluated.

The Cancercare Ontario Practice Guidelines initiative has recently formulated an evidence-based guideline, which recommends the use of a single 8 Gy for palliation of uncomplicated symptomatic bone metastases [19]. Referring physicians and care-givers should be made aware that repeat treatment is feasible and effective. The recommendation does not apply to lesions that involve the skull, hands, or feet, or to lesions that cause cord compression or pathologic fracture. Weight-bearing bones that appear to be at high risk for fracture (lytic lesion in long bone > 2.5 cm or involving > 50% of the circumference of the cortical bone [17]) should be assessed by an orthopedic surgeon but radiotherapy is still indicated post-fixation. Compliance with this practice guideline has yet to be assessed.

Half-body irradiation

For widespread symptomatic metastatic bone disease, half-body irradiation can be used for rapid palliation. A single dose is rapidly effective and provides pain relief as early as 24 hours in one-third of patients [20] and a median onset of relief in 3 days. Maximal pain relief is reported in 8 days [21] and is maintained until death in the majority of cases (median time is 5 months) [20]. A dose of 6 Gy is commonly used for the upper half body (no lung correction) and 8 Gy for the lower half. The major toxicity from upper half-body radiotherapy is upper gastrointestinal (nausea and vomiting); diarrhea and abdominal discomfort are associated with lower half-body treatments. Hematologic toxicity is common for both, and the percent drop in peripheral counts from baseline to nadir (at 1–2 weeks) is 18% for hemoglobin, 48% for white blood cells, and 57% for platelets [21]. Recovery occurs in 4–6 weeks. Effectiveness is similar but may be more durable, and toxicity is reduced with fractionated schemes such as 15 Gy in 5 fractions over 5 days, which minimize the need for pre-medication [22]. The median duration of pain relief for a fractionated course of 25–30 Gy in 9–10 fractions was 8.5 months in one small report of 15 patients [22]. In a comparison of single dose versus a fractionated regimen, Zelefsky [22] reported complete pain relief at 24–48 hours in the single dose group (n = 14) compared with 1–2 weeks in the fractionated group (n = 14). However, complete response was seen in 86% of the fractionated group versus 76% of the single-dose group and re-treatments were eventually required much more often in the single-dose group (71% versus 13%).

Radiopharmaceuticals

Systemic radiopharmaceuticals such as strontium 89, rhenium 188, and samarium 153 also have a role in the management of diffuse symptomatic metastatic disease. Strontium 89 has a longer physical half-life of 50.5 days and decays with a maximum energy beta emission of 1.5 MeV. The range in tissue is about 0.8 cm. It is preferentially taken up in osteoblastic sites; the biologic half-life in healthy bone is about 14 days. Samarium 153 EDTMP (ethylene-diamine-tetra-methylene-phosphonic acid) has a short physical half-life of 46.8 hours and a low energy beta emission of a maximum of 0.81 MeV. Rhenium 188 HEDP (hydroxyethylene diphosphonic acid) has a half-life of 16.9 hours and a higher energy beta emission of 2.1 MeV. Both have a gamma component [23,24]. Bone-seeking radiopharmaceuticals should not be considered when there are extensive soft tissue metastases, impending pathologic fracture or spinal cord compression, recent hemi-body radiotherapy or myelo-suppressive chemotherapy (< 2 months), or platelets < 60,000/mL and white count < 2.5×10^3/mL [17].

Strontium 89

Of the radiopharmaceuticals, Strontium 89 has received the most use for bone pain. The usual dose is 150 MBq (4 mCi). Subjective response rates of about 65% are expected (range: 35%–89%) [25–28] and the duration of response ranges from 3 to 12 months [26,28]. Complete responses may be seen in 10%–31% of patients [27,28]. Complete responses are more common in patients who have fewer than 10 sites on bone scan [27]. A flare in pain has been reported in 23%–50%, usually within a day and lasting 2–4 days [26,27]. Blood counts nadir in 6 weeks and will show a median decrease from baseline of 15% for hemoglobin, 32% for white blood cells, and 40% for platelets [29]. Up to 10 injections have been reported, spaced 3 months apart, with repeat palliative effect. Based on Strontium 85 urine levels, the effective half-life of Strontium 89 is 9.6–20.7 days. Five times the effective half-life leaves < 5% in the body, and this time interval can establish the timing for repeated doses or for administration of chemotherapy. The wide variability in effective half-life requires that treatment schedules be based on individual kinetics rather than fixed intervals [30].

Porter and colleagues [31] randomized 126 men with hormone refractory prostate cancer to receive either Strontium 89 (400 MBq) or placebo following involved field local radiotherapy. Significantly more patients who received strontium were free of new painful metastatic sites at 3 months compared with local field radiotherapy alone (59% versus 34%) [28,31]. At 3 months, more were pain free (40% versus 23%) and more were able to discontinue analgesics (17% versus 2%; P < .05). It should be noted that the dose of strontium in this study was higher than that generally used.

The European Organization for the Research and Treatment of Cancer (EORTC) conducted a randomized comparison of palliative local field radiotherapy (n = 102) versus a single intravenous injection of 4 mCi of Strontium 89 (n = 101) for hormonally resistant prostate cancer [25]. Response was defined as a decrease in pain score by one level, or a reduction in analgesic use by 25%, or an improvement in performance status without increased analgesics. Subjective response was recorded in about one-third of each group; there no difference in toxicity and a lower cost for local field radiotherapy. A significant survival advantage in favor of local field radiotherapy

(11 months versus 7 months; $P = .045$) was an unexpected finding that could not be explained. A previous trial reported by Quilty and coworkers [32], which randomized 284 men who had metastatic prostate cancer to either Strontium 89 or an appropriate form of external radiotherapy (either local field or hemi-body), found pain relief at 3 months in 66% after Strontium as compared with 64% after hemi-body radiotherapy and 61% after local field radiotherapy; there was no difference in survival.

Brundage and colleagues [33] published an evidence-based guideline for the CancerCare Ontario Practice Guideline initiative and recommended that strontium 89 was indicated for men who had hormone-refractory prostate cancer and uncontrolled painful sites on both sides of the diaphragm, for whom multiple involved field radiotherapy was not possible. Systemic radiopharmaceuticals will not treat adjacent soft tissue disease or neurologic compromise, and external beam radiotherapy remains the treatment of choice under these circumstances.

Strontium plus chemotherapy

Low-dose cisplatinum has been reported to act as a radiosensitizer when combined with Strontium [34]. Seventy patients who had metastatic hormone-refractory cancer were randomized to either Strontium 89 alone (148 MBq) or combined with 50 mg/m^2 of cisplatinum in 3 divided doses. Efficacy in terms of pain palliation was assessed at 2 months and bone scan response was assessed at 6 months. Onset of pain relief was at 15 days in both arms but median duration was 120 days in the combined arm and only 60 days for the strontium arm. Progression on bone scan at 6 months was seen in 27% of the combined arm as compared with 64% of the strontium arm.

One small randomized trial (n = 72) reported that the combination of strontium with doxorubicin for patients who have advanced androgen-independent prostate cancer and who have responded to induction chemotherapy (consisting of ketokonazole and doxorubicin alternating with estramustine and vinblastine) for 2 or 3 cycles, may lead to a survival benefit (27.7 months versus 16.8 months; $P = .001$) when compared with doxorubicin alone [35].

Samarium 153

Samarium 153 has been shown to offer pain relief in approximately two-thirds of patients in placebo-controlled, randomized trials. Pain relief occurred within 1–2 weeks and analgesics were reduced by week 3–4 after a single intravenous administration of 1 mCi/kg [36] as an out-patient procedure. The associated myelo-suppression was both mild and reversible [36]. Duration of effect was not described but up to 11 repeated doses have been reported for an individual patient using a dose of 1 mCi/kg (37 MBq/kg) [37]. Liepe [24] reported a response rate of 73% and 13% of the patients were able to discontinue analgesics (n = 15).

Rhenium 188

Recently there have been several reports about the use of Rhenium 188 [23,38]. The usual dose is 2.7–3.5 GBq. Blood counts nadir in 2–4 weeks, and pain relief is maximal in 3–8 weeks [23,24]. Administration requires a 2-day hospital admission [23]. Response rates range from 60% to 75%. One randomized study of 1 injection versus 2 injections 8 weeks apart (n = 64) reported a response rate of 92% and a median time to progression of 7 months in the repeated injection arm [38].

Summary

Multiple large, carefully conducted randomized trials indicate that a single fraction of approximately 8 Gy offers equivalent pain palliation and no increased toxicity when compared with more protracted fractionation schemes. The threshold for re-treatment may be lower after a single fraction but this can be conducted simply and effectively and does not negate the convenience for the patient, or the cost-effectiveness of this approach. A more protracted fractionation scheme may be justified in the occasional patient who is predicted to have a particularly long life expectancy.

For multiple painful sites on the same side of the diaphragm, hemi-body radiotherapy is rapidly effective. Pre-medication with odansetron and steroids will minimize side effects and eliminate the need for hospitalization.

When multiple painful sites exist on both sides of the diaphragm, systemic radiopharmaceuticals can be considered; however, systemic radiopharmaceuticals will not treat adjacent soft tissue disease or neurologic compromise. External radiotherapy remains the treatment of choice under these circumstances.

References

[1] Gaze MN, Kelly CG, Kerr GR, et al. Pain relief and quality of life following radiotherapy for bone metastases: a randomised trial of two fractionation schedules. Radiother Oncol 1997;45(2):109–16.

[2] Di Lorenzo G, Autorino R, Ciardiello F, et al. External beam radiotherapy in bone metastatic prostate cancer: impact on patients' pain relief and quality of life. Oncol Rep 2003;10(2):399–404.

[3] Nielsen OS, Bentzen SM, Sandberg E, et al. Randomized trial of single dose versus fractionated palliative radiotherapy of bone metastases. Radiother Oncol 1998;47(3):233–40.

[4] Rose CM, Kagan AR. The final report of the expert panel for the radiation oncology bone metastasis work group of the American College of Radiology. Int J Radiat Oncol Biol Phys 1998;40(5):1117–24.

[5] Steenland E, Leer JW, van Houwelingen H, et al. The effect of a single fraction compared to multiple fractions on painful bone metastases: a global analysis of the Dutch Bone Metastasis Study. Radiother Oncol 1999;52(2):101–9.

[6] Ben-Josef E, Shamsa F, Williams AO, et al. Radiotherapeutic management of osseous metastases: a survey of current patterns of care. Int J Radiat Oncol Biol Phys 1998;40(4):915–21.

[7] Hartsell WF, Scott CB, Bruner DW, et al. Randomized trial of short- versus long-course radiotherapy for palliation of painful bone metastases. J Natl Cancer Inst 2005;97(11):798–804.

[8] Hartsell WFSC, Bruner DW, Scarantino CW, et al. Phase III radomized trial of 8 Gy in 1 fraction vs. 30 Gy in 10 fractions for palliation of painful bone metastases: preliminary results of RTOG 97–14. Int J Radiat Oncol Biol Phys 2003;57(2):S124.

[9] Wu JS, Wong R, Johnston M, et al. Meta-analysis of dose-fractionation radiotherapy trials for the palliation of painful bone metastases. Int J Radiat Oncol Biol Phys 2003;55(3):594–605.

[10] Price P, Hoskin PJ, Easton D, et al. Prospective randomised trial of single and multifraction radiotherapy schedules in the treatment of painful bony metastases. Radiother Oncol 1986;6(4):247–55.

[11] Tong D, Gillick L, Hendrickson FR. The palliation of symptomatic osseous metastases: final results of the study by the Radiation Therapy Oncology Group. Cancer 1982;50(5):893–9.

[12] Arcangeli G, Giovinazzo G, Saracino B, et al. Radiation therapy in the management of symptomatic bone metastases: the effect of total dose and histology on pain relief and response duration. Int J Radiat Oncol Biol Phys 1998;42(5):1119–26.

[13] Blitzer PH. Reanalysis of the RTOG study of the palliation of symptomatic osseous metastasis. Cancer 1985;55(7):1468–72.

[14] Yarnold JR. 8 Gy single fraction radiotherapy for the treatment of metastatic skeletal pain: randomised comparison with a multifraction schedule over 12 months of patient follow-up. Bone Pain Trial Working Party. Radiother Oncol 1999;52(2):111–21.

[15] van den Hout WB, van der Linden YM, Steenland E, et al. Single- versus multiple-fraction radiotherapy in patients with painful bone metastases: cost-utility analysis based on a randomized trial. J Natl Cancer Inst 2003;95(3):222–9.

[16] Konski A. Radiotherapy is a cost-effective palliative treatment for patients with bone metastasis from prostate cancer. Int J Radiat Oncol Biol Phys 2004;60(5):1373–8.

[17] Chow E, Danjoux C, Wong R, Szumacher E, Franssen E, Fung K, et al. Palliation of bone metastases: a survey of patterns of practice among Canadian radiation oncologists. Radiother Oncol 2000;56(3):305–14.

[18] Roos DE. Continuing reluctance to use single fractions of radiotherapy for metastatic bone pain: an Australian and New Zealand practice survey and literature review. Radiother Oncol 2000;56(3):315–22.

[19] Wu JS, Wong RK, Lloyd NS, et al. Radiotherapy fractionation for the palliation of uncomplicated painful bone metastases - an evidence-based practice guideline. BMC Cancer 2004;4(1):71.

[20] Kuban DA, Delbridge T, el-Mahdi AM, et al. Half-body irradiation for treatment of widely metastatic adenocarcinoma of the prostate. J Urol 1989;141(3):572–4.

[21] Salazar OM, Sandhu T, da Motta NW, et al. Fractionated half-body irradiation (HBI) for the rapid palliation of widespread, symptomatic, metastatic bone disease: a randomized Phase III trial of the International Atomic Energy Agency (IAEA). Int J Radiat Oncol Biol Phys 2001;50(3):765–75.

[22] Zelefsky MJ, Scher HI, Forman JD, et al. Palliative hemiskeletal irradiation for widespread metastatic prostate cancer: a comparison of single dose and fractionated regimens. Int J Radiat Oncol Biol Phys 1989;17(6):1281–5.

[23] Liepe K, Kropp J, Runge R, et al. Therapeutic efficiency of rhenium-188-HEDP in human prostate cancer skeletal metastases. Br J Cancer 2003;89(4):625–9.

[24] Liepe K, Runge R, Kotzerke J. The benefit of bone-seeking radiopharmaceuticals in the treatment of metastatic bone pain. J Cancer Res Clin Oncol 2005;131(1):60–6.

[25] Oosterhof GO, Roberts JT, de Reijke TM, et al. Strontium(89) chloride versus palliative local field radiotherapy in patients with hormonal escaped prostate cancer: a phase III study of the European Organisation for Research and Treatment of Cancer, Genitourinary Group. Eur Urol 2003;44(5):519–26.

[26] Pons F, Herranz R, Garcia A, et al. Strontium-89 for palliation of pain from bone metastases in patients with prostate and breast cancer. Eur J Nucl Med 1997;24(10):1210–4.

[27] Kraeber-Bodere F, Campion L, Rousseau C, et al. Treatment of bone metastases of prostate cancer with strontium-89 chloride: efficacy in relation to the degree of bone involvement. Eur J Nucl Med 2000;27(10):1487–93.

[28] Robinson RG, Preston DF, Schiefelbein M, et al. Strontium 89 therapy for the palliation of pain due to osseous metastases. JAMA 1995;274(5):420–4.

[29] Lee CK, Aeppli DM, Unger J, et al. Strontium-89 chloride (Metastron) for palliative treatment of bony metastases. The University of Minnesota experience. Am J Clin Oncol 1996;19(2):102–7.

[30] Ben-Yosef R, Pelled O, Marko R, et al. Establishing schedules for repeated doses of strontium and for concurrent chemotherapy in hormone-resistant patients with prostate cancer: measurement of blood and urine strontium levels. Am J Clin Oncol 2005; 28(2):138–42.

[31] Porter AT, McEwan AJ, Powe JE, et al. Results of a randomized phase-III trial to evaluate the efficacy of strontium-89 adjuvant to local field external beam irradiation in the management of endocrine resistant metastatic prostate cancer. Int J Radiat Oncol Biol Phys 1993;25(5):805–13.

[32] Quilty PM, Kirk D, Bolger JJ, et al. A comparison of the palliative effects of strontium-89 and external beam radiotherapy in metastatic prostate cancer. Radiother Oncol 1994;31(1):33–40.

[33] Brundage MD, Crook JM, Lukka H. Use of strontium-89 in endocrine-refractory prostate cancer metastatic to bone. Provincial Genitourinary Cancer Disease Site Group. Cancer Prev Control 1998; 2(2):79–87.

[34] Sciuto R, Festa A, Rea S, et al. Effects of low-dose cisplatin on 89Sr therapy for painful bone metastases from prostate cancer: a randomized clinical trial. J Nucl Med 2002;43(1):79–86.

[35] Tu SM, Millikan RE, Mengistu B, et al. Bone-targeted therapy for advanced androgen-independent carcinoma of the prostate: a randomised phase II trial. Lancet 2001;357:336–41.

[36] Sartor O, Reid RH, Hoskin PJ, et al. Samarium-153-Lexidronam complex for treatment of painful bone metastases in hormone-refractory prostate cancer. Urology 2004;63(5):940–5.

[37] Menda Y, Bushnell DL, Williams RD, et al. Efficacy and safety of repeated samarium-153 lexidronam treatment in a patient with prostate cancer and metastatic bone pain. Clin Nucl Med 2000;25(9): 698–700.

[38] Palmedo H, Manka-Waluch A, Albers P, et al. Repeated bone-targeted therapy for hormone-refractory prostate carcinoma: tandomized phase II trial with the new, high-energy radiopharmaceutical rhenium-188 hydroxyethylidenediphosphonate. J Clin Oncol 2003;21(15):2869–75.

ELSEVIER
SAUNDERS

Urol Clin N Am 33 (2006) 227–236

UROLOGIC
CLINICS
of North America

Changing Perspectives of the Role of Chemotherapy in Advanced Prostate Cancer

Earle F. Burgess, MD, Bruce J. Roth, MD*

*Department of Medicine, Division of Hematology/Oncology, Vanderbilt University Medical Center,
Vanderbilt-Ingram Cancer Center, 777 Preston Research Building, Nashville, TN 37232-6307, USA*

The use of cytotoxic chemotherapy in advanced prostate adenocarcinoma has been validated by the recent demonstration of survival benefit in two large randomized phase III trials [1,2]. Before publication of these landmark trials, SWOG 9916 and TAX 327, no chemotherapeutic regimen had shown survival benefit in the treatment of androgen independent prostate cancer (AIPC). These trials provide new encouragement for the use of chemotherapy in all stages of disease. Improved communication between medical and urologic oncologists and early patient referral for clinical trial participation remains essential for identifying new chemotherapeutic regimens with improved activity in AIPC and for defining the role of chemotherapy in earlier-stage disease. This article discusses the role of chemotherapy as the current standard of care for the treatment of AIPC and provides a historical perspective of the trials that preceded the development of current docetaxel-based regimens.

Chemotherapy for AIPC

Trials from the National Prostatic Cancer Project era

In the 1980s, the National Prostatic Cancer Project (NPCP) conducted the largest series to date of phase II trials involving single and combinational cytotoxic agents in AIPC. The results of the NPCP and other early trials have

previously been reviewed and heavily criticized for erroneously concluding that many of the tested agents possessed clinically significant activity [3–6]. Although the trials were not designed to study impact on survival, patient median survival was generally no better than best supportive care, even though the response rates often exceeded 50% with some regimens. The underlying biology and difficulties associated with studying advanced prostate cancer can explain the misleading conclusions drawn from some of the trials. The classic objective criteria for gauging tumor response in phase II trials continue to be bidimensional measurement of solid tumor lesions before and after therapy. Because prostate cancer often metastasizes to bone only, assessment of tumor response after therapy in AIPC has been difficult to achieve in an objective and reproducible manner. Imaging modalities do not provide accurate bidimensional measurement of skeletal lesions, and, before the routine use of serum prostate specific antigen (PSA) as a surrogate marker, the methodologic challenges of measuring tumor response were well recognized. Faced with these limitations, the NPCP-era trial investigators used response criteria that were often subjective and that lacked the specificity to provide accurate assessment of drug activity. For example, the presence of "stable" disease, as defined by the absence of progression on bone scan and acid phosphatase levels after 12 weeks of therapy, was included as one criterion for drug response in the NPCP guidelines [7]. The trials did show that patients who had "stable" disease had longer median survival than those who had progressed, but they did not distinguish whether disease stability was a result of treatment or reflected the underlying biology of

* Corresponding author.
E-mail address: bruce.roth@vanderbilt.edu
(B.J. Roth).

disease in those patients [8]. In the NPCP trials, approximately 90% of the patient responses were classified as "stable disease" [4]. Because this response criterion is hardly specific for drug effect, false "activity" was incorrectly attributed to drugs that ultimately were shown to lack clinical benefit.

Mitoxantrone

After the NPCP and other trials of the 1980s, much debate existed over how best to measure tumor response in AIPC clinical trials. At the time, the general attitude regarding the use of chemotherapy in this setting was pessimistic and shared by urologists and oncologists alike. However, in the 1990s, the use of post-treatment serum PSA decline was validated as a surrogate marker for drug activity, and trialists were hopeful that PSA response could provide a much needed objective criterion that was reproducible and could be used in patients who had isolated skeletal disease [9,10]. Measurement of PSA response, as defined by a >50% decline from pretreatment baseline, solved key problems from earlier trials and established an end point in subsequent trials that more accurately reflected drug activity.

After acknowledgment of limited response criteria before the routine use of PSA decline, investigators considered palliation of symptoms as a primary endpoint in trials of cytotoxic agents. The idea originated in the AIPC setting after low-dose prednisone was shown to improve pain symptoms and quality of life [11]. Although PSA response has limitations, its superiority over historical standards quickly established this criterion as a gold standard for drug activity in phase II trials. Mitoxantrone, a member of the anthracenedione class that interacts with DNA topoisomerase II, was selected for evaluation of palliative ability based on a favorable side effect profile in elderly patients from an earlier phase II study [12–14]. Based on palliative endpoints, two phase III trials established that the addition of mitoxantrone provided superior response over glucocorticoids alone [15–17]. Mitoxantrone subsequently became the first cytotoxic agent approved by the FDA for use in AIPC and was approved for palliative treatment based on these trials. After FDA approval, mitoxantrone remained first-line standard of care in symptomatic patients before the approval of docetaxel.

Mitoxantrone provides effective palliative therapy. Although PSA response rates ranged from 33% to 48% in three phase III trials, a survival advantage over best supportive care has never been shown [16–18]. Additional phase II trials have explored the feasibility of mitoxantrone in combination with other cytotoxic agents or as sequential therapy with docetaxel-based regimens [19–23]. However, many of these studies accrued taxane-naive patients and need to be re-evaluated because docetaxel has been approved as first-line therapy. Recent trials have also studied the use of mitoxantrone in the second-line setting after patients have failed initial taxane therapy, although data suggest limited activity [24–26]. Based on the promise of docetaxel-based regimens (see below), the role of mitoxantrone will likely continue to diminish.

Estramustine

Estramustine is a synthetic conjugate of estradiol and a nitrogen mustard that was rigorously studied in the NPCP trials and found to have modest activity [4,27]. Although the drug was designed to target delivery of the mustard conjugate to malignant cells that overexpressed sex hormone receptors, estramustine acts through binding microtubule-associated proteins and inducing microtubule destabilization [27,28]. Preclinical studies suggest that combination of estramustine with other antimicrotubule agents could potentiate a cytotoxic effect in vivo [29,30]. These observations provided the scientific rationale for a large number of clinical studies of estramustine combined with other antimicrotubule agents. Many of these trials consistently showed that the addition of estramustine improved PSA response rates over single-agent therapy in the phase II setting [31–49]. Finally, the activity of an estramustine-containing doublet was definitively established by the SWOG 9916 phase III trial, which reported a prolongation of survival in patients who had AIPC treated with docetaxel and estramustine (D/E). SWOG 9916 was not designed to evaluate the contribution of each drug to the regimen. The TAX 327 phase III trial evaluating the docetaxel/prednisone (D/P) doublet showed a similar survival benefit in the docetaxel-treated arm. The results from the TAX 327 trial (see below) suggest that the efficacy of estramustine in the D/E doublet is limited and that the survival benefit is primarily due to docetaxel.

Estramustine is associated with the development of thromboembolic events in up to 25% of treated individuals [50]. Despite this risk, interest in combining the drug with other agents persists [19,51–53]. Many of these trials were written before the results of TAX 327 and SWOG 9916 were known. Given the risk for thromboembolism and limited contribution to docetaxel-based regimens, the continued use of estramustine must be questioned.

Taxanes

In the combination phase II studies involving estramustine, the taxanes had some of the highest activity among the classes tested. The early-phase trials involving paclitaxel and docetaxel have previously been reviewed in detail and are summarized here [54]. Single-agent paclitaxel has shown limited activity in AIPC, with PSA response ranging from 0% to 39% and measurable disease responses ranging from 4% to 50% depending on the administration schedule [55,56]. In these studies, weekly dosing provided better response rates than every-3-week administration, although 33% of patients experienced grade 3 neuropathy [55].

Based on the synergism observed in preclinical models [29], multiple phase II studies evaluated response rates of the paclitaxel/estramustine (P/E) doublet [35–38]. One study combined 96-hour paclitaxel infusion every 3 weeks with oral estramustine and reported a 53% PSA response rate without any grade 3 neuropathy [35]. This study provided evidence that optimized paclitaxel dosing combined with estramustine could produce meaningful responses without excess toxicity. Other trials using lower doses of weekly paclitaxel in combination with estramustine observed PSA response rates ranging 42% to 60% with significantly less grade 3 neuropathy than the original single-agent study [37,38]. Higher-dose weekly paclitaxel in combination with estramustine failed to improve outcome in one trial that reported a 62% PSA response accompanied by grade 3 neuropathy in 21% of patients [36].

Docetaxel is a semisynthetic taxane that has been shown to have greater preclinical activity than paclitaxel [57]. Single-agent phase II studies have been conducted using weekly and every-3-week dosing schedules. In two studies, every-3-week dosing resulted in PSA response rates of 38% to 46%, and one of the studies reported a median survival of 27 months [58,59]. Three trials examined weekly administration of docetaxel and reported PSA response rates ranging from 41% to 48%, with median survival ranging from 9 to 20 months [60–62].

In general, single-agent docetaxel phase II studies showed improved activity and toxicity profiles over single-agent paclitaxel. Because the addition of estramustine to paclitaxel improved response rates in phase I/II trials, the combination of estramustine and docetaxel has also been examined. One small trial based on a weekly dosing schedule reported a 72% PSA response rate with median survival of 16 months, which suggested that, like paclitaxel, the addition of estramustine to docetaxel may provide better response rates than docetaxel alone [63]. Grade 1–3 neutropenia was noted to be 17% in this study. Alternatively, phase I/II D/E doublets based on every-3-week dosing have shown PSA responses of 45% to 74%, measurable soft tissue response rates from 20% to 57%, and a median survival reported in two trials to be 20 to 23 months [32,33,64–66]. Grade 3–4 neutropenia ranged from 56% to 75% in these studies. Although greater myelosuppression was observed in studies based on every-3-week docetaxel administration, rates of neutropenic fever were low. These early docetaxel trials seemed to favor every-3-week administration, and the superiority of every-3-week dosing was clearly established in the two pivotal phase III trials discussed below.

SWOG 9916

In October 2004, two randomized phase III trials concurrently reported a modest survival advantage from docetaxel-based therapy in AIPC [1,2]. These trials ushered in a new era of excitement for the use of cytotoxic regimens because they marked the first time any chemotherapeutic agent has demonstrated a survival advantage in this disease setting. SWOG 9916 [2] was the first of these trials that compared D/E against the previous standard of care mitoxantrone and prednisone (M/P). The significant activity of D/E noted in combination phase I/II trials mentioned previously served as the basis for this trial. Overall survival was the primary endpoint, and the trial was powered to detect a 33% survival improvement in the D/E arm over the M/P arm. Progression-free survival, PSA, and measurable response rates were secondary endpoints. Patients were randomized to receive one of the following 21-day regimens: (1) estramustine 280 mg three times a day on days 1 through 5, docetaxel 60 mg/m^2 on day 1 and 60 mg of dexamethasone over three divided doses starting the night before docetaxel; or (2) mitoxantrone 12 mg/m^2 on day 1 plus prednisone 5 mg twice daily. Doses were increased to docetaxel 70 mg/m^2 and mitoxantrone 14 mg/m^2 on subsequent cycles if no grade 3–4 toxicities were noted in the initial cycle.

Of the 674 eligible patients in the study, 338 received D/E, and 336 received M/P. The median patient age was 70 years, and approximately 90% of both arms were SWOG performance status 0 or 1. The median PSA (ng/ml) was 84 and 90 in the D/E and M/P arms, respectively. Bone pain less than grade 2 was reported in 64% of both arms. Although the study did not achieve the primary endpoint of demonstrating a 33% improvement in survival between the two treatment arms, intention-to-treat analysis revealed a median survival of 17.5 months among patients receiving D/E and 15.6 months among patients receiving M/P ($P = .02$). Along with the TAX 327 trial discussed below, the 2-month median survival advantage noted in this study represented the first survival benefit from chemotherapy in patients with AIPC. The hazard ratio for death in this trial was 0.8 (95% confidence interval, 0.67–0.97), so during the study, the risk of death was reduced by 20% in the docetaxel-treated group. Analysis of secondary endpoints further supported the advantage of D/E therapy: Median time to progression was 6.3 months in the D/E arm versus 3.2 months in the M/P arm ($P < .001$). PSA response rates were 50% in D/E group and 27% in M/P group ($P < .001$). Partial response of measurable disease and subjective pain relief rates were not statistically different between the two treatment groups. Withdrawal rates for adverse events were 16% in the D/E arm and 10% in the M/P arm. Eight and four treatment-related deaths occurred in the D/E and M/P arms, respectively. Grade 3–4 neutropenia occurred in 12.5% versus 16.1% of patients in the M/P and D/E arms, respectively, although the difference was not statistically significant ($P = .22$). The rate of severe neutropenia in patients treated with D/E was markedly lower than seen in the earlier-phase trials, and the rate of neutropenic fever was only 5% in this group.

The results from SWOG 9916 showed that combination of docetaxel and estramustine prolongs median survival by 2 months and reduces the risk for death relative to mitoxantrone and prednisone. The median survival of 15.6 months in the control group was approximately 3.5 months longer than reported in earlier phase III trials that studied a similar regimen of mitoxantrone and prednisone [16,17]. Higher tumor burden in the

patients of the earlier trials may account for this difference because the previously studied patients had symptomatic disease and slightly higher median PSA values (150–158 ng/ml). Nonetheless, the SWOG 9916 trial definitively established that docetaxel-based therapy every 3 weeks prolongs median survival and reduces the risk of death. These results were complemented by the TAX 327 trial and immediately set a new standard of care for first-line therapy in patients who have AIPC.

TAX 327

The TAX 327 trial, reported concurrently with SWOG 9916, was a randomized phase III study that compared dose-equivalent docetaxel given on a weekly basis or every 3 weeks with prednisone against mitoxantrone given every 3 weeks [1]. Notable differences of this trial compared with SWOG 9916 include the addition of a weekly docetaxel arm and the absence of estramustine in the docetaxel arms. As in the SWOG trial, the primary endpoint of this study was to detect an overall survival advantage in the docetaxel arm compared with the mitoxantrone control arm. Secondary endpoints in this trial differed slightly and included measurement of pain levels, quality of life (measured by the FACT-P questionnaire), PSA, and measurable soft tissue responses. Like the SWOG trial, inclusion criteria required progressive AIPC measured radiographically and biochemically, ongoing androgen-ablation therapy, and prior cessation of antiandrogen therapy. Patients were randomized to receive one of the following treatment regimens: (1) docetaxel 75 mg/m^2 every 3 weeks (D/P), (2) docetaxel 30 mg/m^2 every week (wD/P), or (3) mitoxantrone 12 mg/m^2 every 3 weeks (M/P). All patients received prednisone 5 mg twice daily, and patients receiving docetaxel were premedicated with dexamethasone. The impact of dexamethasone on treatment response in the docetaxel arms has previously been suggested not to contribute to the treatment response [67].

Of the 1006 patients enrolled in the trial, 332, 330, and 335 were treated with D/P, wD/P, and M/P, respectively. In each of the three arms, the median patient age was 68 to 69 years, and 12% to 14% of patients had Karnofsky performance status <80%. The median serum PSA value in the three treatment arms ranged from 108 to 123 ng/ml, and approximately 45% of patients had pain. Ninety percent of patients had known bone metastases, and 40% had measurable soft-tissue lesions. Based on intention-to-treat analysis, the median durations of survival were 18.9 months in the every-3-week docetaxel arm, 17.4 months in the weekly docetaxel arm, and 16.5 months in the mitoxantrone arm. Only the every-3-week docetaxel regimen was demonstrated to have a statistically significant survival benefit compared with mitoxantrone. The hazard ratio for death using this regimen was 0.76 (95% confidence interval, 0.62–0.94), which confirmed the mortality reduction seen in the SWOG trial with every-3-week docetaxel/estramustine. Analysis of secondary endpoints showed reduced pain in 35% ($P = .01$), 31% ($P = .08$), and 22% of patients treated with D/P, wD/P, and M/P, respectively. Quality of life improvement was noted in 22% ($P = .009$), 23% ($P = .005$), and 13% of patients treated with D/P, wD/P, and M/P, respectively. D/P provided superior palliation relative to the prior standard M/P, whereas, pain reduction in patients treated with weekly D/P was not different from those treated with M/P. Based on these results, the use of weekly D/P for palliative intent only may be appropriate if the toxicity profile precludes use of every-3-week docetaxel. However, based on the survival advantage, every-3-week docetaxel is the preferred first-line standard regimen. The PSA response to treatment was 45% ($P < .001$) in the D/P, 48% ($P < .001$) in the wD/P, and 32% in the M/P arms (see below). Grade 3–4 neutropenia was seen in 32% ($P \leq .05$) of patients treated with D/P, in 2% ($P \leq .0015$) of patients treated with wD/P, and in 35% of patients treated with M/P, although only 3% of D/P-treated patients had febrile neutropenia. Common adverse events with D/P that occurred more frequently with every-3-week administration included fatigue, diarrhea, alopecia, and neuropathy. Three of five treatment-related deaths occurred in the mitoxantrone group.

The results of TAX 327 confirmed the findings of SWOG 9916 by demonstrating a 2-month survival advantage and a 20% mortality reduction over the study period in patients who had AIPC treated with docetaxel every 3 weeks. Weekly docetaxel was not associated with a statistically significant survival advantage, although this regimen demonstrated pain reduction equivalent to the historical standard of mitoxantrone and prednisone. Every-3-week docetaxel was accompanied by a slightly worse toxicity profile than mitoxantrone and prednisone, although treatment-related deaths were essentially the same in all arms. The

survival advantage associated with every-3-week docetaxel reported in the TAX 327 and SWOG 9916 trials represent independent confirmation from two large, randomized phase III trials that cytotoxic chemotherapy with an acceptable toxicity profile can prolong life in patients with AIPC. These two trials provide new excitement for the use of cytotoxic chemotherapy in patients who have AIPC and establish a foundation on which to develop improved regimens. The urologist will continue to play a critical role in defining better cytotoxic regimens by early referral to medical oncologists for participation in clinical trials. Although these trials report a modest survival improvement, they herald greater potential activity with future regimens. Many trials have been designed based on the results of TAX 327 and SWOG 9916, and expectations for future survival gains in AIPC are optimistic.

PSA response as surrogate marker for clinical benefit

Post-treatment serum PSA decline of at least 50% of pretreatment baseline has been suggested as a surrogate marker of survival benefit in phase II trials [9,10,68,69]. One interesting observation from the TAX 327 trial is the failure of PSA response to predict the proven survival advantage. Only 45% of patients in the every-3-week docetaxel arm experienced a post-therapy PSA decline of at least 50% despite a 2.4-month prolongation of survival. Follow-up analysis by the TAX 327 investigators further confirmed that the PSA response only partly explained the observed survival benefit [70]. Because 50% of patients treated with D/E in SWOG trial had at least a 50% reduction in post-treatment PSA, these results suggest that the addition of estramustine serves only to improve PSA response rates without additive survival benefit. This suggestion is supported by a recent randomized phase II study comparing every-3-week docetaxel with docetaxel plus estramustine that showed a PSA response in 68% of patients treated with D/E compared with only 29% of those treated with docetaxel alone [71]. Based on PSA response, results from this phase II trial imply that every-3-week D/E should have far greater clinical benefit than docetaxel alone and that every-3-week docetaxel alone should not produce any survival benefit. The results of TAX 327 prove otherwise and highlight an important limitation with the use of post-treatment PSA decline as a surrogate marker in phase II studies.

The TAX 327 trial showed that PSA response lacks sufficient sensitivity as a marker of survival benefit in phase II trials to exclude drugs from additional phase III testing. Because a better phase II surrogate marker does not exist, the use of post-treatment PSA response should not be abandoned in future trials at this time. However, this marker should not serve as the sole criteria for excluding drugs from further phase III analysis.

Future directions in AIPC

Current and future clinical trials in AIPC are based on two fundamental paradigms. The search for novel agents with improved activity continues, and such agents have been recently reviewed [72]. A larger number of trials seek to use docetaxel as a component of doublet therapy in combination with an investigational agent. An account of all docetaxel-based combinations under investigation is beyond the scope of this article; however, a few examples are mentioned. Bevacizumab is an anti-vascular endothelial growth factor monoclonal antibody that has shown synergistic activity in combination with traditional cytotoxic agents in other solid tumors [73,74]. Encouraging phase II data from patients treated with docetaxel, estramustine, and bevacizumab [75] led to the creation of cooperative group CALGB 90401 trial, which is an open phase III protocol randomizing participants to docetaxel/prednisone with or without bevacizumab. Synergy between docetaxel and antiangiogenic therapies has been further suggested by results from a phase II trial of docetaxel and thalidomide in which 51% of patients receiving combined treatment had a PSA response versus 37% of patients receiving docetaxel alone [76]. The addition of high-dose calcitriol to docetaxel has recently garnered much interest based on favorable preclinical studies and phase II results of weekly docetaxel plus high-dose pulse calcitriol [77,78]. These data led to the creation of the randomized, double-blind, placebo-controlled AS-CENT trial, which asked whether calcitriol adds to the effect of weekly docetaxel on serum PSA response [79]. Recent analysis of the trial showed a failure to achieve its primary goal [80]. Although the data indicated a trend toward improved survival, the study was not powered to detect a survival advantage. Additional studies have examined the impact of calcitriol on alternate docetaxel-based regimens [51], although no benefit has been confirmed in a randomized phase III trial, so clinical use should be limited to the investigational setting. Given the large number of open trials seeking to improve docetaxel-based therapy with novel combinations, oncologists are likely to have multiple active options for the treatment of AIPC in the coming years.

Chemotherapy in the nonmetastatic setting

Strong interest lies in whether earlier stages of disease ranging from the neoadjuvant setting to biochemical failure can gain survival benefit from cytotoxic therapy. Multiple pilot studies have shown that docetaxel-based therapy is safe and active in earlier stages of disease [81–87]. These and other trials have served as the basis for larger randomized phase III trials seeking to define the activity of chemotherapy in earlier stages of disease. For example, the adjuvant TAX 3501 (ATLAS) trial scheduled to open this fall is a large international phase III trial planning to enroll over 2000 patients with high risk for relapse after radical prostatectomy. Patients with a predicted risk of biochemical failure within 3 years of surgery will be randomized to receive 18 months of leuprolide with or without docetaxel or receive deferred treatment after radical prostatectomy. The primary endpoint of the trial is progression-free survival, and secondary endpoints include overall survival and cancer-specific survival.

Progress in the nonmetastatic setting has been hindered by poor accrual to the large, cooperative group studies, which has resulted in the premature termination of the RTOG 0014 and ECOG 1899 trials. These two phase III trials were designed to examine the role of chemotherapy in the setting of PSA relapse after local therapy but only enrolled 2% of target accrual. The anemic participation recently seen in the large cooperative group trials has been a subject of much debate [88]. It is unfortunate that lack of physician interest has plagued the nonmetastatic trials because the pilot studies have shown tolerable drug activity and raise critical clinical questions that require large phase III trials for proper answers. As patients become more savvy and seek other therapies for earlier-stage disease, medical and urologic oncologists have an unprecedented need to communicate and to facilitate enrollment in clinical trials to obtain the much-needed answers to pressing clinical questions.

Summary

This article summarizes the historical perspective of clinical trials in androgen independent prostate cancer. In October of 2004, the results from TAX 327 and SWOG 9916, two large, randomized, phase III trials, independently confirmed that every-3-week docetaxel-based therapy produces a modest survival benefit and immediately established docetaxel as first-line standard treatment. These trials reported the first survival benefit from cytotoxic therapy seen in the treatment of AIPC and led to the FDA approval of docetaxel in this setting. Multiple clinical trials are ongoing in attempts to extend the survival benefits gained from docetaxel in AIPC and to define the role of cytotoxic therapy in earlier stages of disease. Improved collaboration between medical and urologic oncologists is essential to facilitate clinical trial enrollment so that answers can be learned to important clinical questions regarding optimal management of all stages of disease.

References

[1] Tannock IF, de Wit R, Berry WR, et al. Docetaxel plus prednisone or mitoxantrone plus prednisone for advanced prostate cancer. N Engl J Med 2004; 351:1502–12.

[2] Petrylak DP, Tangen CM, Hussain MH, et al. Docetaxel and estramustine compared with mitoxantrone and prednisone for advanced refractory prostate cancer. N Engl J Med 2004;351:1513–20.

[3] Elder JS, Gibbons RP. Results of trials of the USA National Prostatic Cancer Project. Prog Clin Biol Res 1985;185A:221–42.

[4] Eisenberger MA, Simon R, O'Dwyer PJ, et al. A reevaluation of nonhormonal cytotoxic chemotherapy in the treatment of prostatic carcinoma. J Clin Oncol 1985;3:827–41.

[5] Tannock IF. Is there evidence that chemotherapy is of benefit to patients with carcinoma of the prostate? J Clin Oncol 1985;3:1013–21.

[6] Yagoda A, Petrylak D. Cytotoxic chemotherapy for advanced hormone-resistant prostate cancer. Cancer 1993;71(Suppl):1098–109.

[7] Murphy GP, Slack NH. Response criteria for the prostate of the USA National Prostatic Cancer Project. Prostate 1980;1:375–82.

[8] Slack NH, Brady MF, Murphy GP. A reexamination of the stable category for evaluating response in patients with advanced prostate cancer. Cancer 1984;54:564–74.

[9] Kelly WK, Scher HI, Mazumdar M, et al. Prostate-specific antigen as a measure of disease outcome in metastatic hormone-refractory prostate cancer. J Clin Oncol 1993;11:607–15.

[10] Bubley GJ, Carducci M, Dahut W, et al. Eligibility and response guidelines for phase II clinical trials in androgen-independent prostate cancer: recommendations from the Prostate-Specific

[11] Antigen Working Group. J Clin Oncol 1999;17: 3461–7.

[11] Tannock I, Gospodarowicz M, Meakin W, et al. Treatment of metastatic prostatic cancer with low-dose prednisone: evaluation of pain and quality of life as pragmatic indices of response. J Clin Oncol 1989;7:590–7.

[12] Osborne CK, Drelichman A, Von Hoff DD, et al. Mitoxantrone: modest activity in a phase II trial in advanced prostate cancer. Cancer Treat Rep 1983; 67:1133–5.

[13] Koeller J, Eble M. Mitoxantrone: a novel anthracycline derivative. Clin Pharm 1988;7:574–81.

[14] Moore MJ, Osoba D, Murphy K, et al. Use of palliative end points to evaluate the effects of mitoxantrone and low-dose prednisone in patients with hormonally resistant prostate cancer. J Clin Oncol 1994;12:689–94.

[15] Osoba D, Tannock IF, Ernst DS, Neville AJ. Health-related quality of life in men with metastatic prostate cancer treated with prednisone alone or mitoxantrone and prednisone. J Clin Oncol 1999; 17:1654–63.

[16] Tannock IF, Osoba D, Stockler MR, et al. Chemotherapy with mitoxantrone plus prednisone or prednisone alone for symptomatic hormone-resistant prostate cancer: a Canadian randomized trial with palliative end points. J Clin Oncol 1996;14:1756–64.

[17] Kantoff PW, Halabi S, Conaway M, et al. Hydrocortisone with or without mitoxantrone in men with hormone-refractory prostate cancer: results of the cancer and leukemia group B 9182 study. J Clin Oncol 1999;17:2506–13.

[18] Berry W, Dakhil S, Modiano M, et al. Phase III study of mitoxantrone plus low dose prednisone versus low dose prednisone alone in patients with asymptomatic hormone refractory prostate cancer. J Urol 2002;168:2439–43.

[19] Samelis GF, Kalofonos H, Adamou A, et al. The combination of estramustine, vinorelbine, and mitoxantrone in hormone-refractory prostate cancer: a Phase II feasibility study conducted by the Hellenic Cooperative Oncology Group. Urology 2005;66:382–5.

[20] Font A, Murias A, Arroyo FR, et al. Sequential mitoxantrone/prednisone followed by docetaxel/estramustine in patients with hormone refractory metastatic prostate cancer: results of a phase II study. Ann Oncol 2005;16:419–24.

[21] Bernardi D, Talamini R, Zanetti M, et al. Mitoxantrone, vinorelbine and prednisone (MVD) in the treatment of metastatic hormonoresistant prostate cancer–a phase II trial. Prostate Cancer Prostatic Dis 2004;7:45–9.

[22] Samelis GF, Skarlos D, Bafaloukos D, et al. The combination of estramustine and mitoxantrone in hormone-refractory prostate cancer: a phase II feasibility study conducted by the Hellenic Cooperative Oncology Group. Urology 2003;61:1211–5.

[23] Siefker-Radtke A, Poulter V, Mathew P, et al. Preliminary evidence of efficacy and tolerance for weekly intravenous bortezomib plus mitoxantrone in patients with advanced androgen-independent prostate cancer (AIPCa) [abstract]. Proc Am Soc Clin Oncol 2005;23:4567.

[24] Oh WK, Manola J, Babcic V, et al. Response to second-line chemotherapy in patients with hormone refractory prostate cancer (HRPC) receiving two sequences of mitoxantrone (M) and taxanes (T) [abstract]. Proc Am Soc Clin Oncol 2005;23:4616.

[25] Rosenberg JE, Kelly WK, Michaelson MD, et al. A randomized phase II study of ixabepilone (Ix) or mitoxantrone and prednisone (MP) in patients with taxane (T)-resistant hormone refractory prostate cancer (HRPC) [abstract]. Proc Am Soc Clin Oncol 2005;23:4566.

[26] Michels JE, Montemurro T, Kollmannsberger C, et al. First- and second-line chemotherapy with docetaxel or mitoxantrone in patients with hormone-refractory prostate cancer (HRPC): does sequence matter? [abstract]. Proc Am Soc Clin Oncol 2005;23:4611.

[27] Tew KD, Glusker JP, Hartley-Asp B, et al. Preclinical and clinical perspectives on the use of estramustine as an antimitotic drug. Pharmacol Ther 1992;56:323–39.

[28] Stearns ME, Tew KD. Antimicrotubule effects of estramustine, an antiprostatic tumor drug. Cancer Res 1985;45:3891–7.

[29] Speicher LA, Barone L, Tew KD. Combined antimicrotubule activity of estramustine and taxol in human prostatic carcinoma cell lines. Cancer Res 1992;52:4433–40.

[30] Kreis W, Budman DR, Calabro A. Unique synergism or antagonism of combinations of chemotherapeutic and hormonal agents in human prostate cancer cell lines. Br J Urol 1997;79:196–202.

[31] Sweeney CJ, Monaco FJ, Jung SH, et al. A phase II Hoosier Oncology Group study of vinorelbine and estramustine phosphate in hormone-refractory prostate cancer. Ann Oncol 2002;13:435–40.

[32] Savarese DM, Halabi S, Hars V, et al. Phase II study of docetaxel, estramustine, and low-dose hydrocortisone in men with hormone-refractory prostate cancer: a final report of CALGB 9780. Cancer and Leukemia Group B. J Clin Oncol 2001;19:2509–16.

[33] Sinibaldi VJ, Carducci MA, Moore-Cooper S, et al. Phase II evaluation of docetaxel plus one-day oral estramustine phosphate in the treatment of patients with androgen independent prostate carcinoma. Cancer 2002;94:1457–65.

[34] Oh WK, Halabi S, Kelly WK, et al. A phase II study of estramustine, docetaxel, and carboplatin with granulocyte-colony-stimulating factor support in patients with hormone-refractory prostate carcinoma: Cancer and Leukemia Group B 99813. Cancer 2003;98:2592–8.

[35] Hudes GR, Nathan F, Khater C, et al. Phase II trial of 96-hour paclitaxel plus oral estramustine phosphate in metastatic hormone-refractory prostate cancer. J Clin Oncol 1997;15:3156–63.

[36] Vaishampayan U, Fontana J, Du W, et al. An active regimen of weekly paclitaxel and estramustine in metastatic androgen-independent prostate cancer. Urology 2002;60:1050–4.

[37] Vaughn DJ, Brown AW Jr, Harker WG, et al. Multicenter phase II study of estramustine phosphate plus weekly paclitaxel in patients with androgen-independent prostate carcinoma. Cancer 2004;100: 746–50.

[38] Ferrari AC, Chachoua A, Singh H, et al. A phase I/II study of weekly paclitaxel and 3 days of high dose oral estramustine in patients with hormone-refractory prostate carcinoma. Cancer 2001;91:2039–45.

[39] Smith DC, Esper P, Strawderman M, et al. Phase II trial of oral estramustine, oral etoposide, and intravenous paclitaxel in hormone-refractory prostate cancer. J Clin Oncol 1999;17:1664–71.

[40] Meluch AA, Greco FA, Morrissey LH, et al. Weekly paclitaxel, estramustine phosphate, and oral etoposide in the treatment of hormone-refractory prostate carcinoma: results of a Minnie Pearl Cancer Research Network phase II trial. Cancer 2003;98: 2192–8.

[41] Smith MR, Kaufman D, Oh W, et al. Vinorelbine and estramustine in androgen-independent metastatic prostate cancer: a phase II study. Cancer 2000;89:1824–8.

[42] Hudes GR, Greenberg R, Krigel RL, et al. Phase II study of estramustine and vinblastine, two microtubule inhibitors, in hormone-refractory prostate cancer. J Clin Oncol 1992;10:1754–61.

[43] Seidman AD, Scher HI, Petrylak D, et al. Estramustine and vinblastine: use of prostate specific antigen as a clinical trial end point for hormone refractory prostatic cancer. J Urol 1992;147:931–4.

[44] Hudes G, Einhorn L, Ross E, et al. Vinblastine versus vinblastine plus oral estramustine phosphate for patients with hormone-refractory prostate cancer: a Hoosier Oncology Group and Fox Chase Network phase III trial. J Clin Oncol 1999;17:3160–6.

[45] Albrecht W, Van Poppel H, Horenblas S, et al. Randomized phase II trial assessing estramustine and vinblastine combination chemotherapy vs estramustine alone in patients with progressive hormone-escaped metastatic prostate cancer. Br J Cancer 2004;90:100–5.

[46] Pienta KJ, Redman B, Hussain M, et al. Phase II evaluation of oral estramustine and oral etoposide in hormone-refractory adenocarcinoma of the prostate. J Clin Oncol 1994;12:2005–12.

[47] Pienta KJ, Redman BG, Bandekar R, et al. A phase II trial of oral estramustine and oral etoposide in hormone refractory prostate cancer. Urology 1997; 50:401–6 [discussion: 406–7].

[48] Dimopoulos MA, Panopoulos C, Bamia C, et al. Oral estramustine and oral etoposide for hormone-refractory prostate cancer. Urology 1997;50:754–8.

[49] Vaishampayan U, Fontana J, Du W, et al. Phase II trial of estramustine and etoposide in androgen-sensitive metastatic prostate carcinoma. Am J Clin Oncol 2004;27:550–4.

[50] Lubiniecki GM, Weinstein RB, Berlin JA, et al. Thromboembolic events with estramustine phosphate-based chemotherapy in patients with hormone-refractory prostate carcinoma: results of a meta-analysis. Cancer 2004;101:2755–9.

[51] Tiffany NM, Ryan CW, Garzotto M, et al. High dose pulse calcitriol, docetaxel and estramustine for androgen independent prostate cancer: a phase I/II study. J Urol 2005;174:888–92.

[52] Galsky MD, Small EJ, Oh WK, et al. Multi-institutional randomized phase II trial of the epothilone B analog ixabepilone (BMS-247550) with or without estramustine phosphate in patients with progressive castrate metastatic prostate cancer. J Clin Oncol 2005;23:1439–46.

[53] Oh WK, Hagmann E, Manola J, et al. A phase I study of estramustine, weekly docetaxel, and carboplatin chemotherapy in patients with hormone-refractory prostate cancer. Clin Cancer Res 2005;11:284–9.

[54] Petrylak DP. Docetaxel for the treatment of hormone-refractory prostate cancer. Rev Urol 2003;5(Suppl 2):S14–21.

[55] Trivedi C, Redman B, Flaherty LE, et al. Weekly 1-hour infusion of paclitaxel: clinical feasibility and efficacy in patients with hormone-refractory prostate carcinoma. Cancer 2000;89:431–6.

[56] Roth BJ, Yeap BY, Wilding G, et al. Taxol in advanced, hormone-refractory carcinoma of the prostate: a phase II trial of the Eastern Cooperative Oncology Group. Cancer 1993;72:2457–60.

[57] Ringel I, Horwitz SB. Studies with RP 56976 (taxotere): a semisynthetic analogue of taxol. J Natl Cancer Inst 1991;83:288–91.

[58] Friedland D, Cohen J, Miller R Jr, et al. A phase II trial of docetaxel (Taxotere) in hormone-refractory prostate cancer: correlation of antitumor effect to phosphorylation of Bcl-2. Semin Oncol 1999;26(Suppl 17):19–23.

[59] Picus J, Schultz M. Docetaxel (Taxotere) as monotherapy in the treatment of hormone-refractory prostate cancer: preliminary results. Semin Oncol 1999;26(Suppl 17):14–8.

[60] Berry W, Dakhil S, Gregurich MA, et al. Phase II trial of single-agent weekly docetaxel in hormone-refractory, symptomatic, metastatic carcinoma of the prostate. Semin Oncol 2001;28(Suppl 15):8–15.

[61] Gravis G, Bladou F, Salem N, et al. Weekly administration of docetaxel for symptomatic metastatic hormone-refractory prostate carcinoma. Cancer 2003;98:1627–34.

[62] Beer TM, Pierce WC, Lowe BA, et al. Phase II study of weekly docetaxel in symptomatic androgen-independent prostate cancer. Ann Oncol 2001;12:1273–9.

[63] Copur M, Tarantolo S, Hauke R, et al. Weekly estramustine (E) taxotere (T) and dexamethasone (D) in patients with hormone refractory prostate cancer (HRPC) [abstract]. Proc Am Soc Clin Oncol 2000;19:347a.

[64] Petrylak D, Shelton G, England-Owen C, et al. Response and preliminary survival results of a phase ii study of docetaxel (D) + estramustine (E) in patients (Pts) with androgen-independent prostate cancer (AIPCA) [abstract]. Proc Am Soc Clin Oncol 2000;19:334a.

[65] Petrylak DP, Macarthur R, O'Connor J, et al. Phase I/II studies of docetaxel (Taxotere) combined with estramustine in men with hormone-refractory prostate cancer. Semin Oncol 1999;26(Suppl 17):28–33.

[66] Petrylak DP, Macarthur RB, O'Connor J, et al. Phase I trial of docetaxel with estramustine in androgen-independent prostate cancer. J Clin Oncol 1999;17:958–67.

[67] Weitzman AL, Shelton G, Zuech N, et al. Dexamethasone does not significantly contribute to the response rate of docetaxel and estramustine in androgen independent prostate cancer. J Urol 2000;163:834–7.

[68] Smith DC, Dunn RL, Strawderman MS, et al. Change in serum prostate-specific antigen as a marker of response to cytotoxic therapy for hormone-refractory prostate cancer. J Clin Oncol 1998;16:1835–43.

[69] Scher HI, Kelly WM, Zhang ZF, et al. Post-therapy serum prostate-specific antigen level and survival in patients with androgen-independent prostate cancer. J Natl Cancer Inst 1999;91:244–51.

[70] Roessner M, de Wit R, Tannock I, et al. Prostate-specific antigen (PSA) response as a surrogate endpoint for overall survival (OS): analysis of the TAX 327 Study comparing docetaxel plus prednisone with mitoxantrone plus prednisone in advanced prostate cancer [abstract]. Proc Am Soc Clin Oncol 2005;23:4554.

[71] Eymard J, Joly F, Priou F, et al. Phase II randomized trial of docetaxel plus estramustine (DE) versus docetaxel (D) in patients (pts) with hormone-refractory prostate cancer (HRPC): a final report [abstract]. Proc Am Soc Clin Oncol 2004;22:4603.

[72] Strother JM, Beer TM, Dreicer R. Novel cytotoxic and biological agents for prostate cancer: where will the money be in 2005? Eur J Cancer 2005;41:954–64.

[73] Sandler A, Gray R, Brahmer J, et al. Randomized phase II/III trial of paclitaxel (P) plus carboplatin (C) with or without bevacizumab (NSC #704865) in patients with advanced non-squamous non-small cell lung cancer (NSCLC): an Eastern Cooperative Oncology Group (ECOG) Trial - E4599 [abstract]. Proc Am Soc Clin Oncol 2005;23:4.

[74] Hurwitz H, Fehrenbacher L, Novotny W, et al. Bevacizumab plus irinotecan, fluorouracil, and leucovorin for metastatic colorectal cancer. N Engl J Med 2004;350:2335–42.

[75] Picus J, Halabi S, Rini B, et al. The use of bevacizu-mab (B) with docetaxel (D) and estramustine (E) in hormone refractory prostate cancer (HRPC): initial results of CALGB 90006 [abstract]. Proc Am Soc Clin Oncol 2003;22:393.

[76] Dahut W, Arlen P, Gulley J, et al. A randomized phase II trial of docetaxel plus thalidomide in andro-gen-independent prostate cancer [abstract]. Proc Am Soc Clin Oncol 2002;21:183.

[77] Beer TM, Eilers KM, Garzotto M, et al. Weekly high-dose calcitriol and docetaxel in metastatic androgen-independent prostate cancer. J Clin Oncol 2003;21:123–8.

[78] Ahmed S, Johnson CS, Rueger RM, et al. Calcitriol (1,25-dihydroxycholecalciferol) potentiates activity of mitoxantrone/dexamethasone in an androgen in-dependent prostate cancer model. J Urol 2002;168: 756–61.

[79] Beer TM. ASCENT: The androgen-independent prostate cancer study of calcitriol enhancing taxo-tere. BJU Int 2005;96:508–13.

[80] Beer T, Ryan C, Venner P, et al. Interim results from ASCENT: a double-blinded randomized study of DN-101 (high-dose calcitriol) plus docetaxel vs. pla-cebo plus docetaxel in androgen-independent pros-tate cancer (AIPC) [abstract]. Proc Am Soc Clin Oncol 2005;23:4516.

[81] Goodin S, Medina P, Capanna T, et al. Effect of docetaxel in patients with hormone-dependent pros-tate-specific antigen progression after local therapy for prostate cancer. J Clin Oncol 2005;23:3352–7.

[82] Febbo PG, Richie JP, George DJ, et al. Neoadjuvant docetaxel before radical prostatectomy in patients with high-risk localized prostate cancer. Clin Cancer Res 2005;11:5233–40.

[83] Beer TM, Garzotto M, Lowe BA, et al. Phase I study of weekly mitoxantrone and docetaxel before pros-tatectomy in patients with high-risk localized pros-tate cancer. Clin Cancer Res 2004;10:1306–11.

[84] Berger AP, Niescher M, Fischer-Colbrie R, et al. Single-agent chemotherapy with docetaxel signifi-cantly reduces PSA levels in patients with high-grade localized prostate cancers. Urol Int 2004;73:110–2.

[85] Dreicer R, Magi-Galluzzi C, Zhou M, et al. Phase II trial of neoadjuvant docetaxel before radical prosta-tectomy for locally advanced prostate cancer. Urol-ogy 2004;63:1138–42.

[86] Kumar P, Perrotti M, Weiss R, et al. Phase I trial of weekly docetaxel with concurrent three-dimensional conformal radiation therapy in the treatment of un-favorable localized adenocarcinoma of the prostate. J Clin Oncol 2004;22:1909–15.

[87] Rosenbaum E, Kibel A, Roth B, et al. Adjuvant weekly docetaxel (D) for high-risk prostate cancer patients (pts) after radical prostatectomy (RP): pre-liminary data of a multicenter pilot trial. Proc Am Soc Clin Oncol 2004;22:4649.

[88] Carducci MA. What is more exciting? The activity of docetaxel in early prostate cancer or the successful collaboration between urologists and medical oncol-ogists to complete a study in early prostate cancer? [editorial] J Clin Oncol 2005;23:3304–7

ELSEVIER
SAUNDERS

Urol Clin N Am 33 (2006) 237–246

UROLOGIC
CLINICS
of North America

Complementary and Alternative Medicine for Advanced Prostate Cancer

J. Daniell Rackley, MD, Peter E. Clark, MD, M. Craig Hall, MD*

Department of Urology, Wake Forest University School of Medicine, Comprehensive Cancer Center, Medical Center Boulevard, Winston-Salem, NC 27157-1094, USA

According to American Cancer Society statistics, prostate cancer remained the most commonly diagnosed noncutaneous malignancy in men in 2005, with an estimated 232,090 new cases [1]. It is the second leading cause of cancer death in men, with over 30,000 succumbing to the disease in the same year. Although the death rate and stage at diagnosis continues to decline, up to one third of men present with metastatic disease. These patients are typically treated with androgen ablation therapy, which has a finite period of effectiveness before hormone-refractory disease develops. Also, a significant proportion of men who undergo definitive local therapy have disease recurrence first heralded by a rising serum prostate specific antigen (PSA).

With the appreciation that androgen ablation therapy has significant long-term morbidity, there is a growing interest in alternative and complementary forms of therapy that may improve the outcomes of patients who have recurrent or advanced prostate cancer while obviating the need for more toxic forms of therapy [2]. Dietary and nutritional factors have gained much interest in recent years, much of which stems from epidemiologic observations. These include geographic and racial differences, especially the markedly decreased incidence of prostate cancer in Asians compared with other races, and the fact that Asian men who immigrate to America have an increased rate of prostate cancer compared with Asian men living in Asia [3]. It has been suggested that the Asian diet, which is higher in grains, fruits, and vegetables than the standard American diet, has a protective effect on the development of prostate cancer. An additional observation is the inverse relationship of prostate cancer incidence and sunlight exposure, presumably related to increased ergocalciferol (vitamin D) production in areas with greater sunlight exposure [4]. Observations like these have fostered a large interest in vitamin and nutritional supplements that might be used in the prevention or treatment of prostate cancer.

Complementary medicine refers to medical practices that are not within the traditional philosophies of Western medicine but are often used as a supplement to conventional practices. For example, a patient might take a vitamin or herbal supplement with a traditional chemotherapeutic agent. Alternative medicine attempts to specifically treat a disease, forgoing the use of traditional Western therapies. Patients who have advanced prostate cancer often turn to alternative therapies after conventional medicines have failed. Complementary and alternative medicines (CAM) have increased drastically in popularity in the past decade [2,5]. These are largely in the form of nutritional supplements. Other holistic practices, such as yoga, meditation, and acupuncture, fall under the heading of CAM but are outside the scope of this article. Boon and colleagues [2] reported that 27% of a random sample of men diagnosed who had prostate cancer used some form of CAM. Wiygul and colleagues [5] reported that 73% of men diagnosed with prostate cancer in a retrospective study used nutritional supplements. Despite a wealth of information sources

* Corresponding author.

E-mail address: mchall@wfubmc.edu (M.C. Hall).

on the subject, the fundamental problem with CAM therapies is a dearth of evidence-based medicine. In this article, we summarize the use of some of the more common CAM nutritional supplements and review the scientific data that are available to support their use.

Lycopene

Lycopene is the most abundant carotenoid in tomato products and is responsible for giving tomatoes their red color. Its potent antioxidant properties and its high concentration in serum and prostate tissue has generated much interest in this agent as a potential chemopreventive of prostate cancer [6,7]. A prospective cohort study by Giovannucci and colleagues [8] demonstrated a 40% decreased risk of prostate cancer in United States men who consumed four to five servings of tomato products per week. It is well known that reactive oxygen species produced throughout cellular metabolism result in DNA damage, which may play a role in tumorigenesis. Lycopene has been demonstrated to have potent antioxidant effects because it freely binds oxygen free radicals [9] and has been shown to decrease oxidative DNA damage in prostate tissues [10]. We have recently reported that deficient nucleotide excision repair capacity enhances human prostate cancer risk [11]. Numerous in vivo and in vitro studies have since demonstrated an antitumorigenic effect of lycopene on prostate cancer cells [12–15].

Other investigators have demonstrated additional potential anticancer effects of lycopene in addition to its antioxidant effects. The molecule may increase the expression of connexin 43, which enhances gap junction communication, preventing neoplastic transformation [16,17]. Lycopene may decrease eicosanoid metabolism by blocking COX-2 synthesis [18]. It may also induce cellular differentiation and apoptosis and inhibit cell proliferation [14,19,20]. Lycopene's multiple anticancer activities, low cost, ready availability, and apparent lack of systemic side effects have made it attractive for use in strategies against prostate and other cancers.

A few prospective studies have sought to determine if lycopene would alter the course of existent disease. Lycopene is an attractive alternative in the treatment of advanced prostate cancer because it has substantially less toxicity than androgen ablation and chemotherapy. We recently reported on a single patient with poorly

differentiated hormone-refractory prostate cancer whose PSA continued to rise after chemotherapy. The patient's PSA peaked at 365 ng/ml, and he developed extensive nodal disease and skeletal metastasis. He stopped all other treatments and was started on lycopene and saw palmetto supplementation. He had a dramatic PSA response (PSA nadir 3 ng/ml) that was remarkably durable (>12 months) [21].

Kucuk and colleagues [22] performed a phase II randomized clinical trial of lycopene supplementation before radical prostatectomy in 26 men. Participants received 15 mg of lycopene twice daily or no supplementation for 3 weeks before radical prostatectomy. Gleason score, pathologic stage, volume of cancer, and extent of high-grade prostatic intraepithelial neoplasia were evaluated after surgery. Connexin 43 expression was increased significantly in the prostate tissue of the intervention group. The intervention group had positive margins in 2 out of 13 versus 11 out of 13 in the control group. The treatment group had decreased tumor volume compared with the control group, leading the authors to suggest that lycopene supplementation might decrease the growth of prostate cancer.

Another prospective, nonrandomized study was completed by Ansari and colleagues [23] in which 20 patients who had metastatic hormone-refractory prostate cancer with clinical and biochemical evidence of disease progression were treated with 10 mg/d of lycopene for 3 months. One patient had a complete response (PSA <4 ng/ml), six patients had a partial response, 10 patients had stable disease, and disease progressed in three patients. Eastern Cooperative Oncology Group performance status improved in 10 patients, was unchanged in seven patients, and worsened in three patients. Of the 16 patients who had pain at the start of the study, bone pain improved in 10 patients, was stable in five patients, and worsened in one patient. Eleven of eighteen patients had improvement in their lower urinary tract symptoms. Although this was not a randomized, controlled study, lycopene did seem to be effective, and no patient had significant toxicity.

Ansari and colleagues [24] performed a prospective, randomized trial comparing lycopene and orchiectomy versus orchiectomy alone in 54 patients who had advanced prostate cancer. Patients were randomized to an orchiectomy arm or orchiectomy plus lycopene (OL) at a dose of 2 mg twice daily. Patients were evaluated with PSA, bone scan, and uroflowmetry before and every 3 months after intervention. At 6 months, the PSA levels in the control group and OL groups were 26.4 and 9.1 ng/ml, respectively. At 9 months, the PSA levels were 9.02 and 3.01 in the control arm and the OL arm, respectively. Eleven patients in the orchiectomy, versus 21 patients in the OL arm, responded completely. There was disease progression in seven patients in the orchiectomy arm versus two patients in the OL arm. Bone scans demonstrated complete response in four patients in the orchiectomy arm, whereas eight patients in the OL arm had a complete response. There was also a significant improvement in the peak urinary flow rate, with a mean increase of 1.17 ml/s in the OL arm.

We recently completed a dose-escalating phase I/II trial for patients who had biochemical relapse after definitive local therapy [25]. Six consecutive groups of six men received lycopene at a dose of 15, 30, 45, 60, 90, and 120 mg/d for 1 year. Serum PSA levels were monitored before treatment and every 3 months during therapy. There were no observed serum PSA responses (defined as a 50% decrease in serum PSA from baseline). Thirteen out of thirty-six patients had disease progression. Lycopene supplementation was well tolerated, with only one patient withdrawing from the study as a result of diarrhea thought possibly due to the lycopene.

The results of clinical efficacy of lycopene are mixed. Lycopene has some promise as CAM therapy, but until more clinical trials are performed, the degree to which this agent may benefit patients with advanced prostate cancer cannot be predicted.

Silbinin

Silbinin, a polyphenolic flavanoid with strong antioxidant properties, is derived from the seeds of milk thistle (*Silybum marianum*) and has become a popular dietary supplement in the United States and Europe. This agent has minimal toxicity in humans and has demonstrated efficacy and anticancer activity in many epithelial tumors, including prostate cancer [26–28]. The agent has demonstrated an inhibitory growth effect in various human prostate cancer cell lines in vitro [29,30]. It also has a synergistic effect when given in addition to doxorubicin, cisplatin, and carboplatin in prostate cancer cells [31]. There are multiple potential molecular targets through which the compound might exert its antiproliferative

effects by interruption of cell signaling, proapoptotic effects, and antiangiogenesis activity. Singh and colleagues [32] demonstrated inhibition of hormone-resistant prostate cancer xenografts in athymic nude mice. None of the animals demonstrated obvious toxic side effects. Silbinin seems to be well tolerated in humans and causes no obvious adverse effects. No clinical trials have been performed in patients who have advanced prostate cancer.

Shark cartilage

Much interest was generated about shark cartilage as a nutritional supplement to prevent or treat prostate cancer in the 1990s. This stemmed from the fact that sharks rarely develop cancer, and some researchers hypothesized that some element found in the cartilage of sharks might be beneficial in preventing or treating cancer [33]. Little evidence-based medicine has supported this idea. Recently, Loprinzi and colleagues [34] performed a prospective randomized, placebo-controlled trial in which patients who had advanced cancers were treated with a shark cartilage supplement or placebo. There was no difference in overall survival between the two groups.

Vitamin D

Vitamin D is a steroid hormone that has a well-known role in calcium and mineral homeostasis by acting on vitamin D receptors (VDR) located in the intestines, kidney, and bone. Vitamin D is acquired in the diet or can be synthesized in the skin from 7-dehydrocholesterol in response to ultraviolet light. There are several studies that have demonstrated that vitamin D is present in many tissues that have no role in calcium and mineral metabolism, suggesting that the hormone has other functions [35]. Several researchers have shown that vitamin D exposure has antitumorigenic activity in several neoplasms and that VDR ligands have antiproliferative effects on a wide range of cancers [36–38]. In vitro and in vivo studies in animal models and humans on a wide variety of malignancies have demonstrated multiple mechanisms that might result in tumor suppression, including prodifferentiating, antimetastatic, cell cycle arrest, and antiproliferative effects. Calcitriol and other VDR ligands have been shown to arrest the G0/G1 phase of meiosis

[39], to inhibit angiogenesis [40], and to induce apoptosis [41] and multiple other mechanisms.

Interest in the possibility of vitamin D activity in prostate cancer was aroused from epidemiologic studies that have demonstrated that the incidence of prostate cancer is increased in blacks, elderly men, and those who live in northern latitudes [42]. Many researchers have theorized that each group would have decreased levels of vitamin D, which might increase their risk of prostate cancer. Schwarz and colleagues [5] have suggested that a deficiency of vitamin D allows subclinical prostate cancer to progress to clinical disease. Evidence has shown that vitamin D, VDR, and 1α-hydroxylase are present in prostate and prostate cancer cells [43]. In vivo studies in murine models have demonstrated inhibition of prostate cancer tumor growth and decreased metastasis when exposed to vitamin D [44]. Corder and colleagues [45] performed a retrospective analysis of stored sera in 181 men who developed prostate cancer. Controls were taken from same-day blood samples in men who did not have known prostate cancer. A significantly lower level of calcitriol was found in the patients who later developed prostate cancer versus control subjects.

One possible problem of calcitriol therapy is the potential for significant hypercalcemia. Other vitamin D ligands have been developed that are less hypercalcemic yet have similar binding affinity for the VDR [46,47]. These studies have led to several phase I and II clinical trials to determine if vitamin D analogs are safe and efficacious in the treatment of advanced prostate cancer.

Liu and colleagues [48] performed a phase I trial with 1α-hydroxyvitamin D_2 in patients who had hormone-refractory prostate cancer. The drug was given orally at doses ranging from 5 to 15 μg daily to 25 patients who were monitored for toxicity and pharmacokinetics. The drug was well tolerated, with the main toxicities being hypercalcemia in five patients. Four of the five patients were in the 15-μg/d cohort, and only two of the five patients discontinued the treatment due to an increase in creatinine. Both of these patients had return of their creatinine to baseline after drug discontinuation. The same group subsequently performed a phase II trial with 1α-hydroxyvitamin D_2 [49]. Twenty-six patients who had metastatic prostate cancer were given 12.5 μg by mouth daily, with the primary end point being progression-free survival. Patients who had PSA elevations only were excluded from the study. Six patients failed to complete the study, five due to disease progression <8 weeks into the study and one due to toxicity. Of the 20 patients who completed the study, none had an objective response. All but two patients had radiographic evidence of disease progression, and those two patients had increased bony pain. Six patients had stable disease for >6 months.

Schwartz and colleagues [50] have recently completed a phase I/II study using 19-nor-1α-25-dihydroxyvitamin D_2 (Paricalcitol) in patients who had advanced, androgen-insensitive prostate cancer. Eighteen patients were enrolled in this dose-escalation trial; PSA response was the primary endpoint. There were no primary responders (ie, 50% reduction in PSA with confirmatory consecutive measurement at least 4 weeks apart). Overall, the drug was well tolerated, with no patients having to discontinue the drug. The authors noted that participants had significantly decreased parathyroid hormone levels and hypothesized that this could have beneficial effects in this patient population by decreasing the risk of skeletal complications.

Vitamin D has also been used in combination with chemotherapeutic agents. Beer and colleagues [51] recently demonstrated an 81% response rate (30/37 patients) for the combination of docetaxel and calcitriol in advanced prostate cancer. Previously, the highest response rate reported with docetaxel monotherapy was 42% [52]. Confirmation of synergistic activity awaits results from an ongoing prospective randomized trial. Calcitriol has also been combined with platinum-based drugs in vitro and has demonstrated increased antiproliferative activity over either drug alone [53].

Vitamin D to decrease osteoporosis and bone pain

Patients who have advanced prostate cancer suffer significant bone-related morbidity. These may be related to bony metastasis, bony pain secondary to pathologic fractures, and advanced osteoporosis from androgen deprivation therapy. Although patients who have advanced prostate cancer may live for several months or years, their quality of life is often diminished because of these bone complications. Dawson-Hughes and colleagues [54] performed a 3-year, prospective, double-blind study in which 389 men and women over 65 years of age received 500 mg of calcium plus 700 IU of cholecalciferol or placebo [54]. There was significantly improved bone density in the treatment group versus the placebo group. This led to similar studies in patients who had advanced prostate cancer who are at high risk for bony complications. Other studies have demonstrated that vitamin D supplements given to patients on androgen deprivation therapy can result in decreased bony pain and improved muscle strength [55].

Green tea

Evidence for the use of green tea or its extracts has been fueled by epidemiologic studies that demonstrated decreased incidence of cancer in areas where the beverage is highly consumed [56,57]. In fact, China has the lowest worldwide incidence of prostate cancer and the highest consumption rate of green tea [58]. Similar studies have prompted investigators to determine which components of green tea might provide anticancer activity. Multiple biochemical analyses have shown that green tea contains polyphenol compounds called catechins that are potent antioxidants. The major catechin is epigallocatechin-3-gallate (EGCG), which has antioxidant activity that is more potent that vitamins E and C. EGCG has been studied extensively in animal models and has demonstrated reliable anticancer activity among multiple cancer types [59–61]. In vitro studies using prostate cancer cell lines with hormone-sensitive and hormone-refractory cell lines have demonstrated antiproliferative effects with EGCG [61,62].

There have been two clinical trials testing the efficacy and safety of green tea in patients who have advanced prostate cancer. Jatoi and colleagues [63] performed a phase II trial with green tea in the treatment of patients with hormone-refractory metastatic prostate cancer [63]. Forty-two patients who had asymptomatic disease were treated with 6 g of green tea orally each day in six divided doses. Response was defined as a decrease in PSA $\geq 50\%$ of the baseline PSA. Only one patient responded, and this response did not last beyond 2 months. Furthermore, 69% of patients had grade 1 or 2 toxicity, the majority being gastrointestinal side effects (nausea, emesis, diarrhea, and abdominal pain). Six patients had grade 3 toxicity, and one patient had grade 4 toxicity, which manifested as severe confusion.

Another prospective clinical trial was performed by Choan and colleagues [64], who enrolled 19 patients who had HRPC. The primary endpoint was PSA or measurable disease progression by imaging studies after 2 months of therapy. Each patient was treated with 250 mg of green tea extract capsules orally twice daily. The researches deemed this dose to be consistent with dosing that would be realistic in a CAM setting in which patients could buy the supplement over the counter. Efficacy and toxicity were evaluated monthly. In general, the supplement was well tolerated; however, 12 patients reported at least one side effect. The majority was gastrointestinal related or due to caffeine intake found in the extract. Four patients did not complete the minimum 2 months of therapy (two due to intolerance, one due to physician stoppage, and one due to an unrelated cerebrovascular accident). Among the 15 patients who completed the study, nine had progressive disease within 2 months of starting therapy. The remaining six patients had progressive disease within an additional 4 months of therapy.

Based on these two studies, one at a higher dose and one more consistent with a traditional CAM dose, green tea extract does not seem to have any appreciable benefit in patients who have advanced prostate cancer. It is unlikely that a trial using a higher dose would provide any further benefit, and a phase I trial by Pisters and colleagues [65] demonstrated the maximum daily tolerable dose of green tea to be 4.2 g/m^2. This agent may hold more promise as a chemopreventative measure than for treatment of established disease [66].

Selenium and vitamin E

Selenium is a trace mineral found largely in plants but can also be found in the meat of animals raised in geographic locations where selenium is plentiful in the soil. It is known for its antioxidant activity, and observational studies have shown decreased incidences of colorectal, lung, and prostate cancers in patients who have high selenium intake [67]. Growth inhibition has been demonstrated in DU145 prostate cancer cells when exposed to selenium in vitro [68]. The selenium and vitamin E cancer prevention trial (SELECT) is a prospective trial with over 35,000 men randomized to receive selenium, vitamin E, both, or placebo [69]. The final results of this trial are expected in 2013. Several other trials are underway exploring the use of selenium as a chemopreventative agent, but no clinical studies have sought to determine if it has any effect on advanced prostate cancer. Like selenium, vitamin E has potent antioxidant properties. It occurs naturally in the diet (γ-tocopherol) or can be taken as a supplement (α-tocopherol). Laboratory and animal studies have demonstrated apoptotic and antiproliferative effects of vitamin E on prostate cancer cells and tumors, respectively [70–72]. No clinical studies have been done using vitamin E in patients who have advanced prostate cancer.

Selenium may hold some promise as a complementary agent. Several laboratory studies have shown that selenium induces apoptosis of prostate cancer cells [30,73,74]. Many researchers have sought to find a relatively nontoxic agent that can potentiate the activity (and thereby lower the required dose) of more toxic chemotherapies. Hu and colleagues [75] have demonstrated that selenium increases the apoptotic potential of etoposide and paclitaxel against prostate cancer cells when given concomitantly versus selenium or the drugs given alone. This could improve the chemotherapeutic index by allowing increased tumor cell killing while allowing lower doses of these toxic agents.

Grape seed extract

Grapes are rich in polyphenols called procyanidins, which have strong antioxidant activity and are found in abundance in wine. Grape seed extract (GSE) can be purchased as a nutritional supplement. GSE has been shown to inhibit growth and promote apoptosis of prostate cancer cells in vitro [76]. Recently, the same group demonstrated antineoplastic activity of GSE in animal models of hormone-refractory prostate cancer; however, clinical studies are lacking [32].

Modified citrus pectin

Modified citrus pectin (MCP) is a complex carbohydrate from the peel of citrus fruits. Raz and colleagues [77] determined that pectin can prevent cancer cell adhesion by binding to carbohydrate-binding proteins on the surfaces of cancer cells. Theoretically, this prevents cancer cells from organizing into solid tumors and may prevent metastasis by blocking the binding of cancer cells to other tissues. In vitro studies with human androgen independent prostate cancer cells demonstrated significantly decreased growth in culture medium when exposed to MCP [78].

Preclinical studies in a rat prostate cancer model demonstrated no change in the growth of the primary tumor but did show significantly reduced metastatic disease [79]. In a phase II pilot study involving 10 men who had biochemical failure after local treatment who were treated with MCP, 7 out of 10 men demonstrated a significantly increased PSA doubling time compared with pretreatment PSA doubling time [80]. Further work is needed with regard to dosing, safety, and efficacy before this supplement can be recommended to patients who have prostate cancer.

Soy

Soy products are rich in isoflavones and are found in abundance in Asian diets where the prostate cancer incidence is low [81]. The two most prominent isoflavones found in soy are daidzein and genistein [82]. Genistein has been shown to have several antineoplastic properties in laboratory and animal studies [83,84]. The agent has been shown to induce apoptosis and to inhibit protein kinase and functions as a phytoestrogen [85–87]. In an animal model study, LNCaP cells transplanted into nude mice had decreased growth with soy [88]. The authors noted that there was no difference in growth rates once the mice developed palpable tumors and hypothesized that soy exerts antiproliferative effects during an early stage of tumor development.

Jacobsen and colleagues [89] demonstrated a 70% reduction in prostate cancer in a cohort of men who frequently consumed soy milk. Another prospective study demonstrated no PSA reduction in men who had biochemical recurrence or HRPC who were given genistein supplementation [90]. Several trials evaluating the effectiveness of soy protein as a chemopreventative agent are underway. No clinical trials have been performed evaluating the use of soy protein in men who have advanced prostate cancer.

PC-SPES

PC-SPES (PC is short for prostate cancer, and *spes* is Latin for hope) is an herbal supplement that was marketed in the United States until 2002. PC-SPES is a proprietary formulation of eight herbs: *Chrysanthemum morifolium, Isatis indigotica, Glycyrrhiza glabra, Ganoderma lucidum, Panax pseudoginseng, Rabdosia rubescens,*

Serona repens (saw palmetto), and *Scutellaria baicalensis*. Some of the components inhibit 5-alpha reductase, and some have estrogenic activity to which many researchers attribute the agents' antineoplastic activity [91]. Preclinical studies have demonstrated antiproliferative activity against hormone-sensitive and hormone-resistant prostate cancer cell lines [92,93].

The first clinical use in patients who had advanced prostate cancer was a case report by de le Taille and colleagues [94] in which two patients were treated with PC-SPES and had drops in their PSA levels from 100 to 24 and 386 to 114, after which the levels remained stable. Several small phase II trials have also been performed. In one study, 37 patients with hormone-refractory cancer and 33 with hormone-sensitive cancer were treated with nine capsules of PC-SPES daily [95]. Every patient in the hormone-sensitive group had a PSA decline of $\geq 80\%$, with a durability of 57 weeks. Nineteen out of thirty-five patients who had hormone-refractory disease had a PSA decline of $\geq 50\%$, with a median time to progression of 16 weeks. Severe toxicities were thromboembolic events ($n = 3$) and allergic reactions ($n = 3$). Other common side effects were related to the estrogenic effects of the supplement: gynecomastia, gynecodynia, diarrhea, and leg cramps.

In addition to the estrogenic activity in the principle compounds of PC-SPES, batches of the supplement have been found to contain diethylstilbestrol (DES), a synthetic steroid [96]. Many researchers have questioned whether the antiproliferative effect of PC-SPES in prostate cancer was due to the DES instead of the other herbal components. Oh and colleagues [97] performed a randomized, phase II, cross-over study in which 90 patients were randomly assigned to receive DES or PC-SPES. PSA declines of $\geq 50\%$ were noted in 40% of the PC-SPES group versus 24% of the DES group. DES was present in the PC-SPES used in the study. This raises the question of whether some component of PC-SPES contains an active antineoplastic agent other than DES.

PC-SPES has also been fraught with other problems due to contaminants and impurities. Some batches have been found to contain warfarin and indomethacin, and several patients taking the supplement had hemorrhagic complications [96]. Subsequently, the United States Food and Drug Administration advised the discontinuation of this product by all users, and the manufacturer is no longer in business.

Summary

PC-SPES is a paradigm for the clinical gains and the pitfalls that arise with CAM therapies. There is little governmental regulation over these substances in the United States; therefore, manufacturers can continue to produce their products even when evidence of potential toxicities exists. There is also limited scientific data supporting the efficacy, or lack thereof, for most of these products; however, most patients purchase them based only on the potential that they may be beneficial. Although some of these products show some promise as potential treatments for advanced prostate cancer, the data are limited for the most part, and clinical studies are lacking. However, there is abundant information in the media, the internet, and elsewhere touting the benefits of these agents. Patients who have advanced prostate cancer have few alternatives in the way of traditional medicine and are especially vulnerable to experimenting with CAM agents because their physicians often have few traditional treatment options left to offer them. It is incumbent upon clinicians who treat patients who have advanced prostate cancer to be familiar with these forms of therapy so that they may better counsel patients about their use. Furthermore, there must be more carefully designed clinical trials to properly test these compounds in a scientific manner before they are recommended to the public.

References

[1] Jemal A, Murray T, Ward E, et al. Cancer statistics, 2005. CA Cancer J Clin 2005;55:10–30.

[2] Boon H, Westlake K, Stewart M, et al. Use of complementary/alternative medicine by men diagnosed with prostate cancer: prevalence and characteristics. Urology 2003;62:849–53.

[3] Spitz MR, Strom SS, Yamamura Y, et al. Epidemiologic determinants of clinically relevant prostate cancer. Int J Cancer 2000;89:259–64.

[4] Schwartz GG, Hulka BS. Is vitamin D deficiency a risk factor for prostate cancer? (Hypothesis). Anticancer Res 1990;10:1307–11.

[5] Wiygul JB, Evans BR, Peterson BL, et al. Supplement use among men with prostate cancer. Urology 2005;66:161–6.

[6] Zhao Z, Khachik F, Richie JP Jr, et al. Lycopene uptake and tissue disposition in male and female rats. Proc Soc Exp Biol Med 1998;218:109–14.

[7] Khachik F, Spangler CJ, Smith JC Jr, et al. Identification, quantification, and relative concentrations of carotenoids and their metabolites in human milk and serum. Anal Chem 1997;69:1873–81.

[8] Giovannucci E, Ascherio A, Rimm EB, et al. Intake of carotenoids and retinol in relation to risk of prostate cancer. J Natl Cancer Inst 1995;87: 1767–76.

[9] Di Mascio P, Kaiser S, Sies H. Lycopene as the most efficient biological carotenoid singlet oxygen quencher. Arch Biochem Biophys 1989;274:532–8.

[10] Chen L, Stacewicz-Sapuntzakis M, Duncan C, et al. Oxidative DNA damage in prostate cancer patients consuming tomato sauce-based entrees as a whole-food intervention. J Natl Cancer Inst 2001;93: 1872–9.

[11] Hu JJ, Hall MC, Grossman L, et al. Deficient nucleotide excision repair capacity enhances human prostate cancer risk. Cancer Res 2004;64:1197–201.

[12] Pastori M, Pfander H, Boscoboinik D, et al. Lycopene in association with alpha-tocopherol inhibits at physiological concentrations proliferation of prostate carcinoma cells. Biochem Biophys Res Commun 1998;250:582–5.

[13] Kotake-Nara E, Kushiro M, Zhang H, et al. Carotenoids affect proliferation of human prostate cancer cells. J Nutr 2001;131:3303–6.

[14] Hantz HL, Young LF, Martin KR. Physiologically attainable concentrations of lycopene induce mitochondrial apoptosis in LNCaP human prostate cancer cells. Exp Biol Med (Maywood) 2005;230:171–9.

[15] Tang L, Jin T, Zeng X, et al. Lycopene inhibits the growth of human androgen-independent prostate cancer cells in vitro and in BALB/c nude mice. J Nutr 2005;135:287–90.

[16] Bertram JS. Carotenoids and gene regulation. Nutr Rev 1999;57:182–91.

[17] Aust O, Ale-Agha N, Zhang L, et al. Lycopene oxidation product enhances gap junctional communication. Food Chem Toxicol 2003;41:1399–407.

[18] Cohen LA. Nutrition and prostate cancer: a review. Ann N Y Acad Sci 2002;963:148–55.

[19] Hwang ES, Bowen PE. Cell cycle arrest and induction of apoptosis by lycopene in LNCaP human prostate cancer cells. J Med Food 2004;7:284–9.

[20] McCarty MF. Targeting multiple signaling pathways as a strategy for managing prostate cancer: multifocal signal modulation therapy. Integr Cancer Ther 2004;3:349–80.

[21] Matlaga BR, Hall MC, Stindt D, et al. Response of hormone refractory prostate cancer to lycopene. J Urol 2001;166:613.

[22] Kucuk O, Sarkar FH, Sakr W, et al. Phase II randomized clinical trial of lycopene supplementation before radical prostatectomy. Cancer Epidemiol Biomarkers Prev 2001;10:861–8.

[23] Ansari MS, Gupta NP. Lycopene: a novel drug therapy in hormone refractory metastatic prostate cancer. Urol Oncol 2004;22:415–20.

[24] Ansari MS, Gupta NP. A comparison of lycopene and orchidectomy vs orchidectomy alone in the management of advanced prostate cancer. BJU Int 2003;92:375–8 [discussion: 378].

[25] Borden L, Clark P, Miller A, et al. Prospective dose-escalation trial of lycopene in men with recurrent prostate cancer following definitive local therapy. J Urol 2005;173:275.

[26] Katiyar SK, Korman NJ, Mukhtar H, et al. Protective effects of silymarin against photocarcinogenesis in a mouse skin model. J Natl Cancer Inst 1997;89: 556–66.

[27] Lahiri-Chatterjee M, Katiyar SK, Mohan RR, et al. A flavonoid antioxidant, silymarin, affords exceptionally high protection against tumor promotion in the SENCAR mouse skin tumorigenesis model. Cancer Res 1999;59:622–32.

[28] Zi X, Agarwal R. Silibinin decreases prostate-specific antigen with cell growth inhibition via G1 arrest, leading to differentiation of prostate carcinoma cells: implications for prostate cancer intervention. Proc Natl Acad Sci USA 1999;96:7490–5.

[29] Zi X, Grasso AW, Kung HJ, et al. A flavonoid antioxidant, silymarin, inhibits activation of erbB1 signaling and induces cyclin-dependent kinase inhibitors, G1 arrest, and anticarcinogenic effects in human prostate carcinoma DU145 cells. Cancer Res 1998;58:1920–9.

[30] Jiang C, Hu H, Malewicz B, et al. Selenite-induced p53 Ser-15 phosphorylation and caspase-mediated apoptosis in LNCaP human prostate cancer cells. Mol Cancer Ther 2004;3:877–84.

[31] Tyagi AK, Singh RP, Agarwal C, et al. Silibinin strongly synergizes human prostate carcinoma DU145 cells to doxorubicin-induced growth Inhibition, G2-M arrest, and apoptosis. Clin Cancer Res 2002;8:3512–9.

[32] Singh RP, Sharma G, Dhanalakshmi S, et al. Suppression of advanced human prostate tumor growth in athymic mice by silibinin feeding is associated with reduced cell proliferation, increased apoptosis, and inhibition of angiogenesis. Cancer Epidemiol Biomarkers Prev 2003;12:933–9.

[33] Ernst E. Shark cartilage for cancer? Lancet 1998; 351:298.

[34] Loprinzi CL, Levitt R, Barton DL, et al. Evaluation of shark cartilage in patients with advanced cancer: a North Central Cancer Treatment Group trial. Cancer 2005;104:176–82.

[35] Stumpf WE, Sar M, Reid FA, et al. Target cells for 1,25-dihydroxyvitamin D3 in intestinal tract, stomach, kidney, skin, pituitary, and parathyroid. Science 1979;206:1188–90.

[36] Abe E, Miyaura C, Sakagami H, et al. Differentiation of mouse myeloid leukemia cells induced by 1 alpha, 25-dihydroxyvitamin D3. Proc Natl Acad Sci USA 1981;78:4990–4.

[37] Colston KW, Chander SK, Mackay AG, et al. Effects of synthetic vitamin D analogues on breast cancer cell proliferation in vivo and in vitro. Biochem Pharmacol 1992;44:693–702.

[38] Higashimoto Y, Ohata M, Nishio K, et al. 1 alpha, 25-dihydroxyvitamin D3 and all-trans-retinoic acid

inhibit the growth of a lung cancer cell line. Anticancer Res 1996;16:2653–9.

[39] Campbell MJ, Koeffler HP. Toward therapeutic intervention of cancer by vitamin D compounds. J Natl Cancer Inst 1997;89:182–5.

[40] Mantell DJ, Owens PE, Bundred NJ, et al. 1 alpha, 25-dihydroxyvitamin D(3) inhibits angiogenesis in vitro and in vivo. Circ Res 2000;87:214–20.

[41] Park WH, Seol JG, Kim ES, et al. Induction of apoptosis by vitamin D3 analogue EB1089 in NCI-H929 myeloma cells via activation of caspase 3 and p38 MAP kinase. Br J Haematol 2000;109:576–83.

[42] Hanchette CL, Schwartz GG. Geographic patterns of prostate cancer mortality: evidence for a protective effect of ultraviolet radiation. Cancer 1992;70:2861–9.

[43] Schwartz GG, Whitlatch LW, Chen TC, et al. Human prostate cells synthesize 1,25-dihydroxyvitamin D3 from 25-hydroxyvitamin D3. Cancer Epidemiol Biomarkers Prev 1998;7:391–5.

[44] Getzenberg RH, Light BW, Lapco PE, et al. Vitamin D inhibition of prostate adenocarcinoma growth and metastasis in the Dunning rat prostate model system. Urology 1997;50:999–1006.

[45] Corder EH, Guess HA, Hulka BS, et al. Vitamin D and prostate cancer: a prediagnostic study with stored sera. Cancer Epidemiol Biomarkers Prev 1993; 2:467–72.

[46] Schwartz GG, Oeler TA, Uskokovic MR, et al. Human prostate cancer cells: inhibition of proliferation by vitamin D analogs. Anticancer Res 1994;14:1077–81.

[47] Skowronski RJ, Peehl DM, Feldman D. Actions of vitamin D3, analogs on human prostate cancer cell lines: comparison with 1,25-dihydroxyvitamin D3. Endocrinology 1995;136:20–6.

[48] Liu G, Oettel K, Ripple G, et al. Phase I trial of 1alpha-hydroxyvitamin d(2) in patients with hormone refractory prostate cancer. Clin Cancer Res 2002;8:2820–7.

[49] Liu G, Wilding G, Staab MJ, et al. Phase II study of 1alpha-hydroxyvitamin D(2) in the treatment of advanced androgen-independent prostate cancer. Clin Cancer Res 2003;9:4077–83.

[50] Schwartz GG, Hall MC, Stindt D, et al. Phase I/II study of 19-nor-1alpha-25-dihydroxyvitamin D2 (paricalcitol) in advanced, androgen insensitive prostate cancer. Clin Cancer Res 2005;11:8680–5.

[51] Beer TM, Eilers KM, Garzotto M, et al. Weekly high-dose calcitriol and docetaxel in metastatic androgen-independent prostate cancer. J Clin Oncol 2003;21:123–8.

[52] Berry W, Dakhil S, Gregurich MA, et al. Phase II trial of single-agent weekly docetaxel in hormone-refractory, symptomatic, metastatic carcinoma of the prostate. Semin Oncol 2001;28(Suppl 15):8–15.

[53] Moffatt KA, Johannes WU, Miller GJ. 1Alpha, 25dihydroxyvitamin D3 and platinum drugs act synergistically to inhibit the growth of prostate cancer cell lines. Clin Cancer Res 1999;5:695–703.

[54] Dawson-Hughes B, Harris SS, Krall EA, et al. Effect of calcium and vitamin D supplementation on bone density in men and women 65 years of age or older. N Engl J Med 1997;337:670–6.

[55] Van Veldhuizen PJ, Taylor SA, Williamson S, et al. Treatment of vitamin D deficiency in patients with metastatic prostate cancer may improve bone pain and muscle strength. J Urol 2000;163:187–90.

[56] Zhang M, Lee AH, Binns CW, et al. Green tea consumption enhances survival of epithelial ovarian cancer. Int J Cancer 2004;112:465–9.

[57] Yu GP, Hsieh CC, Wang LY, et al. Green-tea consumption and risk of stomach cancer: a population-based case-control study in Shanghai, China. Cancer Causes Control 1995;6:532–8.

[58] Gupta S, Ahmad N, Mohan RR, et al. Prostate cancer chemoprevention by green tea: in vitro and in vivo inhibition of testosterone-mediated induction of ornithine decarboxylase. Cancer Res 1999;59:2115–20.

[59] Katiyar SK, Agarwal R, Mukhtar H. Protection against malignant conversion of chemically induced benign skin papillomas to squamous cell carcinomas in SENCAR mice by a polyphenolic fraction isolated from green tea. Cancer Res 1993;53:5409–12.

[60] Xu Y, Ho CT, Amin SG, et al. Inhibition of tobacco-specific nitrosamine-induced lung tumorigenesis in A/J mice by green tea and its major polyphenol as antioxidants. Cancer Res 1992;52:3875–9.

[61] Liao S, Umekita Y, Guo J, et al. Growth inhibition and regression of human prostate and breast tumors in athymic mice by tea epigallocatechin gallate. Cancer Lett 1995;96:239–43.

[62] Paschka AG, Butler R, Young CY. Induction of apoptosis in prostate cancer cell lines by the green tea component, (-)-epigallocatechin-3-gallate. Cancer Lett 1998;130:1–7.

[63] Jatoi A, Ellison N, Burch PA, et al. A phase II trial of green tea in the treatment of patients with androgen independent metastatic prostate carcinoma. Cancer 2003;97:1442–6.

[64] Choan E, Segal R, Jonker D, et al. A prospective clinical trial of green tea for hormone refractory prostate cancer. An evaluation of the complimentary/alternative approach. Urol Oncol 2005 Mar-Apr;23(2):108–13.

[65] Pisters KM, Newman RA, Coldman B, et al. Phase I trial of oral green tea extract in adult patients with solid tumors. J Clin Oncol 2001;19:1830–8.

[66] Adhami VM, Ahmad N, Mukhtar H. Molecular targets for green tea in prostate cancer prevention. J Nutr 2003;133(Suppl):2417S–24S.

[67] Combs GF Jr, Clark LC, Turnbull BW. An analysis of cancer prevention by selenium. Biofactors 2001; 14:153–9.

[68] Webber MM, Perez-Ripoll EA, James GT. Inhibitory effects of selenium on the growth of DU-145 human prostate carcinoma cells in vitro. Biochem Biophys Res Commun 1985;130:603–9.

[69] Klein EA. Selenium and vitamin E cancer prevention trial. Ann N Y Acad Sci 2004;1031:234–41.

[70] Gunawardena K, Murray DK, Meikle AW. Vitamin E and other antioxidants inhibit human prostate cancer cells through apoptosis. Prostate 2000;44:287–95.

[71] Israel K, Yu W, Sanders BG, et al. Vitamin E succinate induces apoptosis in human prostate cancer cells: role for Fas in vitamin E succinate-triggered apoptosis. Nutr Cancer 2000;36:90–100.

[72] Heinonen OP, Albanes D, Virtamo J, et al. Prostate cancer and supplementation with alpha-tocopherol and beta-carotene: incidence and mortality in a controlled trial. J Natl Cancer Inst 1998;90:440–6.

[73] Jiang C, Wang Z, Ganther H, et al. Caspases as key executors of methyl selenium-induced apoptosis (anoikis) of DU-145 prostate cancer cells. Cancer Res 2001;61:3062–70.

[74] Jiang C, Wang Z, Ganther H, Lu J. Distinct effects of methylseleninic acid versus selenite on apoptosis, cell cycle, and protein kinase pathways in DU145 human prostate cancer cells. Mol Cancer Ther 2002;1:1059–66.

[75] Hu H, Jiang C, Ip C, et al. Methylseleninic acid potentiates apoptosis induced by chemotherapeutic drugs in androgen-independent prostate cancer cells. Clin Cancer Res 2005;11:2379–88.

[76] Agarwal C, Singh RP, Agarwal R. Grape seed extract induces apoptotic death of human prostate carcinoma DU145 cells via caspases activation accompanied by dissipation of mitochondrial membrane potential and cytochrome c release. Carcinogenesis 2002;23:1869–76.

[77] Inohara H, Raz A. Effects of natural complex carbohydrate (citrus pectin) on murine melanoma cell properties related to galectin-3 functions. Glycoconj J 1994;11:527–32.

[78] Hsieh TC, Wu JM. Changes in cell growth, cyclin/kinase, endogenous phosphoproteins and nm23 gene expression in human prostatic JCA-1 cells treated with modified citrus pectin. Biochem Mol Biol Int 1995;37:833–41.

[79] Pienta KJ, Naik H, Akhtar A, et al. Inhibition of spontaneous metastasis in a rat prostate cancer model by oral administration of modified citrus pectin. J Natl Cancer Inst 1995;87:348–53.

[80] Guess BW, Scholz MC, Strum SB, et al. Modified citrus pectin (MCP) increases the prostate-specific antigen doubling time in men with prostate cancer: a phase II pilot study. Prostate Cancer Prostatic Dis 2003;6:301–4.

[81] Parkin DM, Pisani P, Ferlay J. Global cancer statistics. CA Cancer J Clin 1999;49:33–64, 1.

[82] Fournier DB, Erdman JW Jr, Gordon GB. Soy, its components, and cancer prevention: a review of the in vitro, animal, and human data. Cancer Epidemiol Biomarkers Prev 1998;7:1055–65.

[83] Mentor-Marcel R, Lamartiniere CA, Eltoum IA, et al. Dietary genistein improves survival and reduces expression of osteopontin in the prostate of transgenic mice with prostatic adenocarcinoma (TRAMP). J Nutr 2005;135:989–95.

[84] Pollard M, Wolter W, Sun L. Prevention of induced prostate-related cancer by soy protein isolate/isoflavone-supplemented diet in Lobund-Wistar rats. In Vivo 2000;14:389–92.

[85] Davis JN, Singh B, Bhuiyan M, et al. Genistein-induced upregulation of p21WAF1, downregulation of cyclin B, and induction of apoptosis in prostate cancer cells. Nutr Cancer 1998;32:123–31.

[86] Messina MJ, Persky V, Setchell KD, et al. Soy intake and cancer risk: a review of the in vitro and in vivo data. Nutr Cancer 1994;21:113–31.

[87] Zand RS, Jenkins DJ, Diamandis EP. Steroid hormone activity of flavonoids and related compounds. Breast Cancer Res Treat 2000;62:35–49.

[88] Bylund A, Zhang JX, Bergh A, et al. Rye bran and soy protein delay growth and increase apoptosis of human LNCaP prostate adenocarcinoma in nude mice. Prostate 2000;42:304–14.

[89] Jacobsen BK, Knutsen SF, Fraser GE. Does high soy milk intake reduce prostate cancer incidence? The Adventist Health Study (United States). Cancer Causes Control 1998;9:553–7.

[90] deVere White RW, Hackman RM, Soares SE, et al. Effects of a genistein-rich extract on PSA levels in men with a history of prostate cancer. Urology 2004;63:259–63.

[91] DiPaola RS, Zhang H, Lambert GH, et al. Clinical and biologic activity of an estrogenic herbal combination (PC-SPES) in prostate cancer. N Engl J Med 1998;339:785–91.

[92] Kubota T, Hisatake J, Hisatake Y, et al. PC-SPES: a unique inhibitor of proliferation of prostate cancer cells in vitro and in vivo. Prostate 2000;42:163–71.

[93] de la Taille A, Buttyan R, Hayek O, et al. Herbal therapy PC-SPES: in vitro effects and evaluation of its efficacy in 69 patients with prostate cancer. J Urol 2000;164:1229–34.

[94] de la Taille A, Hayek OR, Burchardt M, et al. Role of herbal compounds (PC-SPES) in hormone-refractory prostate cancer: two case reports. J Altern Complement Med 2000;6:449–51.

[95] Small EJ, Frohlich MW, Bok R, et al. Prospective trial of the herbal supplement PC-SPES in patients with progressive prostate cancer. J Clin Oncol 2000;18:3595–603.

[96] Sovak M, Seligson AL, Konas M, et al. Herbal composition PC-SPES for management of prostate cancer: identification of active principles. J Natl Cancer Inst 2002;94:1275–81.

[97] Oh WK, Kantoff PW, Weinberg V, et al. Prospective, multicenter, randomized phase II trial of the herbal supplement, PC-SPES, and diethylstilbestrol in patients with androgen-independent prostate cancer. J Clin Oncol 2004;22:3705–12.

ELSEVIER
SAUNDERS

Urol Clin N Am 33 (2006) 247–272

UROLOGIC
CLINICS
of North America

Future Innovations in Treating Advanced Prostate Cancer

Pratik Desai, MD[a], Juan A. Jiménez[a], Chinghai Kao, PhD[b],
Thomas A. Gardner, MD[b],*

[a]Department of Urology, Indiana University School of Medicine, 535 Barnhill Drive,
#420 Indianapolis, IN 46202, USA
[b]Walther Oncology Center, Department of Urology, Indiana University School of Medicine,
535 Barnhill Drive, #420, Indianapolis, IN 46202, USA

In 2005, it was estimated that prostate cancer will account for the second most new cancer diagnoses (skin cancer will account for the most) and will effect 232,090 men in the United States. It will be the second most common cause of cancer deaths and will claim 30,350 lives. A steady decline in the annual age-adjusted prostate cancer death rates over the past 5 years as recorded in the Surveillance Epidemiology and End Results Cancer Statistics Review would suggest improvements in early detection and treatment of locally confined prostate cancer [1]. Current treatment options prolong life; however, most patients will eventually experience local recurrence or develop advanced disease. Androgen ablation therapy slows the dissemination of the disease but, once the cancer changes its androgen status, tumors become refractory to hormonal treatment. A greater understanding of the molecular events underlying cancer and the subsequent development of metastatic disease has enabled investigators to explore gene therapy approaches that are targeted against these molecular events. The focus of study may be grouped into three broad topics: (1) antiangiogenic therepy, (2) immune based therapy, and (3) gene therapy. Each group is unique in its design and approach to the treatment of prostate cancer.

This work is supported by NIH grant K08 CA079544-01A2 and the Department of Defense grant DAMD 17-03-1-0077.

* Corresponding author.
E-mail address: thagardn@iupui.edu (T.A. Gardner).

Antiangiogenic therapy

Antiangiogenic therapy is a promising adjuvant to conventional therapies that should help to overcome their current limitations and enhance their antitumor effect [2]. Antiangiogenic therapy targets endothelial cells rather than cancer cells. The resulting loss of tumor vasculature limits the nutrient supply to the tumor and inhibits growth or induces apoptosis in surrounding cancer cells [3]. Several antiangiogenic agents are currently under investigation in phase I, II, and III clinical trials and the early results are promising. One advantage of antiangiogenic therapy over conventional therapy is the low frequency of drug resistance mutations in endothelial cells. Current antiangiogenic strategies target endothelial cells either directly, by inhibiting their proliferation and migration or inducing apoptosis, or indirectly, by inhibiting the production of angiogenic factors by tumor cells. Therapeutic strategies include the delivery of endogenous inhibitors of angiogenesis, agents that prevent the degradation of the basement membrane or extracellular membrane (ECM), agents that interfere with or block the action of proangiogenic factors, and small molecule inhibitors of angiogenic factor receptors found in prostate cancer. The hopes of antiangiogenic therapy are to transform prostate cancer to a chronic disease state.

Angiogenesis in prostate cancer

As first suggested by Dr. Folkman in 1971, tumor growth is dependent on nutritional support derived from the local blood supply [4], and tumors are limited in size by the diffusion capacity of oxygen and nutrients from the existing vasculature. Further growth requires the induction of neovascularization and invasion of capillaries from surrounding vessels. This tightly regulated process, called angiogenesis, is depicted in Fig. 1 and involves the degradation of the existing endothelial basement membrane, migration of endothelial cells into the ECM of the tumor, proliferation and structural reorganization of endothelial cells, and fusion of the endothelial cells into tubular vessels [5]. Angiogenesis is involved in wound healing and regrowth of the endometrial lining, where it is controlled by a balance of angiogenic inducers and inhibitors. Prostate tumors remain dormant and clinically undetectable until they begin to secrete angiogenic factors and downregulate the expression of angiogenic inhibitors [6], a defined early event in tumor development known as the angiogenic switch [7]. The result is an imbalance of angiogenic factors leading to growth of new vessels and the tumor.

Fig. 2 lists the common endogenous angiogenic promoters and inhibitors found in prostate cancer.

Surface antigens on newly formed tumor vessels differ from those of the existing normal vasculature and can be used to quantify the tumor vasculature. Vascular endothelial growth factor (VEGF) receptors are upregulated in neovasculature [8], and prostate-specific membrane antigen (PSMA) is associated with tumor vasculature, including non-prostate tumors, but not normal vasculature [9]. Using immunohistochemistry for endothelial-specific antigens such as CD31 and CD34, microvessel density (MVD) in prostate tumors can be measured. Several studies have shown that MVD correlates with disease progression and may function as a prognostic factor for prostate cancer. MVD was nearly twofold higher in patients with metastatic disease compared with patients with organ-confined disease, and MVD was shown to increase in higher grade tumors [10]. Clearly, angiogenic switch is critical to the tumorigenesis of prostate cancer.

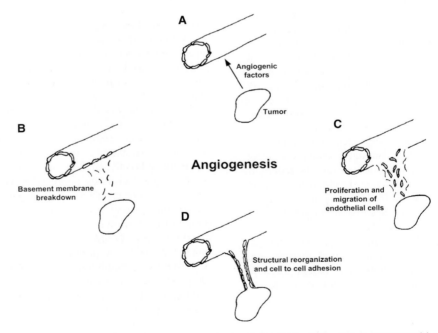

Fig. 1. Angiogenesis and the progression of tumor growth. An angiogenic switch results in a tumor with an angiogenic factor-secreting phenotype (A). Angiogenic factors cause the permeabilization and break-down of the basement membrane in the surrounding vasculature (B). Endothelial cells are stimulated to proliferate and migrate toward the angiogenic factor-secreting tumor (C). Microvascular endothelial networks composed of loosely connected cellular cords differentiate into capillary tubules. Structural reorganization and penetration of the capillary sprouts into the tumor provides blood flow to the growing tumor (D).

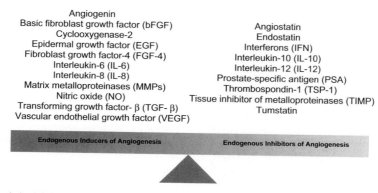

Angiogenin
Basic fibroblast growth factor (bFGF)
Cyclooxygenase-2
Epidermal growth factor (EGF)
Fibroblast growth factor-4 (FGF-4)
Interleukin-6 (IL-6)
Interleukin-8 (IL-8)
Matrix metalloproteinases (MMPs)
Nitric oxide (NO)
Transforming growth factor- β (TGF- β)
Vascular endothelial growth factor (VEGF)

Angiostatin
Endostatin
Interferons (IFN)
Interleukin-10 (IL-10)
Interleukin-12 (IL-12)
Prostate-specific antigen (PSA)
Thrombospondin-1 (TSP-1)
Tissue inhibitor of metalloproteinases (TIMP)
Tumstatin

Endogenous Inducers of Angiogenesis   **Endogenous Inhibitors of Angiogenesis**

Fig. 2. Angiogenesis is tightly controlled by a balance of endogenous inducers and inhibitors of angiogenesis. Primary tumors cannot grow larger than 2–3 mm without inducing neovascularization. Early in tumor progression, an imbalance of angiogenesis regulators occurs, which favors an angiogenic environment. This angiogenic switch results in the over-secretion of angiogenesis inducers such as VEGF and the subsequent neovascularization and growth of the tumor.

Vascular endothelial growth factor

VEGF is perhaps the most important factor that induces angiogenesis in prostate cancer. It was first characterized by Senger and coworkers [11] as a mitogenic factor for endothelial cells. The gene encoding VEGF is found on chromosome 6p21.3 [12] and comprises eight exons [13]. Through alternative splicing of the VEGF transcripts, six VEGF isoforms exist and are named for their length in amino acids: $VEGF_{121}$, $VEGF_{145}$, $VEGF_{165}$, $VEGF_{183}$, $VEGF_{189}$, and $VEGF_{206}$ [14]. All six isoforms are secreted from VEGF-producing tumor cells; however, $VEGF_{121}$, $VEGF_{165}$, and $VEGF_{189}$ appear to be preferentially secreted. In response to hypoxia, transcription of VEGF is activated by the hypoxia-induced transcription factor 1 (HIF-1) [15]. VEGF may also be regulated by the hypoxia-induced activation of NF-κB, as blockade of the NF-κB pathway resulted in inhibition of angiogenesis in PC-3M human prostate cancer cells [16]. Consistent with an early molecular switch in oncogenesis, overexpression of *ras* and *raf* stimulate the expression and secretion of VEGF [17]. Normal prostate tissue expresses minimal to no VEGF [18], unlike prostate cancer tissue which stained positively for VEGF in areas of increased MVD [19]. Recently, a correlation between elevated serum VEGF levels and hormone-refractory prostate cancer was discovered, which suggests the potential clinical usefulness for VEGF as a prognostic factor in prostate cancer [20]. Of interest, recent studies have shown that VEGF expression is stimulated in the presence of androgens. In this regard, androgen ablation therapy is a clinical means of suppressing tumor angiogenesis in vivo [21].

The function of VEGF during embryogenesis is to promote de novo vascularization from endothelial precursor cells. In fact, loss of a single *VEGF* allele in mouse embryos leads to vascular deformities and an embryonic-lethal phenotype [22]. During tumor angiogenesis, VEGF induces the expression of proteases by endothelial cells which facilitates the digestion of the endothelial basement membrane, release from anchorage and migration [23]. VEGF is also a permeability factor which causes leakage of plasma from capillaries into the surrounding tissue matrix [11]. In addition, it stimulates the elongation, branching, and proliferation of endothelial cells [24,25]. As new vessels are formed, VEGF functions as a survival factor for the emerging endothelial cells [26]. The angiogenic effect of VEGF is mediated by two receptors on which VEGF binds as a homodimer [27]. The first receptor to be identified, VEGF receptor-1 (VEGFR-1) or fms-like tyrosine kinase receptor (Flt-1), has the highest affinity for VEGF [28]; however, tyrosine phosphorylation of VEGF-1 results in only minor endothelial proliferation or migration [29]. VEGF receptor-2 (VEGFR-2), also known as kinase insert domain-containing receptor or fetal liver kinase-1 (Flk-1) [30,31], mediates the major VEGF response in endothelial cells [32].

Basic fibroblast growth factor

Another growth factor with the ability to induce proliferation and migration of endothelial cells in prostate cancer is basic fibroblast growth factor (bFGF) or fibroblast growth factor-2 (FGF-2). Like VEGF, bFGF stimulates the release and activity of collagenases, proteases, and integrins on the ECM to form nascent microvascular networks [33]. The angiogenic effects of FGF-2 and VEGF were found to be synergistic in three-dimensional endothelial cell cultures [34]. In addition, FGF-2 is a strong autocrine mitogen for prostate stromal fibroblasts and induces paracrine growth stimulation on prostate epithelial cells. This is further supported by the discovery of FGF-2 receptor (FGFR-1) on both endothelial and prostate cancer cells [35]. Similar to VEGF, FGF-2 expression varies with the grade of prostate cancer. Primary specimens of high-grade, metastatic prostate cancer express more FGF-2 than low-grade, organ-confined prostate cancers [36]. In addition, androgen-independent prostate cancer cell lines, such as PC-3 and DU-145, express higher levels of FGF-2 than androgen-dependent LNCaP cells, which indicates a relationship between FGF-2 status and prostate cancer progression [37].

Matrix metalloproteinases

Interactions between endothelial cells and the vascular basement membrane or the tumor ECM are a critical component of angiogenesis. The degradation of the vascular basement membrane, which is required for endothelial cell migration, is performed by type IV collagenases called matrix metalloproteinases (MMPs) [38]. In a study to evaluate the expression of MMPs in prostate cancer, MMP-2 and MMP-9 were identified at the leading tumor margins in prostate cancer specimens, and demonstrated a positive correlation to Gleason score [39]. MMPs are regulated by tissue inhibitors of matrix metalloproteinases. Other proteases are implicated in prostate cancer angiogenesis. Urokinase plasminogen activator (uPA) is expressed by aggressive prostate cancers and highly metastatic PC-3 and DU-145 cell lines [40]. Blockade of the uPA receptor inhibited tumor angiogenesis and prostate cancer growth in the rat Dunning MATLyLu model [41]. uPA also negatively regulates angiogenesis by catalyzing the conversion of plasminogen to the angiogenesis inhibitor, angiostatin [42].

Other proangiogenic factors in prostate cancer

Several other factors contribute to the promotion of angiogenesis in prostate cancer. Transforming growth factor-β (TGF-β) is a negative regulator of prostate epithelial growth whose expression correlated with increased vascularity and angiogenesis in prostate cancer specimens [43]. Cyclooxygenase-2 (COX-2), an enzyme responsible for converting arachidonic acid to prostaglandins, is also a positive regulator of angiogenesis through its major product, prostaglandin E2 [44]. The COX-2 inhibitor, NS-938, was shown to suppress angiogenesis and the growth of PC-3 tumors in nude mouse xenograft models [45]. Another potent mediator of angiogenesis is angiogenin [46]. Inhibition of angiogenin by monoclonal antibodies resulted in lower frequencies of established PC-3M tumors and metastases in nude mice [47].

Antiangiogenic agents

An understanding of the basic science of angiogenesis has led to the development of several antiangiogenic therapies which have only recently been introduced into clinical practice. By the inhibition of tumor neovascularization, tumor growth is suppressed. For this reason, most antiangiogenic compounds were traditionally considered cytostatic; however, preclinical and clinical data have demonstrated cytotoxic effects as well. Antiangiogenic drugs have been discovered to block nearly every step in the angiogenic cascade and include large molecules, small molecule inhibitors, protein fragments, monoclonal antibodies, and chemotherapeutic agents.

Thrombospondin-1

Good [48] and colleagues identified the first endogenous inhibitor of angiogenesis, Thrombospondin-1 (TSP-1), from a culture of normal fibroblasts. TSP-1 is a major antiangiogenic protein in prostate cells. Doll and coworkers [36] found that normal prostate epithelial cells secrete high levels of TSP-1, and prostate cancer cells secrete significantly lower levels of the inhibitor, which supports a switch to a proangiogenic phenotype. TSP-1 is a large ECM protein of 450 kDa which inhibits endothelial cell proliferation and capillary network formation by binding to endothelial cell matrix proteins [49]. This inhibition was potentiated by angiocidin, a TSP-1 binding protein [50]. The large size and instability of TSP-1 limits its clinical utility as an intravenous pharmaceutical agent; however, delivery and expression by gene therapy remains feasible. cDNA encoding TSP-1 was transfected into

DU-145 prostate cancer cell lines. Although expression of TSP-1 did not affect the growth of DU-145 cells in culture, overexpression of TSP-1 inhibited the growth of DU-145 xenografts in nude mice [51].

TNP-470

Ingber and coworkers [52] observed a ring of inhibition around *Asperigillus fumigatus* contaminants in endothelial cell cultures which led to the discovery of the antiangiogenic properties of the secreted antibiotic, fumagillin. Fumagillin retained its antiangiogenic activity in vivo and suppressed tumor growth; however, it was extremely toxic to mice. The synthetic fumagillin analog, O-(chloroacetyl-carbamoyl) fumagillol (TNP-470), was found to be 50-fold more potent than fumagillin and generally well tolerated. The antiangiogenic effect of TNP-470 appears to be mediated by the perturbation of endothelial cell cycle regulators or the promotion of TSP-1 production [53]. TNP-470 inhibited androgen-independent PC-3 xenografts in nude mice by 96%, and had an additive antitumor effect when combined with cisplatin treatment. In addition, TNP-470 demonstrated slight inhibitory activity against PC-3 cells in culture, which suggested a direct inhibitory effect on prostate cancer cells in addition to the antiangiogenic effect [54]. Combined therapy with docetaxel and TNP-470 demonstrated a synergistic effect against murine subcutaneous and orthotopic PC-3 tumors. In addition, this therapy reduced the incidence of lymph node metastases [55]. Despite the great preclinical success of TNP-470, a phase I clinical trial conducted by Logothetis and colleagues [56] demonstrated no definite antitumor activity against androgen-independent prostate cancer in 33 men. In addition, dose-limiting neuropsychiatric toxicities which resolved 14 weeks after treatment cessation were observed in several patients.

Thalidomide

Once marketed in Europe as an over-the-counter sedative and antimimetic for pregnant women, thalidomide was withdrawn because of reports of dysmyelia and severe teratogenic effects. Today, it is approved for the treatment of certain autoimmune disorders including AIDS, tuberculosis, and malignancies. D'Amato [57] first described the antiangiogenic properties of thalidomide against the neovascularization of a bFGF-stimulated rabbit cornea model. In humans, thalidomide is antiangiogenic only when metabolized to its active product [58]. Figg and colleagues [59] tested the clinical utility of thalidomide in men who had metastatic prostate cancer and who had failed multiple therapies. Sixty-three patients were given either low or high dose thalidomide; 27% of all patients responded with a decline in serum prostate-specific antigen (PSA) $\geq$ 40%. This treatment regimen was well tolerated. A second clinical trial investigated the effect of combination docetaxel and thalidomide therapy. Thirty-five percent of patients who received docetaxel therapy alone responded with a PSA decrease of at least 50%, and 53% of the patients who received both docetaxel and thalidomide responded with a serum PSA decrease of at least 50% [60]. The median progression-free survival was higher in the combined group (5.9 months) than in the docetaxel-alone group (3.7 months). In addition, at 18 months, the overall survival was higher in the combined group (68.2%) than in the docetaxel-alone group (42.9%) [61]. Data from these clinical trials are very promising. Currently, thalidomide analogs are being developed with higher antiangiogenic activities and wider therapeutic windows [62,63].

Angiostatin

The most potent and specific inhibitors of angiogenesis are the products of proteolytic cleavage of larger proteins. Angiostatin, a 38 kDa fragment of plasminogen, was first characterized by O'Reilly and colleagues [64] as a circulating antiangiogenic factor discovered in a murine Lewis lung carcinoma model. Gately and coworkers [65] demonstrated that serine protease activity in PC-3, DU-145 and LNCaP prostate cancer cells was required for the generation of bioactive angiostatin from purified plasminogen. In several murine tumor models, systemic administration of angiostatin resulted in dormancy of metastases [66]. Galaup and colleagues [67] developed a combined therapy to target both the epithelial and endothelial components of prostate cancer. The kringle 1-3 domain of angiostatin was delivered to prostate cancer cells via AdK3, a replication-deficient adenovirus, in association with the chemotherapeutic agent, docetaxel. In vitro, human endothelial cells were up to 100-fold more sensitive to docetaxel than PC-3, LNCaP, or DU-145 prostate cancer cells. Furthermore, the cytotoxic effect of angiostatin was enhanced by the administration of docetaxel. In vivo, total regression was observed in 83% of PC-3 nude mouse xenograft tumors receiving the combination therapy [67].

Receptor tyrosine kinase inhibitors

VEGF and its receptors play a key role in angiogenesis as well as tumor growth and spread. Activated VEGF receptors initiate their signaling cascade in endothelial cells through autophosphorylation on tyrosine residues. Small molecule inhibitors of receptor tyrosine kinases (RTKs) have been discovered with high potency and specificity for the VEGF receptors. These low molecular weight proteins are orally active which simplifies the administration to patients. ZD6474 is an RTK inhibitor with specificity for VEGFR-2 tyrosine kinase ($IC_{50} = 40nM$). In vitro, ZD6474 inhibited the VEGF-stimulated proliferation of human umbilical vein endothelial cells (HUVECs) ($IC_{50} = 60nM$), and oral administration of ZD6474 to nude mice bearing PC-3 xenografts resulted in growth inhibition and profound regression in larger tumors [68]. KRN633 is another RTK inhibitor that shows higher inhibition of VEGF-2 tyrosine phosphorylation ($IC_{50} = 1.16nM$) in HUVECs. Oral administration of KRN633 was well tolerated and inhibited tumor growth in nude mice prostate cancer xenografts [69]. CEP-7055 is an RTK inhibitor that has broad VEGF receptor activity. CEP-7055 demonstrated inhibition of VEGFR-1 ($IC_{50} = 12nM$), VEGFR-2 ($IC_{50} = 18nM$), and VEGFR-3 ($IC_{50} = 17nM$) phosphorylation in biochemical kinase assays. Inhibition of VEGFR-2 autophosphorylation in HUVECs was even higher ($IC_{50} = 10nM$). In male nude mouse LNCaP orthotopic models, p.o. administration of CEP-7055 significantly inhibited the formation of metastases. CEP-7055 is currently in phase I clinical evaluation [70]. AEE788 is a dual family RTK, that shows inhibitory action against VEGFR-1 ($IC_{50} = 59nM$), VEGFR-2 ($IC_{50} = 77nM$) and epidermal growth factor (EGF) receptor ($IC_{50} = 2nM$) tyrosine kinases. In addition to the antiangiogenic effect of AEE788, it directly inhibits prostate cancer cell growth, because EGF is a potent growth stimulatory signal for prostate epithelium [71].

Antiangiogenic properties of chemotherapeutic agents

At low doses, some cytotoxic chemotherapy drugs inhibit tumor-associated angiogenesis. Of course, at sufficiently high doses, any chemotherapeutic drug will kill endothelial cells; however, because of the narrow therapeutic windows of such agents, these drugs cannot be used clinically for their antiangiogenic properties. Miller and colleagues [72] defined the criteria to properly classify chemotherapeutic drugs as antiangiogenic agents. To qualify, a drug must by toxic to endothelial cells at lower doses than those needed to achieve cytotoxicity against cancer cells. In addition, the drug should inhibit angiogenesis by interfering with angiogenic cascade rather than killing endothelial cells. Finally, these effects should be observed in vivo. The most widely investigated chemotherapeutics with antiangiogenic properties are the microtubule-stabilizing taxanes. Docetaxel, used for hormone-refractory prostate cancer, targets the microtubule cytoskeleton of endothelial cells and decreases the frequency of reorientation of endothelial cell centrosomes, which leads to a decrease in cell migration without the disruption of microtubule gross structure [73]. Endothelial cells are 10- to 100-fold more sensitive to taxanes than cancer cells. Comparative studies have shown docetaxel to be 10-times stronger than paclitaxel at inhibiting angiogenesis [74]. Other compounds such as the alpha-blocker doxazosin have been shown to suppress tumor vascularity in pathological specimens. In addition, doxazosin successfully inhibited the VEGF- and bFGF-mediated migration of HUVECs in vitro [75]. Continuously administered low-dose chemotherapeutics carry great potential as well-tolerated antiangiogenic agents.

VEGF inhibitors

Several agents including large synthetic molecules and monoclonal antibodies have been discovered that block the direct binding of VEGF to its receptor. GFA-116 is a synthetic cyclohexapeptidomimetic calixarene that has high affinity and selectivity for Flk-1, which inhibits prostate tumor-derived VEGF binding ($IC_{50} = 750nM$), which prevents Flk-1 tyrosine phosphorylation. In vitro, GFA-116 inhibited migration and formation of tubular vessels from HUVECs as well as microvessel outgrowth from rat aortic rings. In vivo, GFA-116 was effective at inhibiting tumor growth and metastasis formation in nude mice [76]. DC101 is a monoclonal antibody against Flk-1. Orthotopic PC-3 and LNCaP prostate cancer models were treated with paclitaxel alone, DC101 alone, or DC101 plus paclitaxel. Tumors were greatly inhibited in the combination group compared with untreated or single-treatment group tumors. In addition, the incidence of lymph node metastases was greatly reduced (2 of 11 animals) in the combined group, compared with paclitaxel alone (5 of 9 mice) or DC101 alone (5 of 12 mice). Early tumors were more successfully treated than late tumors, which suggests that tumor burden at the initiation of treatment is a critical factor in determining response to DC101 [77]. A4.6.1 is a neutralizing anti-VEGF antibody that completely inhibited the neovascularization and growth of subcutaneous DU-145 prostate cancer tumors in nude mice [78]. A4.6.1 also inhibited the formation of pulmonary metastases. Even when treatment with A4.6.1 was delayed, metastatic progression was inhibited [79]. Recently, bevacizumab, a humanized monoclonal antibody against VEGF, was approved for use in patients who have metastatic colon cancer. Clinical studies are ongoing to evaluate its efficacy in patients who have advanced prostate cancer.

Immune based therapies for prostate cancer

Immune based therapies can be classified as either active or passive therapies. Passive therapies require the administration of effector cells or molecules to the patient. These therapies are not reliant on any activity of the patient's immune system. Passive immunotherapies include cytokines, antibodies, and lymphocytes. Active immunotherapies attempt to elicit a host anti-tumor immune response. Prime examples of active therapies are vaccines. Both active and passive immunotherapy strategies may be specific or nonspecific. Specificity is related to tumor-specific antigens that are presented to T cells or antibodies. Nonspecific strategies induce inflammation or augmentation of an already present immune response.

Passive immunotherapy

Nonspecific passive immunotherapy

Passive nonspecific immunotherapy generally involves the administration of cytokines, which act directly on the tumor cell. Cytokines are produced by host stromal and immune cells, in response to molecules secreted by the cancer cells or as part of inflammation that frequently accompanies tumor growth.

One model hypothesizes that dendritic cells act as sentinel cells that may modulate immune response. Signals such as heat-shock proteins,

pro-inflammatory factors (including cytokines), and reactive host cells such as macrophages and natural killer cells may initiate the response of dendritic cells. These signals are released as a result of tumor cell damage or necrosis. Cytokines, such as interleukin-1 (IL-1), tumor necrosis factor (TNF), type I interferon (IFN), granulocyte–macrophage colony-stimulating factor (GM-CSF), and IL-15, can promote dendritic cell differentiation and activity by multiple mechanisms. Dendritic cells may then interact with tumor-associated antigens and in turn acquire a mature activated phenotype. These mature dendritic cells may then migrate to lymph nodes where the tumor-associated antigens are presented to CD4 + and CD8 + T cells. Additionally, B cells may also be activated. These complex interactions may attack tumors with both cellular and humoral responses.

Strategies exploiting the activity cytokines have been investigated, but often are limited by unacceptable systemic toxicities as seen with IFN or TNF-α. Newer delivery strategies, such as intra-tumoral injection may decrease the systemic effects of these agents. In a study by Kramer and coworkers [80] 10 patients who had locally advanced, hormone-resistant prostate cancer, were treated with recombinant TNF-α injected locally into prostate tumor tissue at 4-week intervals (maximum of 4 cycles) combined with intermittent subcutaneous administration of IFN-α2b. TNF-α induced prostate tumor cell necrosis in all patients, which led to a significant reduction of prostate volume in 9 of 10 cases and subsequent PSA decreases that ranged from 18% to 87%. Even though objective responses were not seen, the TNF-α was well tolerated with only World Health Organization grade 1–2 toxicity.

GM-CSF, an immunostimulatory growth protein, has been investigated for its activity against prostate cancer. It has been given as a single agent and has shown direct antitumor activity. Dreicer and colleagues [81] performed a small phase II trial in which 16 patients with metastatic prostate cancer were treated with 250g GM-CSF three times per week for up to 6 months. This yielded a serum PSA decline in some patients; however, they could not report any objective responses Additionally, GM-CSF is also being investigated as a vaccine adjuvant. As such, cytokines may play an important role in a multifaceted anti-tumor intervention.

Specific passive immunotherapy

The generation of a directed immune response that is fulcrum of specific passive immunotherapy involves multiple factors. Antigens direct interaction with cells (such as B lymphocytes, antigen presenting cells, and dendritic cells) that allow for recognition by the immune system. T lymphocytes also play a key role in recognition of antigens, and with CD4 + cells stimulate cytotoxic T lymphocytes and B lymphocytes. This entire process of recognition begins a cascade of events that involves cytokine production, B lymphocyte proliferation, and ultimately the production of antibodies.

Many tumor-associated antigens have been identified which include over-expressed or selectively expressed normal molecules (such as differentiation and oncofetal antigens), and viral- and tumor-specific antigens including mutated products. These antigens, which differentiate tumor from normal cells, have been the targets of investigation for many novel therapies using antibodies.

Antibodies may have several mechanisms that may be exploited for immunotherapeutic benefits. There may be direct induction of apoptosis or the blocking a necessary growth factor. Indirectly, the interaction of antibody to the cell can signal cellular cytotoxicity by an effector cell (lymphocyte, macrophage, monocyte, etc.). These interactions of antibodies are often not sufficient to provide effective cytotoxicity.

To increase the potential of antibody directed therapy, the ability of an antibody to recognize a malignant cell may be used to carry a toxic substance directly to a desired cell. This toxic substance may be in the form a radioactive moiety or an inhibitor of growth pathways.

Milowsky and colleagues [82] treated 29 patients who had androgen independent prostate cancer with yttrium-90-labeled anti-prostate specific membrane antigen monoclonal antibody J591. This was a phase I trial; however, it provided some exciting data about the potential of this immunotherapy. Prostate antibody mediated therapy has been limited in part by the lack of identification of a good prostate specific antigen to target. Although there were significant toxicities at doses required for response, prostate specific membrane antigen did show potential as a unique antigen for target of further research In other malignancies such as breast cancer, Herceptin, a monoclonal antibody directed at HER-2/neu, is currently used as standard treatment. There has been evidence that prostate tissue also has expression of this protein. Currently animal investigations of Herceptin activity against prostate cancer are underway.

Active immunotherapy

The goal of vaccine mediated therapy is to stimulate an immune mediated anti-tumor associated antigen response resulting in the destruction of tumor cell. The approaches to this goal are diverse, and often involve the generation of cytotoxic T lymphocytes. The antigen may be a whole cell, a protein, immune stimulatory components, or different epitopes of the target antigen.

Whole cell vaccines

Live whole tumor cells inactivated by radiation were the first types of antitumor vaccines investigated. This strategy has some intuitive appeal because a whole cell vaccine has a large array of tumor-associated antigens that may be potential targets for the immune system. Furthermore, the whole tumor cells may be isolated from individuals and so employ tumor-associated antigens that are unique to that patient. This theory of whole cell vaccines, however, has produced only limited successes.

A phase I trial performed by Simons and coworkers [83] pioneered autologous tumor vaccination with prostate cancer cells that had been transfected to express GM-CSF. Although the trial did not have notable results in tumor response, it did readily demonstrate "both T-cell and B-cell immune responses to human PCA can be generated by treatment with irradiated, GM-CSF gene-transduced PCA vaccines."

Peptides and recombinant proteins

Processing tumor cells results in the identification of many different peptides that are present on the surface of the cell along with major histocompatibility complex (MHC) molecules. Many of these are tumor- specific antigens to be presented to T lymphocytes. One of the limitations peptide-based vaccines face is the fact that these complexes are restricted by HLA typing. This introduces great variation in the efficiency of recognition by the immune system based on the HLA type, as HLA molecules expressed by an individual restricts the repertoire of peptides that are presented.

Use of recombinant proteins instead of peptide approaches facilitates the delivery of all possible epitopes to the cells of the immune system that recognize antigens. As a result, vaccines based on recombinant protein technology can be administered regardless of the individual tissue type.

Harris and colleagues [84] reported phase I results of a vaccine consisting of liposome-encapsulated recombinant PSA and lipid A. In preliminary reports, they reported that although immunologic tolerance was disrupted, some subjects were able to generate CD4 + cells.

Tumor associated carbohydrate vaccines

Some membrane-bound carbohydrates are epitopes of tumor-associated antigens. These have been found to be preferentially expressed by cancer cells, or they may be unique tumor-associated antigens associated with the alteration of normally occurring carbohydrate by the tumor cell. These carbohydrates may be targeted as tumor-associated antigens.

Naked DNA vaccines

Specific genes that code for tumor-specific antigens can be cloned into plasmids. This plasmid can then be injected directly to the host (in many cases directly into muscle). The tumor specific antigen gene then uses the host cell to produce the antigenic protein. Additionally, all of this can be done fairly easily, in large quantities, and easily delivered.

Kim and colleagues [85,86] used DNA-based PSA vaccine to elicit PSA-specific host immune responses in rodent and rhesus monkeys. They also used cytokine gene adjuvants to modulate vaccine-induced immune responses. In addition to inducing PSA specific immunity, they were also able to identify that coimmuniztion with cDNA coding for certain cytokines (IL-2) resulted in a greater PSA-specific response.

Recombinant viral vaccines

Viral infections result in the presentation of viral peptides complexed with HLA molecules on the surface of infected cells. As such, viruses may be an ideal vector to deliver tumor-associated antigens. The advantage of these vaccines is that proteins are endogenously synthesized from viral DNA by host cells, and the result is that an array of peptides are produced, processed, and presented on the cell surface in conjunction with MHC class I molecules. Such a system poses no restriction on patient HLA genotypes.

Kaufman and coworkers [87] conducted a phase II clinical trail with the Eastern Cooperative Oncology Group for patients who had early metastatic prostate cancer. Sixty-four eligible patients were randomly assigned to receive four vaccinations with fowlpox-PSA (rF-PSA), three rF-PSA vaccines followed by one vaccinia-PSA (rV-PSA) vaccine, or one rV-PSA vaccine followed by three rF-PSA vaccines. Although the study design was not powered for outcome comparisons of the cohorts, the treatment group that received a priming dose of rV-PSA was favored. This outcome was measured by PSA-specific immune responses and inhibition of progressive tumor growth.

Dendritic cell vaccines

Autologous dendritic cells may prove to be an important tool in the delivery of vaccines. These cells are derived from bone marrow and are uniquely capable of sensitizing naïve T lymphocytes to protein antigens. The dendritic cell can be isolated in vitro and then loaded with tumor antigen. The antigen bearing dendritic cell is then injected as a cancer vaccine.

To this end, Fong and coworkers [88,89] administered two monthly vaccinations of xenoantigen-loaded dendritic cells pulsed with recombinant mouse prostatic acid phosphatase (PAP) to 21 patients who had metastatic prostate cancer. Although all 21 patients developed T cell immunity to the mouse PAP after immunization, disease stabilized in 6 of the 21 patients who had previously progressing disease.

Small and coworkers [90] immunized 31 hormone-refractory prostate cancer patients with autologous dendritic cells loaded ex vivo with a recombinant fusion protein that consisted of PAP linked to granulocyte-macrophage colony-stimulating factor. The infusions were very well tolerated. Patients who achieved T cell response (38% of patients) were found to have a significantly prolonged time to progression [90]. This very exciting result has resulted in a multi-institutional, randomized, placebo controlled, phase III trial.

Gene therapy

The ultimate goal of molecular therapies is an efficient oncologic treatment without adverse effects on nontarget cells. Gene therapy develops from strategy that carefully uses our understanding of the genetic code and the use of vectors to manipulate it. The genetic material for transfer is determined by the objective of the therapy. For example, gene therapy for prostate cancer can provide corrective therapy for genetic alterations that give the cancer a survival advantage such as those affecting tumor suppressors or growth-promoting oncogenes; however, because multiple mutations occur in the pathogenesis and progression of cancer, correction of one genetic insult may not be sufficient to change the cancer cell phenotype. Nevertheless, in vivo correction of single gene defects has been successful in several preclinical studies [91–94]. Targets for corrective therapy include the proto-oncogenes *p53, p21, p16, retinoblastoma (Rb)*, and certain cell adhesion molecules as well as the oncogenes *ras, myc,* and *bcl-2*. A second objective of molecular therapy for prostate cancer is to deliver genes that are capable of destroying tumor cells either directly or indirectly. Such cytoreductive therapies include the direct killing of prostate cancer cells by replication-competent oncolytic viruses, and the indirect killing of cancer cells through the delivery of suicide genes such as pro-drug enzyme and apoptosis-inducing genes. The final objective of the ideal gene therapy for prostate cancer is to enhance the body's antitumor immune response. Current approaches involve (1) ex vivo gene therapy of autologous tumor cells and subsequent vaccination with the irradiated cells that now express cytokines such as IL-2 and GM-CSF, (2) ex vivo gene transfer of genes that encode tumor antigens and subsequent vaccination which leads to enhanced induction of T-cell immunity, (3) in vivo intratumoral gene transfer of cytokine genes, and (4) delivery of naked tumor DNA or RNA and the subsequent uptake and expression by antigen presenting cells such as dendrites [95]. Table 1 summarizes these objectives the way they appear in clinical trials registered with the Office of Biologic Activities (OBA).

The ideal method of delivery would transfer the genetic material efficiently and specifically to the targeted organ, not be harmful to the patient, and be inexpensive to produce and administer. Each vector has advantages and disadvantages as couriers of genetic information. Adenovirus, perhaps the most commonly administered vector, clearly has its advantages and disadvantages. For example, adenovirus can efficiently deliver large amounts of genetic information regardless of the cell cycle status; however, it is highly immunogenic. To further compound this issue, it is believed that up to 75% of the population has innate immunity to several serotypes of adenovirus because of prior infection. Efforts have been made to create less immunogenic forms of the virus as well as gutless forms of the virus that

Table 1
Current approaches for prostate cancer gene therapy

Strategy	Vector(s)	DNA transferred
Corrective	Retrovirus	p53
	Adenovirus	p16
		c-myc
Cytoreductive (suicide)	Adenovirus	TK
		CD
		TK/CD
		NIS
(oncolytic)		OC promoter
		PB/PSA promoter
		PB/PSE promoter
		PSES promoter
Immunotherapy	Retrovirus	GM-CSF
	Vaccinia/fowl	MUC-1/IL-2
		PSA
	Liposome	PSA
		hTERT
		PSMA
		IL-2
	RNA	Tumor RNA
	AAV	GM-CSF
	Adenovirus	IL-12
		Inf-β

are incapable of replicating in immunocompromised patients. Such replication-deficient adenoviruses are achieved by deleting the early genes responsible for the control of viral replication [96].

Finally, the route of administration is determined by a combination of the previous three factors. Now most prostate cancer gene therapy trials involve the intratumoral injection of the vector, which is suitable because of the prostate can be visualized using ultrasound and its convenient transrectal access. Ultimately, to target metastatic prostate cancer, the desired route of administration is systemic intravenous transfusion of the vector. Limiting factors include vector half-life, hematologic inactivation of the vector, and infection of non-target organs. The main concentration at our laboratory has been on the development of tissue-specific promoters to overcome a number of these limitations (eg, **PSA**, osteocalcin, prostate-specific enhancer sequence, and β-hcg). As prostate-specific promoter systems become more effective, gene therapy may become the silver-bullet that seeks and destroys cancer cells in the prostate and distant metastatic sites.

Tissue-specific promoters

Recently, much effort has been made to develop tissue-specific delivery systems that eliminate the threat of harm to the patient. Several studies have demonstrated the importance of tissue-specific vectors, and revealed systemic toxicity with the administration of high doses of nonspecific vectors [97,98]. Essentially, viral vectors can transfer their therapeutic genes to any cell in the body, provided that it expresses the correct receptor for the virus. Through the use of prostate-specific promoters and enhancers, the expression of a therapeutic gene can be limited to cells that contain the appropriate activators and transcription factors. One limitation to this technology is low level leaky activation of prostate-specific promoters in non-prostatic tissues; however, the development of chimeric promoters promises greater prostate-specificity.

Osteocalcin promoter

Osteocalcin (OC) is a highly conserved bone gamma-carboxyglutamic acid protein that has been shown to be transcriptionally regulated by 1,25-dihydroxyvitamin D_3 [99]. This noncollagenous bone protein constitutes 1%–2% of the total protein in bone, and its expression is limited to differentiated osteoblasts and osteotropic tumors [100]. The osteoblastic nature of osseous prostate cancer metastases is well characterized [101], and the mechanism is believed to be via its osteomimetic properties, specifically its ability to express bone-related proteins such as OC [102]. The human OC promoter contains numerous regulatory elements including a vitamin D-responsive element (VDRE), which makes it inducible by vitamin D_3 administration [103,104]; a glucocorticoid response element; an AP-1 binding site [105]; and an AML-1 binding site, which has been shown to be responsible for 75% of OC expression [106]. The OC promoter retains its tissue specificity in a recombinant OC promoter-driven thymidine kinase (TK)-expressing adenoviral vector. Following infection with Ad-OC-TK, only cells of osteoblastic lineage expressed TK; furthermore, Ko and co-workers [107] demonstrated that the addition of acyclovir (ACV) resulted in osteoblast-specific cell toxicity. A similar strategy has been developed for the intralesional injection of Ad-OC-TK to osseous prostate cancer metastases followed by administration of valcyclovir (VAL). In clinical trials this approach induced treatment in lesions treated without serious adverse effects to the patients [108,109]. A phase II trial is currently underway in Japan with continued promising results [110].

Prostate-specific enhancer sequence

Prostate-specific proteins such as PSA and PSMA are released into the bloodstream when prostatic basement membrane is compromised, which occurs in prostate cancer, and therefore is used as a sensitive marker for diagnosis and progression of prostate cancer [111]. PSA expression is androgen receptor (AR)-dependent, and its transcript levels are significantly reduced in the absence of androgen [112]. AR regulates PSA expression by binding to an androgen-responsive enhancer core (AREc) in the upstream 5′ flanking region of the PSA gene [113,114]. This promoter confers high tissue specificity and has been used in several gene therapy studies [115–117]; however, its utility in men undergoing androgen ablation therapy is limited. On the other hand, PSMA expression is upregulated under androgen-depleted conditions [118]. Its expression is elevated higher in prostate cancer than in benign hyperplasia or normal prostate [119]. In addition, serum PSMA levels are highest in patients who have metastatic disease, which suggests enhanced PSMA expression as prostate cancer progresses [120]. Recently, the PSMA enhancer (PSME) was discovered within the third intron of the PSMA gene, FOLH1 [121] and has been used for prostate-specific gene delivery under low androgen levels [122]. Investigators at our laboratory hypothesized that AREc and PSME could function synergistically and developed a novel chimeric promoter, prostate-specific enhancer sequence (PSES) that has high transcriptional activity and strong prostate specificity.

Through deletion and linker scan mutagenesis, PSES was developed by locating the minimal sequences, AREc3 and PSME(del2) in AREc and PSME respectively, and by placing AREc3 upstream from PSME(del2). AREc3 contains six GATA transcription factor binding sites and three AR binding sites that lead to high enhancer activity once surrounding silencer regions are deleted. PSME(del2) contains eight AP-1 and three AP-3 [123] binding sites which act as positive regulators in the absence of androgen and a downstream deletion of an Alu repeat that functions as a transcriptional silencer. PSES drives luciferase activity fivefold higher than universal promoter Rous sarcoma virus (RSV) and slightly higher than cytomegalovirus (CMV) promoter.

Luciferase expression was detected in several PSA- and PSMA-positive prostate cancer cell lines, but not in PSA- and PSMA-negative prostate cells or non-prostate cell lines. PSES retains its prostate-specific nature in recombinant adenoviral vector as well. Fig. 3 shows the results after injection of *BALB/c* nude mice with Ad-CMV-luc and Ad-PSES-luc. Because of its small size, high level of tissue specificity, and strong promoter activity in the presence or absence of androgen, PSES is an ideal promoter for use in prostate cancer gene therapy.

Human telomerase promoter

Telomeres are tandem repeat structures found at the terminal end of chromosomes that maintain chromosomal integrity by preventing DNA rearrangements, degradation, and end-to-end fusions. In most normal somatic cells, the telomeric cap is shortened with each cycle of DNA replication and cell division. When telomeres shorten to a critical length, cells progress toward irreversible arrest of growth and cellular senescence [124]. In contrast, tumor cells have evolved a means to prevent telomere shortening through the activation of the catalytic component of human telomerase reverse transcriptase (hTERT) [125]. The *hTERT* promoter region has been cloned and characterized, and contains a high GC content. Unlike most promoters, it does not contain TATA or CAAT boxes [126]. Importantly, the *hTERT* promoter is active in most cancer cells including prostate cancer [127] and inactive in normal cells, and thereby provides a unique tool to target cancer cells. Promising results have been reported using the *hTERT* promoter to deliver TRAIL, an inducer of apoptosis [128] and to control the replication of an oncolytic adenovirus [129]. Researchers at our laboratory are investigating the use of the *hTERT* promoter in conjunction with our prostate-specific promoter to control adenoviral replication in a prostate cancer-specific manner.

Past approaches

Over the past 10 years, two strategies of gene therapy approaches for prostate cancer have emerged: corrective gene therapy and cytoreductive gene therapy. Each molecular therapy has a strong foundation of preclinical data which facilitates the approval of several clinical studies. Currently, 56 gene transfer protocols registered with the OBA are targeted against prostate cancer. This accounts for 15% of all cancer protocols listed to date [130]. Table 2 highlights the details of the prostate cancer trials registered with the OBA. Prostate cancer research will remain a focus for laboratories because of the limited availability of treatments for advanced disease and the large population that is affected.

Corrective gene therapy

This approach repairs inherited or acquired genetic defects that affect the regulation of the cell

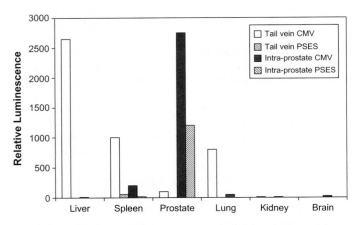

Fig. 3. Comparision of PSES and universal promoter delivered by both intravenous and intraprostatic injection. Recombinant adenoviruses Ad-CMV-luc and Ad-PSES-luc were injected into male athymic mice, 7×10^{10} virus particles by tail vein injection or 1.4×10^{10} virus particles by intra-prostate injection. Mice were sacrificed and organs were harvested for luciferase activity 2 days post injection. After systemic injection, negligible levels of PSES-driven luciferase activity were detected in organs expected to take up adenovirus, mainly liver, spleen, and lung. To overcome the low infectivity of the prostate, intraprostatic injections were administered and revealed high PSES activity in the prostate.

Table 2
Prostate cancer gene therapy trials (OBA protocol list September 20, 2005)

Principal investigator	Institution	Vector	Genetic material	Year reviewed
Simons, JW	Johns Hopkins, MD	Retrovirus	GM-CSF	1994
Steiner, MS	Vanderbilt Univ., TN	Retrovirus	c-myc	1995
Chen, AP	Nat. Naval Med., MD	Vaccinia/fowl pox	PSA	1995
Paulson, DF	Duke Univ., NC	Liposome	IL-2	1995
Scardino, PT	MSKCC, NY	Adenovirus	HSV-TK	1996
Eder, JP	Dana-Farber, MD	Vaccinia/fowl pox	PSA	1996
Sanda, MG	Univ. of Michigan, MI	Vaccinia/fowl pox	PSA	1997
Belldegrun, AS	UCLA, CA	Liposome	IL-2	1997
Hall, SJ	Mt. Sinai, NY	Adenovirus	HSV-TK	1997
Belldegrun, AS	UCLA, CA	Adenovirus	p53	1997
Simons, JW	Johns Hopkins, MD	Retrovirus	GM-CSF	1997
Logothetis, CJ	MD Anderson, TX	Adenovirus	p53	1997
Kadmon, D	Baylor College, TX	Adenovirus	HSV-TK	1998
Simons, JW	Johns Hopkins, MD	Adenovirus	PSA	1998
Figlin, RA	UCLA, CA	Vaccinia/fowl pox	MUC-1/IL-2	1998
Gardner, TA	Univ. of Virginia, VA	Adenovirus	OC-HSV-TK	1998
Eder, JP	Dana-Farber, MD	Vaccinia/fowl pox	PSA	1999
Small, EJ	UCSF, CA	Retrovirus	GM-CSF	1999
Kaufman, HL	Albert Einstein, NY	Vaccinia/fowl pox	PSA	1999
Vieweg, J	Duke Univ., NC	RNA	PSA	1999
Belldegrun, AS	UCLA, CA	Liposome	IL-2	1999
Small, EJ	UCSF, CA	Retrovirus	GM-SCF	1999
Kim, JH	Henry Ford Hosp., MI	Adenovirus	CD/TK	1999
Aguilar-Cordova, E	Harvard Univ., MA	Adenovirus	TK	1999
Gingrich, JR	Univ. of Tenn., TN	Adenovirus	p16	1999
Terris, MK	Stanford Univ., CA	Adenovirus	PSA	1999
Wilding, G	Univ. Of Wisc., WI	Adenovirus	PSA	1999
Belldegrun, AS	UCLA, CA	Liposome	IL-2	1999
Dahut, WL	NIH/NCI, MD	Vaccinia/fowl pox	PSA	1999
Arlen, PM	NIH/NCI, MD	Vaccinia/fowl pox	PSA	2000
Vieweg, J	Duke Univ., NC	RNA	Tumor RNA	2000
Pollack, A	Univ. of Texas, TX	Adenovirus	p53	2000
Gardner, TA	Indiana Univ., IN	Adenovirus	OC promoter	2000
Freytag, SO	Henry Ford Hosp., MI	Adenovirus	CD/TK	2000
Lubaroff, DM	Univ. of Iowa, IA	Adenovirus	PSA	2001
Miles, BJ	Baylor College, TX	Adenovirus	IL-12	2001
DeWeese, TL	Johns Hopkins, MD	Adenovirus	PB/PSE promoter	2001
Small, EJ	UCSF, CA	Adenovirus	PB/PSE promoter	2001
Dula, E	West Coast Clin. Res., CA	AAV	GM-CSF	2001
Freytag, SO	Henry Ford Hosp., MI	Adenovirus	CD/TK	2001
Scher, H	MSKCC, NY	Liposome	PSMA	2001
Corman, J	VA Puget Sound, WA	AAV	GM-CSF	2001
Pantuck, AJ	UCLA, LA	Vaccinia/fowl pox	MUC-1/IL-2	2001
Vieweg, J	Duke, NC	RNA	hTERT	2001
Corman, J	VA Puget Sound, WA	Adenovirus	PSE promoter	2001
Vieweg, J	Duke, NC	RNA	PSA	2001
Dinney, CP	MD Anderson, TX	Adenovirus	Inf-β	2002
Dahut, W	NIH/NCI, MD	Vaccinia/fowl pox	PSA	2002
Morris, J	Mayo Clinic, MN	Adenovirus	NIS	2002
Kaufman, HL	Columbia, NY	Vaccinia/fowl pox	PSA	2002
Zanetti, M	Univ. of Calif., CA	Liposome	hTERT	2002
Malkowicz, SB	Univ. of Penn., PA	Liposome	PSA	2002
Arlen, PM	NIH/NCI, MD	Vaccinia/fowlpox	PSA	2002
Corman, J	Virginia Mason, WI	Adenovirus	PSA	2003

(continued on next page)

Table 2 (*continued*)

Principal investigator	Institution	Vector	Genetic material	Year reviewed
Freytag, S	Henry Ford Hosp., MI	Adenovirus	HSV-TK	2003
Kantoff, P	Dana-Farber, MD	Vaccinia/fowl pox	PSA	2003
Hall, S	Mt Sinai, NY	Adenovirus	IL-2	2003
Konety, B	Univ. of Iowa, IA	Adenovirus	TRAIL	2003
Viewtag, J	Duke Univ., NC	Adenovirus	hTERT	2004
Small, E	UCSF, CA	Adenovirus	PSA	2004
Gulley, J	NIH/NCI, MD	Vaccinia/fowl pox	PSA	2004
Agarwal, M	Univ. of Ark., AR	Adenovirus	GM-CSF	2004
Hamstreet, G	Univ. of Neb., NE	Adenovirus	Tumor RNA	2005
Junghans, R	Boston Univ., MA	Adenovirus	PSMA	2005

growth cycle. A single prostate cancer cell may harbor several such mutations, which gives it a survival advantage. The replacement of a damaged gene with the wild-type is often sufficient to suppress the growth of the cancer or lead to apoptosis, as evidenced in the pre-clinical and clinical trials outlined below.

p53

Tumor suppressor p53 is referred to as the molecular gatekeeper because it protects the integrity of the genome [131]. When cellular DNA damage occurs, wild type p53 is activated and stimulates the expression of *GADD45* (growth arrest and DNA damage) and the cyclin-dependent kinase (CDK) inhibitor, *p21*. p21 inhibits the CDK-cyclin D complex required to phosphorylate Rb, thereby halting the cell at the G_1/S checkpoint to facilitate DNA repair. If GADD45-mediated DNA repair is unsuccessful, p53 activates *bax* which mediates apoptosis [132]. p53 mutations occur in approximately one-third of early prostate cancers [133], and this increases in patients who have advanced and metastatic disease [134]. Replacement of wild-type *p53* with recombinant adenoviral vectors (Ad-p53) has resulted in growth inhibition and induction of apoptosis in prostate cancer both in vitro [93,135] and in vivo [136]. In addition, intratumoral administration of Ad-p53 has been shown to slow the progression of prostate cancer to metastatic disease [137]. Perhaps the most powerful use of *p53* replacement is in combination with conventional therapies. Ad-p53 has been shown to sensitize prostate cancer cells in vitro and in vivo to chemotherapeutic agents [138] and in vitro to radiation therapy [139]. Clinical trials are ongoing to determine the safety of such therapies [140,141]. Ad-p53 is the first gene therapeutic approved in the world (China).

p16

Similar to p53, tumor suppressor p16 is a negative regulator of the cell growth cycle, and prevents the phosphorylation of Rb by sequestering CDK4 of the CDK-cyclin D complex. Underphosphorylated Rb arrests the cell at G_1, and loss of normal p16 function is common in prostate cancer [132]. Small homozygous deletions have been identified as the major mechanism of inactivation of *p16*, which occurs in 40% of primary prostate cancers and 71% of advanced androgen-independent prostate cancers [142–144]. Replacement of *p16* using adenoviral vectors suppressed cell growth and induced senescence in several prostate cancer cell lines including LNCaP (androgen-dependent) and C4-2, DU-145, PPC-1, and PC-3 (androgen-independent) [91,145,146]. Furthermore, intratumoral injection of Ad-CMV-p16 inhibited the growth of PC-3 tumor xenografts in experimental animal models and prolonged the animals' survival [145]. Currently, one clinical trial using *p16* is in progress.

c-myc

The oncogene *c-myc* plays an important role in the progression of the cell cycle. As a transcription factor, it regulates the expression of CDC25 phosphatases that control CDK activity [147]. c-myc amplification is a common mutation in prostate cancer and its levels correlate with increasing tumor grade [148]. The approach developed to suppress the overexpression of oncogenes delivers antisense RNA complimentary to the sense strand for that gene. This approach not only inhibits cancer cell growth, but also induces apoptosis through the down-regulation of *bcl-2* which results from *c-myc* suppression. Steiner and colleagues [94] developed a replication-incompetent retroviral vector to deliver antisense *c-myc* transcripts intratumorily in DU-145 nude mice xenografts. Reduction in tumor size and even complete tumor obliteration were observed. One *c-myc* clinical trial is in progress.

Cytoreductive gene therapy

This approach to the molecular therapy of prostate cancer results in the direct or indirect killing of prostate cancer cells by replication-competent oncolytic viruses such as Ad-OC-E1a, pro-drug enzyme genes such as thymidine kinase, and apoptosis-inducing genes such as tumor necrosis factor-related apoptosis-inducing ligand (TRAIL). This is perhaps one of the most successful approaches to the molecular therapy of prostate cancer and several clinical trials are ongoing to explore cytoreductive treatments.

Oncolytic virus therapy

Previous studies have shown that a replication-competent adenovirus injected intra-organ is sufficient to kill prostate cancer cells [149]. Although this therapy alone might be effective, adenovirus is taken up by the liver and lungs. This has the potential to cause hepatic and respiratory distress in immune-compromised cancer patients [150]. When the replication of adenovirus is controlled solely to prostate cancer cells, the safety of this tumor-eliminating therapy increases. The replication of adenovirus can be controlled by placing the early gene, *E1a*, a transcriptional activator of adenoviral late genes, under the control of a tissue-specific promoter. Without the expression of the essential late genes, the virus cannot reassemble and propagate in the host cell [151]. Recently, Henderson and colleagues [152] demonstrated the ability to conditionally drive the replication of adenovirus by a prostate-specific enhancer (PSE) which resulted in regression of in vivo androgen-independent LNCaP tumors.

Investigators at our laboratory have developed a conditional replication-competent adenoviral vector (Ad-OC-E1a) that uses the mouse *OC* promoter to restrict the expression of *E1a* to prostate epithelia and its supporting bone stroma, in osseous metastases of prostate cancer. This virus appears to be more effective than the PSE-controlled virus at killing a broader spectrum of prostate cancer cells including LNCaP, C4-2, and ARCaP (PSA-positive) as well as PC-3 and DU-145 (PSA-negative). Intratumoral injection of Ad-OC-E1a was effective at obliterating subcutaneous androgen-independent PC-3 tumors in athymic mice. In addition, intraosseous C4-2 prostate cancer xenografts responded very well

to the systemic administration of Ad-OC-E1a. All (100%) of the treated mice responded with a drop in the serum PSA below detectable levels. At the conclusion of the study, 40% of the treated mice were cured of prostate cancer and no PSA rebound or prostate cancer cells in the skeleton were detected [153]. Fig. 4 shows the radiograph of a mouse that has a C4-2 bone tumor before and after treatment with Ad-OC-E1a.

It has been shown that controlling the expression of the early gene *E1b* in addition to *E1a* results in better viral replication control [154]. For this reason, we developed a second replication-competent adenoviral vector, Ad-hOC-E1, which contains a single bidirectional human *OC* promoter to control the expression of both *E1a* and *E1b*. Under the control of this VDRE-containing promoter, viral replication is induced 10-fold higher than wild-type viral replication and cytotoxicity is enhanced by the administration of vitamin D [155]. Although still controversial [156], some preclinical studies indicate that vitamin D has an antiproliferative effect on androgen-independent prostate cancer [157,158]. In our preclinical studies, administration of vitamin D_3 in nude mice with subcutaneous DU-145 xenografts demonstrated a therapeutic effect; however, the systemic administration of Ad-hOC-E1 in combination with vitamin D showed marked repression of the tumors, which indicates the potential for clinical use [159]. The previously outlined preclinical findings have translated into a phase I clinical trial of *OC*-driven oncolytic adenoviral intratumoral therapy for androgen-independent prostate cancer.

Pro-drug enzyme gene therapy

The efficacy of this approach depends on the conversion of a non-toxic pro-drug to an active cytotoxic drug by the enzymatic product of a delivered gene not normally expressed in human cells. After systemic administration of the pro-drug, high concentrations of the lethal metabolite are only found locally at the tumor site and avoid systemic toxicity. Fortunately, the toxic effect is not limited to the cells that produced the cytotoxic drug, but extends to neighboring cells by way of the bystander effect. This bystander effect is mediated by intercellular gap junctions and phagocytosis of debris from dying cells. By these means, the cytotoxic effect is amplified and compensates for low gene transfer efficiencies. The most widely applied pro-drug gene therapy in prostate cancer uses thymidine kinase from the

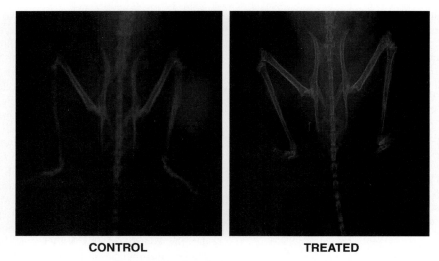

CONTROL   **TREATED**

Fig. 4. Results of systemic administration of oncolytic therapy on prostate bone tumors. C4-2 prostate cancer cells were injected into the bone marrow space of the right tibia in mice with severe combined immune deficiency. The left panel shows the radiograph of the untreated mouse which has a large mass and deformed tibia. The right panel shows the radiograph of a mouse after intravenous administration of Ad-OC-E1a.

herpes simplex virus (HSV-TK) and any one of several anti-herpetic agents such as ganciclovir (GCV), acyclovir (ACV), or valacyclovir (VAL). These nucleoside analogs are phosphorylated specifically by HSV-TK. The phosphorylated forms of the drugs are incorporated into cellular DNA during DNA replication, which results in chain termination and ultimately cell death.

The TK/pro-drug system is widely favored because it is a safe approach for cancer gene therapy for a number of reasons. First, apoptosis is induced in the transduced cell only when it divides and so the gene therapist is able to target cancer cells which divide more rapidly than non-cancerous cells. Second, the toxic effect only occurs when the pro-drug is administered; therefore, treatment can be stopped in the event of adverse effects. Third, several anti-herpetic nucleoside analog drugs are clinically available, which simplifies the approval process for the use of the pro-drug in clinical trials. Finally, the bystander effect greatly increases the killing efficiency of the therapy.

Previously, Eastham and colleagues [160] demonstrated the sensitivity of human prostate cancer cells PC-3 and DU-145 to GCV cytotoxicity following the in vitro transduction of the cells with *HSV-TK* using a recombinant replication-deficient adenoviral vector. Similar results were obtained in vivo in subcutaneous xenografts of

murine and human cancer models following the intralesional injection of Ad-RSV-TK and Ad-CMV-TK [159–161]. When *TK* is under the control of universal promoters such as RSV or CMV, it facilitates the potential of *TK* activation in any cell without discrimination between normal and cancer cells. Therefore, intratumoral injection of the vector is required to prevent systemic dissemination of the virus. Scardino and colleagues developed the initial TK clinical trial in which a replication-deficient adenoviral vector was injected intralesionally to deliver *HSV-TK* preceding the administration of GCV in men with locally recurrent prostate cancer one or more years after definitive external beam radiotherapy [98]. This trial demonstrated the tumoricidal activity of this TK/GCV therapy as evidenced by sustained decreases in serum PSA and improved biopsies. As a result of adenoviral leakage from the injection site through the bloodstream and tracking to the liver, several of the patients experienced a self-limiting hepato-toxicity and one patient experienced moderate but reversible hepatic dysfunction and thrombocytopenia [98]. To circumvent toxicity to the patient, Gotoh and coworkers [115] developed a replication-deficient adenovirus to deliver *HSV-TK* driven by the *PSA* promoter.

Researchers at our laboratory developed a clinical protocol to test the hypothesis that the *OC*

promoter can regulate *HSV-TK* expression specifically within a prostate cancer cell and the supportive stroma of a metastasis. We performed
a phase I clinical trial and enrolled 11 patients
who had locally recurrent or metastatic prostate
cancer. Two post-surgical local recurrences and
nine metastatic lesions (five osseous, four lymph
node) were injected with replication-defective
Ad-OC-TK vector followed by the administration
of oral valacyclovir [108]. All patients tolerated
this therapy with no severe adverse effects. Of
the 11 men, local cancer cell death was observed
in 7 patients; however, the treated lesions of all
11 men showed histological changes as a result
of the treatment. One patient demonstrated regression and stabilization of the treated lesion
for 317 days post-treatment without alternative
treatments, as demonstrated in Fig. 5 [109]. This
trial opened the door to the development of future
adenoviral vectors for the systemic treatment of
osseous and visceral prostate cancer metastases.

Suicide gene therapy

TRAIL, also known as Apo-2 ligand, is a member of the TNF family and has been shown to
preferentially kill tumor cells. Originally discovered because of its similarity to Fas-ligand, TRAIL
is a 32 kDa type II transmembrane protein, whose
C-terminal extracellular domain (amino acids 114–
281) is homologous with other members of the
TNF family [162,163]. TRAIL induces apoptosis
by binding to the death domain-containing receptors DR4 and DR5; however, the death signal is
not transduced via the adaptor molecule FADD.
Instead, the death protease FLICE2 is believed to
be engaged, which cleaves the initiating caspase 8
to begin the caspase cascade [164].

The selectivity of TRAIL for cancer cells over
normal cells makes it a prime candidate for
anticancer therapy. TRAIL expression has been
detected in several normal human tissues which
suggests that TRAIL is not toxic to those cells in
vivo [165]. In essence, these cells are protected
from the apoptotic effects of TRAIL by an antagonistic decoy receptor, TRID, which lacks an intracellular domain and is found on the surface
membrane of TRAIL-resistant cells [164]. Many
prostate cancer cell lines including ALVA-31,
Du-145, and PC-3 are extremely sensitive to
TRAIL and undergo apoptosis when exposed;
however, other cell lines such as LNCaP are
highly resistant [166]. This resistance has been
shown to be reversed by simultaneous administration of the chemotherapeutic agents doxorubicin,
cisplatin, or etoposide [167] or by infection of
those cells with adenovirus [168]. For this reason,
TRAIL is a promising suicide gene to consider for
prostate cancer gene therapy; however, recent
studies suggest that cultured human hepatocytes
may be sensitive to TRAIL [169]. Recombinant
forms of TRAIL with reduced hepatotoxicity are
being investigated [170] in addition to monoclonal

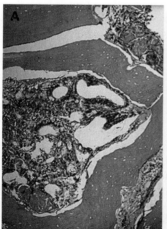 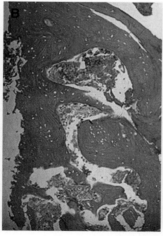 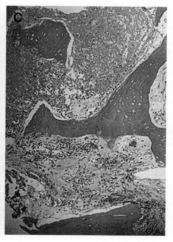

Fig. 5. Prostate cancer bone metastases treated with Ad-OC-TK in phase I trial. Tissue biopsies were collected from one
patient and stained with hematoxylin and eosin before (*A*), during (day 8) (*B*), and after (day 30) (*C*) treatment with Ad-
OC-TK and VAL. Malignant prostate cancer cells surround healthy bone tissue before treatment (*A*). During treatment,
cancer cells are replaced and fibrosis occurs (*B*). By day 30, malignant cells disappear and are replaced completely by
fibrosis and inflammatory cells (*C*).

antibodies that antagonize the TRAIL receptor in hepatocytes [171].

Antiangiogenic gene therapy

Researchers in our laboratory have recently developed several adenoviral vectors that target prostate tumor neovasculature to develop proof of principle. We hypothesized that the combination of multiple antiangiogenic factors delivered by adenoviral vectors would be more effective than the delivery of a single factor and result in viral dose reduction. Similar to angiostatin, endostatin is another potent angiogenesis inhibitor derived endogenously by proteolytic activity. It is a 20 kDa C-terminal fragment of collagen XVIII discovered by O'Reilly and colleagues [100] in the medium of cultured hemangioendothelioma cells. The antiproliferative effect on endothelial cells is mediated by the direct binding of endostatin to VEGFR-2, which blocks the VEGF signaling pathway [87]. A virus, Ad-hEndo-angio, that expresses a novel endostatin-angiostatin fusion protein was developed and its antiangiogenic effects were compared with a previously characterized antiangiogenic virus, Ad-sTie2, which expresses solubilized Tie-2, an endothelium-specific tyrosine kinase receptor [172].

In vitro, Ad-hEndo-angio significantly inhibited microvessel tubular network formation and rat aortic ring capillary sprouting compared with Ad-sTie2. Both viruses were evaluated in vivo in subcutaneous PC-3 nude mouse models. Ad-hEndo-angio when injected intratumorally resulted in 86% tumor growth inhibition compared with the mock-treated group. Similarly, the contralateral untreated tumor was reduced in volume by 87%. Ad-sTie2-treated tumors showed no growth inhibition. An even greater reduction in tumor volume was observed when half the dose of both viruses was co-injected into tumors. Ninety-nine percent tumor volume reduction was achieved at the primary injection site and 98% tumor reduction in the contralateral tumor as compared with the mock-treatment group. Prolonged tumor-free survival was observed in 80% of the animals treated [75]. Fig. 6 depicts representative mice in each treatment group. These results show potential for the clinical translation of a multi-factor antiangiogenesis therapy for advanced prostate cancer.

Future directions in gene therapy

Among clinical trials that have been launched to demonstrate the safety and efficacy of adenoviral-based gene therapy on prostate cancer in the past few years, the most exciting results have come from the study of tumor and tissue-restricted replicative adenovirus (TRRA). This strategy facilitates the viral vector to propagate from a limited number of infected cells to the whole tumor mass, and thereby overcomes the problem of inadequate in vivo infectivity or biodistribution of the vector. TRRA-based therapy, however, is not without its limitations. One of the major limitations of this therapy is the induction of the host immune system, targeted to eliminate the adenovirus from the body.

It will become critical to temporarily suppress the host's immune system or enhance the killing activity of the virus so that it can eliminate tumors within a shorter period of time, so that it can escape from host immune attack. Among immune regulators, TGF-β and Fas-ligand are likely the best candidates for incorporation into TRRA for cancer gene therapy. There are five members reported in the TGF-β family; three of them (TGF-β1, TGF-β2, and TGF-β3) are expressed in mammals. These three isoforms share a high degree of sequence homology in the mature domain, and have similar actions on cells in tissue culture. Suppression of the immune response includes the inhibition of T and B cell proliferation, the down-regulation of natural killer cell activity and cytotoxic T lymphocytes response, and the regulation of macrophage activation [173]. TGF-β is a mediator of immune suppression that allows tumors to escape from immune surveillance, and its use has been explored to suppress the inflammatory and alloreactive immune responses in liver transplantation [174]. Besides TGF-β, Fas-ligand is another immune modulator that has been explored for use in kidney transplant patients to suppress alloreactive lymphocytes [172]. Fas-ligand, also known as CD95 or APO-1, is a membrane-bound protein of the TNF family, and it is expressed in several cell types including tumors, T cells, and B cells. Cells that express the Fas receptor undergo apoptosis when they encounter Fas-ligand [170]. In addition to their immune modulation function, TGF-β and Fas-ligand are also strong growth inhibitors and induce apoptosis in a variety of cancers, including prostate cancer [175]. Therefore, incorporating TGF-β or Fas-ligand into a TRRA will potentially enhance the tumoricidal activity of the vector and blanket the tumor site from the immune system, which will enable the TRRA to complete its mission.

When the TRRA is armed with immune suppressors, there is increased need for tight

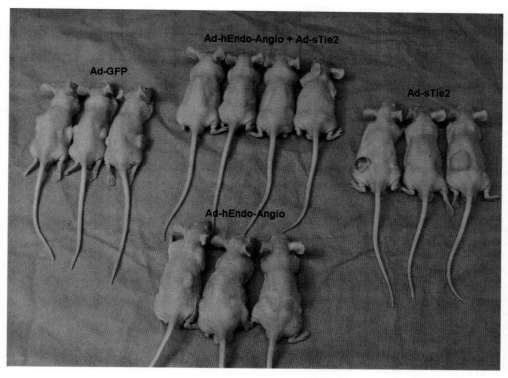

Fig. 6. Combination treatment with Ad-hEndo-Angio and Ad-sTie2 results in complete growth inhibition of co-injected and distant androgen-independent PC-3 subcutaneous tumors. Three replication-deficient adenoviral vectors were injected into flank-induced prostate cancer tumors. Growth inhibition was compared with the mock-treatment group, Ad-GFP (*left*). Ad-hEndo-Angio alone resulted in 86% growth inhibition at the site of injection and 87% inhibition at the contralateral site (*bottom*). Ad-sTie2 alone resulted in no inhibition of tumor growth compared with Ad-GFP-treated mice (*right*). Combined treatment with half doses of each respective virus resulted in 99% growth inhibition at the injection site and 98% inhibition in the contralateral site (*top*).

regulation of viral replication. In addition to controlling *E1a* and *E1b* with prostate-specific promoters, *E4* should be considered. The *E4* transcription unit encodes regulatory genes that are critical for viral replication, which involves the shut-down of host gene expression and the facilitation of late viral gene expression [176]. Mutant adenoviral vectors that lack the *E4* region are severely replication defective and can only propagate in *E4*-expressing cells [177]. If *E4* is placed under the control of a prostate-specific promoter, it should provide additional safety. TK should also be considered for incorporation into a TRRA. TK enhances the tumor-killing activity of a TRRA, and makes it possible for a gene therapist to monitor adenoviral replication in vivo by using positron emission tomography imaging [178].

Finally, because all tissue-specific promoters have basal activity levels in non-target tissues, the potential exists for accumulation of adenovirus in the liver, which results in undesirable toxic effects caused by significant expression of therapeutic genes in the liver. Modification of the adenoviral fiber knob can increase viral tropism toward cancers and away from the liver and other vital organs [179,180]. This is also beneficial in non-prostate cancers because it is well known that expression of the coxsackievirus-adenovirus receptor (CAR) is frequently down regulated in these non-prostate cancers cancers. However, analysis of specimens from our phase I trial demonstrated sufficient CAR. Others are investigating antibodies to redirect viral tropism.

Summary

Many novel techniques for the treatment of prostate cancer are being aggressively investigated for two reasons: (1) prostate cancer is prevalent in the population, and (2) the current treatments for advanced prostate cancer are woefully inadequate.

Antiangiogenesis has great potential as stand-alone therapy to transform prostate cancer into a chronic disease or, in combination with the available therapies, to provide curative approaches with decreased treatment-related morbidities. Further understanding of the angiogenic cascade will reveal additional molecular targets and advancements in molecular delivery approaches, such as gene therapy, will lead to the development of safe and effective treatment strategies.

There are many complex interactions between the immune system and prostate cancer. Although our understanding of these interactions is improving, further understanding will lead to novel treatment strategies. These include the idea that manipulation of cellular pathways, such as the work with growth factor receptors, can lead to tumor stabilization and eventually cytoreduction with continued cell turnover. The adjuvant use of immunotherapy for prostate cancer could also help increase efficacy of current oncologic treatments. This may be even more significant when used in conjuction with nomograms that may predict men who are at particularly high risk for failure of local treatment, and who would be better served with adjuvent immune therapy.

The safety and efficacy of gene therapy for prostate cancer has been demonstrated through various preclinical and clinical trials, and potentially holds the greatest promise. In recent years, interest in this field has expanded and will continue to do so. Because it is conveniently administered through ultrasound-guided transrectal injection, it is also conceivable that gene therapy applied in an outpatient clinic may someday replace current therapy to treat early prostate cancer. As a therapy, it is the culmination of the work of many disciplines that will result in an elegant targeted, efficient, and versatile strategy against prostate cancer.

It is conceivable that, in the near future, any of these experimental modalities will be developed to replace hormone ablation therapy which causes unpleasant side effects, decreases the quality of life of the patient, and only temporarily controls the disease. Factors that limit the disseminated use of these advanced therapies as standards of care include time, funding, and fear from the general public; however, these should diminish as the number of successful clinical trials increase.

References

[1] Jemal A, Murray T, Ward E, et al. Cancer statistics, 2005. CA Cancer J Clin 2005;55:10.

[2] Garcia-Barros M, Paris F, Cordon-Cardo C, et al. Tumor response to radiotherapy regulated by endothelial cell apoptosis. Science 2003;300:1155.

[3] Bergers G, Javaherian K, Lo KM, et al. Effects of angiogenesis inhibitors on multistage carcinogenesis in mice. Science 1999;284:808.

[4] Folkman J. Tumor angiogenesis: therapeutic implications. N Engl J Med 1971;285:1182.

[5] Folkman J, Watson K, Ingber D, et al. Induction of angiogenesis during the transition from hyperplasia to neoplasia. Nature 1989;339:58.

[6] Folkman J, Klagsbrun M. Angiogenic factors. Science 1987;235:442.

[7] Hanahan D, Folkman J. Patterns and emerging mechanisms of the angiogenic switch during tumorigenesis. Cell 1996;86:353.

[8] Feng D, Nagy JA, Brekken RA, et al. Ultrastructural localization of the vascular permeability factor/vascular endothelial growth factor (VPF/VEGF) receptor-2 (FLK-1, KDR) in normal mouse kidney and in the hyperpermeable vessels induced by VPF/VEGF-expressing tumors and adenoviral vectors. J Histochem Cytochem 2000;48:545.

[9] Chang SS, O'Keefe DS, Bacich DJ, et al. Prostate-specific membrane antigen is produced in tumor-associated neovasculature. Clin Cancer Res 1999; 5:2674.

[10] Weidner N, Carroll PR, Flax J, et al. Tumor angiogenesis correlates with metastasis in invasive prostate carcinoma. Am J Pathol 1993;143:401.

[11] Senger DR, Galli SJ, Dvorak AM, et al. Tumor cells secrete a vascular permeability factor that promotes accumulation of ascites fluid. Science 1983; 219:983.

[12] Vincenti V, Cassano C, Rocchi M, et al. Assignment of the vascular endothelial growth factor gene to human chromosome 6p21.3. Circulation 1996;93:1493.

[13] Tischer E, Mitchell R, Hartman T, et al. The human gene for vascular endothelial growth factor. Multiple protein forms are encoded through alternative exon splicing. J Biol Chem 1991;266:11947.

[14] Robinson CJ, Stringer SE. The splice variants of vascular endothelial growth factor (VEGF) and their receptors. J Cell Sci 2001;114:853.

[15] Forsythe JA, Jiang BH, Iyer NV, et al. Activation of vascular endothelial growth factor gene transcription by hypoxia-inducible factor 1. Mol Cell Biol 1996;16:4604.

[16] Huang S, Pettaway CA, Uehara H, et al. Blockade of NF-kappaB activity in human prostate cancer cells is associated with suppression of angiogenesis, invasion, and metastasis. Oncogene 2001;20:4188.

[17] Grugel S, Finkenzeller G, Weindel K, et al. Both v-Ha-Ras and v-Raf stimulate expression of the

vascular endothelial growth factor in NIH 3T3 cells. J Biol Chem 1995;270:25915.

[18] Ferrer FA, Miller LJ, Andrawis RI, et al. Angiogenesis and prostate cancer: in vivo and in vitro expression of angiogenesis factors by prostate cancer cells. Urology 1998;51:161.

[19] Ferrer FA, Miller LJ, Andrawis RI, et al. Vascular endothelial growth factor (VEGF) expression in human prostate cancer: in situ and in vitro expression of VEGF by human prostate cancer cells. J Urol 1997;157:2329.

[20] George DJ, Halabi S, Shepard TF, et al. Prognostic significance of plasma vascular endothelial growth factor levels in patients with hormone-refractory prostate cancer treated on Cancer and Leukemia Group B 9480. Clin Cancer Res 2001;7:1932.

[21] Cheng L, Zhang S, Sweeney CJ, et al. Androgen withdrawal inhibits tumor growth and is associated with decrease in angiogenesis and VEGF expression in androgen-independent CWR22Rv1 human prostate cancer model. Anticancer Res 2004;24:2135.

[22] Ferrara N, Carver-Moore K, Chen H, et al. Heterozygous embryonic lethality induced by targeted inactivation of the VEGF gene. Nature 1996;380:439.

[23] Unemori EN, Ferrara N, Bauer EA, et al. Vascular endothelial growth factor induces interstitial collagenase expression in human endothelial cells. J Cell Physiol 1992;153:557.

[24] Helmlinger G, Endo M, Ferrara N, et al. Formation of endothelial cell networks. Nature 2000;405:139.

[25] Leung DW, Cachianes G, Kuang WJ, et al. Vascular endothelial growth factor is a secreted angiogenic mitogen. Science 1989;246:1306.

[26] Alon T, Hemo I, Itin A, et al. Vascular endothelial growth factor acts as a survival factor for newly formed retinal vessels and has implications for retinopathy of prematurity. Nat Med 1995;1:1024.

[27] Muller YA, Christinger HW, Keyt BA, et al. The crystal structure of vascular endothelial growth factor (VEGF) refined to 1.93 A resolution: multiple copy flexibility and receptor binding. Structure 1997;5:1325.

[28] de Vries C, Escobedo JA, Ueno H, et al. The fms-like tyrosine kinase, a receptor for vascular endothelial growth factor. Science 1992;255:989.

[29] Seetharam L, Gotoh N, Maru Y, et al. A unique signal transduction from FLT tyrosine kinase, a receptor for vascular endothelial growth factor VEGF. Oncogene 1995;10:135.

[30] Quinn TP, Peters KG, de Vries C, et al. Fetal liver kinase 1 is a receptor for vascular endothelial growth factor and is selectively expressed in vascular endothelium. Proc Natl Acad Sci USA 1993;90:7533.

[31] Terman BI, Dougher-Vermazen M, Carrion ME, et al. Identification of the KDR tyrosine kinase as a receptor for vascular endothelial cell growth factor. Biochem Biophys Res Commun 1992;187:1579.

[32] Waltenberger J, Claesson-Welsh L, Siegbahn A, et al. Different signal transduction properties of KDR and Flt1, two receptors for vascular endothelial growth factor. J Biol Chem 1994;269:26988.

[33] Ingber D. Extracellular matrix and cell shape: potential control points for inhibition of angiogenesis. J Cell Biochem 1991;47:236.

[34] Pepper MS, Ferrara N, Orci L, et al. Potent synergism between vascular endothelial growth factor and basic fibroblast growth factor in the induction of angiogenesis in vitro. Biochem Biophys Res Commun 1992;189:824.

[35] Levine AC, Ren M, Huber GK, et al. The effect of androgen, estrogen, and growth factors on the proliferation of cultured fibroblasts derived from human fetal and adult prostates. Endocrinology 1992;130:2413.

[36] Doll JA, Reiher FK, Crawford SE, et al. Thrombospondin-1, vascular endothelial growth factor and fibroblast growth factor-2 are key functional regulators of angiogenesis in the prostate. Prostate 2001;49:293.

[37] Nakamoto T, Chang CS, Li AK, et al. Basic fibroblast growth factor in human prostate cancer cells. Cancer Res 1992;52:571.

[38] Hiraoka N, Allen E, Apel IJ, et al. Matrix metalloproteinases regulate neovascularization by acting as pericellular fibrinolysins. Cell 1998;95:365.

[39] Wood M, Fudge K, Mohler JL, et al. In situ hybridization studies of metalloproteinases 2 and 9 and TIMP-1 and TIMP-2 expression in human prostate cancer. Clin Exp Metastasis 1997;15:246.

[40] Hoosein NM, Boyd DD, Hollas WJ, et al. Involvement of urokinase and its receptor in the invasiveness of human prostatic carcinoma cell lines. Cancer Commun 1991;3:255.

[41] Evans CP, Elfman F, Parangi S, et al. Inhibition of prostate cancer neovascularization and growth by urokinase-plasminogen activator receptor blockade. Cancer Res 1997;57:3594.

[42] Gately S, Twardowski P, Stack MS, et al. The mechanism of cancer-mediated conversion of plasminogen to the angiogenesis inhibitor angiostatin. Proc Natl Acad Sci USA 1997;94:10868.

[43] Wikstrom P, Stattin P, Franck-Lissbrant I, et al. Transforming growth factor beta1 is associated with angiogenesis, metastasis, and poor clinical outcome in prostate cancer. Prostate 1998;37:19.

[44] Yoshimura R, Sano H, Masuda C, et al. Expression of cyclooxygenase-2 in prostate carcinoma. Cancer 2000;89:589.

[45] Liu XH, Kirschenbaum A, Yao S, et al. Inhibition of cyclooxygenase-2 suppresses angiogenesis and the growth of prostate cancer in vivo. J Urol 2000;164:820.

[46] Fett JW, Strydom DJ, Lobb RR, et al. Isolation and characterization of angiogenin, an angiogenic

protein from human carcinoma cells. Biochemistry 1985;24:5480.

[47] Olson KA, Byers HR, Key ME, et al. Inhibition of prostate carcinoma establishment and metastatic growth in mice by an antiangiogenin monoclonal antibody. Int J Cancer 2002;98:923.

[48] Good DJ, Polverini PJ, Rastinejad F, et al. A tumor suppressor-dependent inhibitor of angiogenesis is immunologically and functionally indistinguishable from a fragment of thrombospondin. Proc Natl Acad Sci USA 1990;87:6624.

[49] Vailhe B, Feige JJ. Thrombospondins as anti-angiogenic therapeutic agents. Curr Pharm Des 2003;9:583.

[50] Zhou J, Rothman VL, Sargiannidou I, et al. Cloning and characterization of angiocidin, a tumor cell binding protein for thrombospondin-1. J Cell Biochem 2004;92:125.

[51] Jin RJ, Kwak C, Lee SG, et al. The application of an anti-angiogenic gene (thrombospondin-1) in the treatment of human prostate cancer xenografts. Cancer Gene Ther 2000;7:1537.

[52] Ingber D, Fujita T, Kishimoto S, et al. Synthetic analogues of fumagillin that inhibit angiogenesis and suppress tumour growth. Nature 1990;348:555.

[53] Abe J, Zhou W, Takuwa N, et al. A fumagillin derivative angiogenesis inhibitor, AGM-1470, inhibits activation of cyclin-dependent kinases and phosphorylation of retinoblastoma gene product but not protein tyrosyl phosphorylation or proto-oncogene expression in vascular endothelial cells. Cancer Res 1994;54:3407.

[54] Yamaoka M, Yamamoto T, Ikeyama S, et al. Angiogenesis inhibitor TNP-470 (AGM-1470) potently inhibits the tumor growth of hormone-independent human breast and prostate carcinoma cell lines. Cancer Res 1993;53:5233.

[55] Muramaki M, Miyake H, Hara I, et al. Synergistic inhibition of tumor growth and metastasis by combined treatment with TNP-470 and docetaxel in a human prostate cancer PC-3 model. Int J Oncol 2005;26:623.

[56] Logothetis CJ, Wu KK, Finn LD, et al. Phase I trial of the angiogenesis inhibitor TNP-470 for progressive androgen-independent prostate cancer. Clin Cancer Res 2001;7:1198.

[57] D'Amato RJ, Loughnan MS, Flynn E, et al. Thalidomide is an inhibitor of angiogenesis. Proc Natl Acad Sci USA 1994;91:4082.

[58] Bauer KS, Dixon SC, Figg WD. Inhibition of angiogenesis by thalidomide requires metabolic activation, which is species-dependent. Biochem Pharmacol 1998;55:1827.

[59] Figg WD, Dahut W, Duray P, et al. A randomized phase II trial of thalidomide, an angiogenesis inhibitor, in patients with androgen-independent prostate cancer. Clin Cancer Res 2001;7:1888.

[60] Figg WD, Arlen P, Gulley J, et al. A randomized phase II trial of docetaxel (taxotere) plus thalidomide in androgen-independent prostate cancer. Semin Oncol 2001;28:62.

[61] Dahut WL, Gulley JL, Arlen PM, et al. Randomized phase II trial of docetaxel plus thalidomide in androgen-independent prostate cancer. J Clin Oncol 2004;22:2532.

[62] Capitosti SM, Hansen TP, Brown ML. Thalidomide analogues demonstrate dual inhibition of both angiogenesis and prostate cancer. Bioorg Med Chem 2004;12:327.

[63] Ng SS, MacPherson GR, Gutschow M, et al. Antitumor effects of thalidomide analogs in human prostate cancer xenografts implanted in immunodeficient mice. Clin Cancer Res 2004;10:4192.

[64] O'Reilly MS, Holmgren L, Shing Y, et al. Angiostatin: a novel angiogenesis inhibitor that mediates the suppression of metastases by a Lewis lung carcinoma. Cell 1994;79:315.

[65] Gately S, Twardowski P, Stack MS, et al. Human prostate carcinoma cells express enzymatic-activity that converts human plasminogen to the angiogenesis inhibitor, angiostatin. Cancer Res 1996;56:4887.

[66] O'Reilly MS, Holmgren L, Chen C, et al. Angiostatin induces and sustains dormancy of human primary tumors in mice. Nat Med 1996;2:689.

[67] Galaup A, Opolon P, Bouquet C, et al. Combined effects of docetaxel and angiostatin gene therapy in prostate tumor model. Mol Ther 2003;7:731.

[68] Wedge SR, Ogilvie DJ, Dukes M, et al. ZD6474 inhibits vascular endothelial growth factor signaling, angiogenesis, and tumor growth following oral administration. Cancer Res 2002;62:4645.

[69] Nakamura K, Yamamoto A, Kamishohara M, et al. KRN633: a selective inhibitor of vascular endothelial growth factor receptor-2 tyrosine kinase that suppresses tumor angiogenesis and growth. Mol Cancer Ther 2004;3:1639.

[70] Ruggeri B, Singh J, Gingrich D, et al. CEP-7055: a novel, orally active pan inhibitor of vascular endothelial growth factor receptor tyrosine kinases with potent antiangiogenic activity and antitumor efficacy in preclinical models. Cancer Res 2003;63:5978.

[71] Traxler P, Allegrini PR, Brandt R, et al. AEE788: a dual family epidermal growth factor receptor/ErbB2 and vascular endothelial growth factor receptor tyrosine kinase inhibitor with antitumor and antiangiogenic activity. Cancer Res 2004;64:4931.

[72] Miller KD, Sweeney CJ, Sledge GW Jr. Redefining the target: chemotherapeutics as antiangiogenics. J Clin Oncol 2001;19:1195.

[73] Hotchkiss KA, Ashton AW, Mahmood R, et al. Inhibition of endothelial cell function in vitro and angiogenesis in vivo by docetaxel (Taxotere): association with impaired repositioning of the microtubule organizing center. Mol Cancer Ther 2002;1:1191.

[74] Grant DS, Williams TL, Zahaczewsky M, et al. Comparison of antiangiogenic activities using

paclitaxel (taxol) and docetaxel (taxotere). Int J Cancer 2003;104:121.

[75] Keledjian K, Garrison JB, Kyprianou N. Doxazosin inhibits human vascular endothelial cell adhesion, migration, and invasion. J Cell Biochem 2005;94:374.

[76] Sun J, Blaskovich MA, Jain RK, et al. Blocking angiogenesis and tumorigenesis with GFA-116, a synthetic molecule that inhibits binding of vascular endothelial growth factor to its receptor. Cancer Res 2004;64:3586.

[77] Sweeney P, Karashima T, Kim SJ, et al. Anti-vascular endothelial growth factor receptor 2 antibody reduces tumorigenicity and metastasis in orthotopic prostate cancer xenografts via induction of endothelial cell apoptosis and reduction of endothelial cell matrix metalloproteinase type 9 production. Clin Cancer Res 2002;8:2714.

[78] Borgstrom P, Bourdon MA, Hillan KJ, et al. Neutralizing anti-vascular endothelial growth factor antibody completely inhibits angiogenesis and growth of human prostate carcinoma micro tumors in vivo. Prostate 1998;35:1.

[79] Melnyk O, Zimmerman M, Kim KJ, et al. Neutralizing anti-vascular endothelial growth factor antibody inhibits further growth of established prostate cancer and metastases in a pre-clinical model. J Urol 1999;161:960.

[80] Kramer G, Steiner GE, Sokol P, et al. Local intratumoral tumor necrosis factor-alpha and systemic IFN-alpha 2b in patients with locally advanced prostate cancer. J Interferon Cytokine Res 2001; 21:475.

[81] Dreicer R, See WA, Klein EA. Phase II trial of GM-CSF in advanced prostate cancer. Invest New Drugs 2001;19:261.

[82] Milowsky MI, Nanus DM, Kostakoglu L, et al. Phase I trial of yttrium-90-labeled anti-prostate-specific membrane antigen monoclonal antibody J591 for androgen-independent prostate cancer. J Clin Oncol 2004;22:2522.

[83] Simons JW, Mikhak B, Chang JF, et al. Induction of immunity to prostate cancer antigens: results of a clinical trial of vaccination with irradiated autologous prostate tumor cells engineered to secrete granulocyte-macrophage colony-stimulating factor using ex vivo gene transfer. Cancer Res 1999;59:5160.

[84] Harris DT, Matyas GR, Gomella LG, et al. Immunologic approaches to the treatment of prostate cancer. Semin Oncol 1999;26:439.

[85] Kim JJ, Trivedi NN, Wilson DM, et al. Molecular and immunological analysis of genetic prostate specific antigen (PSA) vaccine. Oncogene 1998;17: 3125.

[86] Kim JJ, Yang JS, Dang K, et al. Engineering enhancement of immune responses to DNA-based vaccines in a prostate cancer model in rhesus macaques through the use of cytokine gene adjuvants. Clin Cancer Res 2001;7:882s.

[87] Kaufman HL, Wang W, Manola J, et al. Phase II randomized study of vaccine treatment of advanced prostate cancer (E7897): a trial of the Eastern Cooperative Oncology Group. J Clin Oncol 2004;22:2122.

[88] Fong L, Brockstedt D, Benike C, et al. Dendritic cell-based xenoantigen vaccination for prostate cancer immunotherapy. J Immunol 2001;167:7150.

[89] Fong L, Brockstedt D, Benike C, et al. Dendritic cells injected via different routes induce immunity in cancer patients. J Immunol 2001;166:4254.

[90] Small EJ, Fratesi P, Reese DM, et al. Immunotherapy of hormone-refractory prostate cancer with antigen-loaded dendritic cells. J Clin Oncol 2000; 18:3894.

[91] Allay JA, Steiner MS, Zhang Y, et al. Adenovirus p16 gene therapy for prostate cancer. World J Urol 2000;18:111.

[92] Bookstein R, Shew JY, Chen PL, et al. Suppression of tumorigenicity of human prostate carcinoma cells by replacing a mutated RB gene. Science 1990;247:712.

[93] Eastham JA, Hall SJ, Sehgal I, et al. In vivo gene therapy with p53 or p21 adenovirus for prostate cancer. Cancer Res 1995;55:5151.

[94] Steiner MS, Anthony CT, Lu Y, et al. Antisense c-myc retroviral vector suppresses established human prostate cancer. Hum Gene Ther 1998;9:747.

[95] Wei C, Willis RA, Tilton BR, et al. Tissue-specific expression of the human prostate-specific antigen gene in transgenic mice: implications for tolerance and immunotherapy. Proc Natl Acad Sci USA 1997;94:6369.

[96] Hay RT. The origin of adenovirus DNA replication: minimal DNA sequence requirement in vivo. EMBO J 1985;4:421.

[97] Brand K, Arnold W, Bartels T, et al. Liver-associated toxicity of the HSV-tk/GCV approach and adenoviral vectors. Cancer Gene Ther 1997;4:9.

[98] Herman JR, Adler HL, Aguilar-Cordova E, et al. In situ gene therapy for adenocarcinoma of the prostate: a phase I clinical trial. Hum Gene Ther 1999;10:1239.

[99] Pan LC, Price PA. The effect of transcriptional inhibitors on the bone gamma-carboxyglutamic acid protein response to 1,25-dihydroxyvitamin D3 in osteosarcoma cells. J Biol Chem 1984;259: 5844.

[100] Jung C, Ou YC, Yeung F, et al. Osteocalcin is incompletely spliced in non-osseous tissues. Gene 2001;271:143.

[101] Wu TT, Sikes RA, Cui Q, et al. Establishing human prostate cancer cell xenografts in bone: induction of osteoblastic reaction by prostate-specific antigen-producing tumors in athymic and SCID/bg mice using LNCaP and lineage-derived metastatic sublines. Int J Cancer 1998;77:887.

[102] Koeneman KS, Yeung F, Chung LW. Osteomimetic properties of prostate cancer cells: a hypothesis

supporting the predilection of prostate cancer metastasis and growth in the bone environment. Prostate 1999;39:246.

[103] Bortell R, Owen TA, Bidwell JP, et al. Vitamin D-responsive protein-DNA interactions at multiple promoter regulatory elements that contribute to the level of rat osteocalcin gene expression. Proc Natl Acad Sci USA 1992;89:6119.

[104] Lian JB, Stein GS, Stein JL, et al. Regulated expression of the bone-specific osteocalcin gene by vitamins and hormones. Vitam Horm 1999;55:443.

[105] Banerjee C, Stein JL, Van Wijnen AJ, et al. Transforming growth factor-beta 1 responsiveness of the rat osteocalcin gene is mediated by an activator protein-1 binding site. Endocrinology 1996;137: 1991.

[106] Banerjee C, Hiebert SW, Stein JL, et al. An AML-1 consensus sequence binds an osteoblast-specific complex and transcriptionally activates the osteocalcin gene. Proc Natl Acad Sci USA 1996;93:4968.

[107] Ko SC, Cheon J, Kao C, et al. Osteocalcin promoter-based toxic gene therapy for the treatment of osteosarcoma in experimental models. Cancer Res 1996;56:4614.

[108] Koeneman KS, Kao C, Ko SC, et al. Osteocalcin-directed gene therapy for for prostate-cancer bone metastasis. World J Urol 2000;18:102.

[109] Kubo H, Gardner TA, Wada Y, et al. Phase I dose escalation clinical trial of adenovirus vector carrying osteocalcin promoter-driven herpes simplex virus thymidine kinase in localized and metastatic hormone-refractory prostate cancer. Hum Gene Ther 2003;14:227.

[110] Shirakawa T, Hinata N, Terao S, et al. Phase I/II clinical trial of Ad-OC-TK plus Val for patients with metastatic or locally recurrent prostate cancer. Initial experience in Japan. Mol Ther 2004;9(Suppl 1):S228.

[111] Stamey TA, Yang N, Hay AR, et al. Prostate-specific antigen as a serum marker for adenocarcinoma of the prostate. N Engl J Med 1987;317:909.

[112] Cleutjens KB, van der Korput HA, van Eekelen CC, et al. An androgen response element in a far upstream enhancer region is essential for high, androgen-regulated activity of the prostate-specific antigen promoter. Mol Endocrinol 1997;11:148.

[113] Pang S, Dannull J, Kaboo R, et al. Identification of a positive regulatory element responsible for tissue-specific expression of prostate-specific antigen. Cancer Res 1997;57:495.

[114] Schuur ER, Henderson GA, Kmetec LA, et al. Prostate-specific antigen expression is regulated by an upstream enhancer. J Biol Chem 1996;271:7043.

[115] Gotoh A, Ko SC, Shirakawa T, et al. Development of prostate-specific antigen promoter-based gene therapy for androgen-independent human prostate cancer. J Urol 1998;160:220.

[116] Lu Y, Carraher J, Zhang Y, et al. Delivery of adenoviral vectors to the prostate for gene therapy. Cancer Gene Ther 1999;6:64.

[117] Wu L, Matherly J, Smallwood A, et al. Chimeric PSA enhancers exhibit augmented activity in prostate cancer gene therapy vectors. Gene Ther 2001;8: 1416.

[118] Wright GL Jr, Grob BM, Haley C, et al. Upregulation of prostate-specific membrane antigen after androgen-deprivation therapy. Urology 1996;48: 326.

[119] Xiao Z, Adam BL, Cazares LH, et al. Quantitation of serum prostate-specific membrane antigen by a novel protein biochip immunoassay discriminates benign from malignant prostate disease. Cancer Res 2001;61:6029.

[120] Sweat SD, Pacelli A, Murphy GP, et al. Prostate-specific membrane antigen expression is greatest in prostate adenocarcinoma and lymph node metastases. Urology 1998;52:637.

[121] Watt F, Martorana A, Brookes DE, et al. A tissue-specific enhancer of the prostate-specific membrane antigen gene, FOLH1. Genomics 2001;73:243.

[122] Uchida A, O'Keefe DS, Bacich DJ, et al. In vivo suicide gene therapy model using a newly discovered prostate-specific membrane antigen promoter/enhancer: a potential alternative approach to androgen deprivation therapy. Urology 2001;58:132.

[123] Lee SJ, Lee K, Yang X, et al. NFATc1 with AP-3 site binding specificity mediates gene expression of prostate-specific-membrane-antigen. J Mol Biol 2003;330:749.

[124] Chiu CP, Harley CB. Replicative senescence and cell immortality: the role of telomeres and telomerase. Proc Soc Exp Biol Med 1997;214:99.

[125] Kim NW, Piatyszek MA, Prowse KR, et al. Specific association of human telomerase activity with immortal cells and cancer. Science 1994;266:2011.

[126] Horikawa I, Cable PL, Afshari C, et al. Cloning and characterization of the promoter region of human telomerase reverse transcriptase gene. Cancer Res 1999;59:826.

[127] Sommerfeld HJ, Meeker AK, Piatyszek MA, et al. Telomerase activity: a prevalent marker of malignant human prostate tissue. Cancer Res 1996;56: 218.

[128] Lin T, Huang X, Gu J, et al. Long-term tumor-free survival from treatment with the GFP-TRAIL fusion gene expressed from the hTERT promoter in breast cancer cells. Oncogene 2002;21:8020.

[129] Lanson NA Jr, Friedlander PL, Schwarzenberger P, et al. Replication of an adenoviral vector controlled by the human telomerase reverse transcriptase promoter causes tumor-selective tumor lysis. Cancer Res 2003;63:7936.

[130] Office of Biotechnology Activities. Recombinant DNA and gene transfer. Available at: http://www4.od.nih.gov/oba/rdna.htm. Accessed November 25, 2005.

[131] Levine AJ. p53, the cellular gatekeeper for growth and division. Cell 1997;88:323.

[132] Sherr CJ. Cancer cell cycles. Science 1996;274:1672.

[133] Downing SR, Russell PJ, Jackson P. Alterations of p53 are common in early stage prostate cancer. Can J Urol 2003;10:1924.

[134] Eastham JA, Stapleton AM, Gousse AE, et al. Association of p53 mutations with metastatic prostate cancer. Clin Cancer Res 1995;1:1111.

[135] Yang C, Cirielli C, Capogrossi MC, et al. Adenovirus-mediated wild-type p53 expression induces apoptosis and suppresses tumorigenesis of prostatic tumor cells. Cancer Res 1995;55:4210.

[136] Ko SC, Gotoh A, Thalmann GN, et al. Molecular therapy with recombinant p53 adenovirus in an androgen-independent, metastatic human prostate cancer model. Hum Gene Ther 1996;7:1683.

[137] Eastham JA, Grafton W, Martin CM, et al. Suppression of primary tumor growth and the progression to metastasis with p53 adenovirus in human prostate cancer. J Urol 2000;164:814.

[138] Gurnani M, Lipari P, Dell J, et al. Adenovirus-mediated p53 gene therapy has greater efficacy when combined with chemotherapy against human head and neck, ovarian, prostate, and breast cancer. Cancer Chemother Pharmacol 1999;44:143.

[139] Colletier PJ, Ashoori F, Cowen D, et al. Adenoviral-mediated p53 transgene expression sensitizes both wild-type and null p53 prostate cancer cells in vitro to radiation. Int J Radiat Oncol Biol Phys 2000;48:1507.

[140] Pantuck AJ, Zisman A, Belldegrun AS. Gene therapy for prostate cancer at the University of California, Los Angeles: preliminary results and future directions. World J Urol 2000;18:143.

[141] Sweeney P, Pisters LL. Ad5CMVp53 gene therapy for locally advanced prostate cancer–where do we stand? World J Urol 2000;18:121.

[142] Isaacs WB. Molecular genetics of prostate cancer. Cancer Surv 1995;25:357.

[143] Jarrard DF, Bova GS, Ewing CM, et al. Deletional, mutational, and methylation analyses of CDKN2 (p16/MTS1) in primary and metastatic prostate cancer. Genes Chromosomes Cancer 1997;19:90.

[144] Liggett WH Jr, Sidransky D. Role of the p16 tumor suppressor gene in cancer. J Clin Oncol 1998;16:1197.

[145] Gotoh A, Kao C, Ko SC, et al. Cytotoxic effects of recombinant adenovirus p53 and cell cycle regulator genes (p21 WAF1/CIP1 and p16CDKN4) in human prostate cancers. J Urol 1997;158:636.

[146] Steiner MS, Zhang Y, Farooq F, et al. Adenoviral vector containing wild-type p16 suppresses prostate cancer growth and prolongs survival by inducing cell senescence. Cancer Gene Ther 2000;7:360.

[147] Galaktionov K, Chen X, Beach D. Cdc25 cell-cycle phosphatase as a target of c-myc. Nature 1996;382: 511.

[148] Jenkins RB, Qian J, Lieber MM, et al. Detection of c-myc oncogene amplification and chromosomal anomalies in metastatic prostatic carcinoma by fluorescence in situ hybridization. Cancer Res 1997;57:524.

[149] Deng J, Xia W, Hung MC. Adenovirus 5 E1A-mediated tumor suppression associated with E1A-mediated apoptosis in vivo. Oncogene 1998;17: 2167.

[150] van der Eb MM, Cramer SJ, Vergouwe Y, et al. Severe hepatic dysfunction after adenovirus-mediated transfer of the herpes simplex virus thymidine kinase gene and ganciclovir administration. Gene Ther 1998;5:451.

[151] Robbins PD, Tahara H, Ghivizzani SC. Viral vectors for gene therapy. Trends Biotechnol 1998;16:35.

[152] Rodriguez R, Schuur ER, Lim HY, et al. Prostate attenuated replication competent adenovirus (ARCA) CN706: a selective cytotoxic for prostate-specific antigen-positive prostate cancer cells. Cancer Res 1997;57:2559.

[153] Matsubara S, Wada Y, Gardner TA, et al. A conditional replication-competent adenoviral vector, Ad-OC-E1a, to cotarget prostate cancer and bone stroma in an experimental model of androgen-independent prostate cancer bone metastasis. Cancer Res 2001;61:6012.

[154] Yu DC, Sakamoto GT, Henderson DR. Identification of the transcriptional regulatory sequences of human kallikrein 2 and their use in the construction of calydon virus 764, an attenuated replication competent adenovirus for prostate cancer therapy. Cancer Res 1999;59:1498.

[155] Hsieh CL, Yang L, Miao L, et al. A novel targeting modality to enhance adenoviral replication by vitamin D(3) in androgen-independent human prostate cancer cells and tumors. Cancer Res 2002;62: 3084.

[156] Konety BR, Johnson CS, Trump DL, et al. Vitamin D in the prevention and treatment of prostate cancer. Semin Urol Oncol 1999;17:77.

[157] Getzenberg RH, Light BW, Lapco PE, et al. Vitamin D inhibition of prostate adenocarcinoma growth and metastasis in the Dunning rat prostate model system. Urology 1997;50:999.

[158] Zhao XY, Feldman D. The role of vitamin D in prostate cancer. Steroids 2001;66:293.

[159] Cheon J, Kim HK, Moon DG, et al. Adenovirus-mediated suicide-gene therapy using the herpes simplex virus thymidine kinase gene in cell and animal models of human prostate cancer: changes in tumour cell proliferative activity. BJU Int 2000; 85:759.

[160] Eastham JA, Chen SH, Sehgal I, et al. Prostate cancer gene therapy: herpes simplex virus thymidine kinase gene transduction followed by ganciclovir in mouse and human prostate cancer models. Hum Gene Ther 1996;7:515.

[161] Hall SJ, Mutchnik SE, Chen SH, et al. Adenovirus-mediated herpes simplex virus thymidine kinase gene and ganciclovir therapy leads to systemic activity against spontaneous and induced metastasis in an orthotopic mouse model of prostate cancer. Int J Cancer 1997;70:183.

[162] Pitti RM, Marsters SA, Ruppert S, et al. Induction of apoptosis by Apo-2 ligand, a new member of the tumor necrosis factor cytokine family. J Biol Chem 1996;271:12687.

[163] Wiley SR, Schooley K, Smolak PJ, et al. Identification and characterization of a new member of the TNF family that induces apoptosis. Immunity 1995;3:673.

[164] Pan G, Ni J, Wei YF, et al. An antagonist decoy receptor and a death domain-containing receptor for TRAIL. Science 1997;277:815.

[165] Pan G, O'Rourke K, Chinnaiyan AM, et al. The receptor for the cytotoxic ligand TRAIL. Science 1997;276:111.

[166] Nesterov A, Lu X, Johnson M, et al. Elevated AKT activity protects the prostate cancer cell line LNCaP from TRAIL-induced apoptosis. J Biol Chem 2001;276:10767.

[167] Munshi A, McDonnell TJ, Meyn RE. Chemotherapeutic agents enhance TRAIL-induced apoptosis in prostate cancer cells. Cancer Chemother Pharmacol 2002;50:46.

[168] Voelkel-Johnson C, King DL, Norris JS. Resistance of prostate cancer cells to soluble TNF-related poptosis-inducing ligand (TRAIL/Apo2L) can be overcome by doxorubicin or adenoviral delivery of full-length TRAIL. Cancer Gene Ther 2002;9:164.

[169] Jo M, Kim TH, Seol DW, et al. Apoptosis induced in normal human hepatocytes by tumor necrosis factor-related apoptosis-inducing ligand. Nat Med 2000;6:564.

[170] Lawrence D, Shahrokh Z, Marsters S, et al. Differential hepatocyte toxicity of recombinant Apo2L/TRAIL versions. Nat Med 2001;7:383.

[171] Mori E, Thomas M, Motoki K, et al. Human normal hepatocytes are susceptible to apoptosis signal mediated by both TRAIL-R1 and TRAIL-R2. Cell Death Differ 2004;11:203-7.

[172] Ke B, Coito AJ, Kato H, et al. Fas ligand gene transfer prolongs rat renal allograft survival and down-regulates anti-apoptotic Bag-1 in parallel with enhanced Th2-type cytokine expression. Transplantation 2000;69:1690.

[173] Huang X, Lee C. From TGF-beta to cancer therapy. Curr Drug Targets 2003;4:243.

[174] Narumoto K, Saibara T, Maeda T, et al. Transforming growth factor-beta 1 derived from biliary epithelial cells may attenuate alloantigen-specific immune responses. Transpl Int 2000;13:21.

[175] Norris JS, Hyer ML, Voelkel-Johnson C, et al. The use of Fas Ligand, TRAIL and Bax in gene therapy of prostate cancer. Curr Gene Ther 2001;1:123.

[176] Tauber B, Dobner T. Molecular regulation and biological function of adenovirus early genes: the E4 ORFs. Gene 2001;278:1.

[177] Krougliak V, Graham FL. Development of cell lines capable of complementing E1, E4, and protein IX defective adenovirus type 5 mutants. Hum Gene Ther 1995;6:1575.

[178] Pantuck AJ, Berger F, Zisman A, et al. CL1–SR39: a noninvasive molecular imaging model of prostate cancer suicide gene therapy using positron emission tomography. J Urol 2002;168:1193.

[179] Campbell M, Qu S, Wells S, et al. An adenoviral vector containing an arg-gly-asp (RGD) motif in the fiber knob enhances protein product levels from transgenes refractory to expression. Cancer Gene Ther 2003;10:559.

[180] Vigne E, Dedieu JF, Brie A, et al. Genetic manipulations of adenovirus type 5 fiber resulting in liver tropism attenuation. Gene Ther 2003;10:153.

ELSEVIER SAUNDERS

Urol Clin N Am 33 (2006) 273–278

UROLOGIC CLINICS of North America

Index

Note: Page numbers of article titles are in **boldface** type.